Learning Disabilities Sourcebook, 3rd Edition

Leukemia Sourcebook

Liver Disorders Sourcebook

Lung Disorders Sourcebook

Medical Tests Sourcebook, 3rd Edition

Men's Health Concerns Sourcebook, 2nd Edition

Mental Health Disorders Sourcebook, 4th Edition

Mental Retardation Sourcebook

Movement Disorders Sourcebook, 2nd Edition

Multiple Sclerosis Sourcebook

Muscular Dystrophy Sourcebook

Obesity Sourcebook

Osteoporosis Sourcebook

Pain Sourcebook, 3rd Edition

Pediatric Cancer Sourcebook

Physical & Mental Issues in Aging Sourcebook

Podiatry Sourcebook, 2nd Edition

Pregnancy & Birth Sourcebook, 2nd Edition

Prostate & Urological Disorders Sourcebook

Prostate Cancer Sourcebook

Reconstructive & Cosmetic Surgery Sourcebook

Rehabilitation Sourcebook

Respiratory Disorders Sourcebook, 2nd Edition

Sexually Transmitted Diseases Sourcebook,
3rd Edition

Sleep Disorders Sourcebook, 3rd Edition

Smoking Concerns Sourcebook

Sports Injuries Sourcebook, 3rd Edition

Stress-Related Disorders Sourcebook, 2nd Edition

Stroke Sourcebook, 2nd Edition

Surgery Sourcebook, 2nd Edition

Thyroid Disorders Sourcebook

Transplantation Sourcebook

Traveler's Health Sourcebook

Urinary Tract & Kidney Diseases & Disorders
Sourcebook, 2nd Edition

Vegetarian Sourcebook

Women's Health Concerns Sourcebook, 3rd Edition

Workplace Health & Safety Sourcebook

Worldwide Health Sourcebook

Teen Health Series

Abuse & Violence Information for
Teens

Accident & Safety Information for
Teens

Alcohol Information for Teens, 2nd
Edition

Allergy Information for Teens

Asthma Information for Teens, 2nd
Edition

Body Information for Teens

Cancer Information for Teens

Complementary & Alternative
Medicine Information for Teens

Diabetes Information for Teens

Diet Information for Teens, 2nd Edition

Drug Information for Teens, 3rd Edition

Eating Disorders Information for Teens,
2nd Edition

Fitness Information for Teens, 2nd
Edition

Learning Disabilities Information for
Teens

Mental Health Information for Teens,
3rd Edition

Pregnancy Information for Teens

Sexual Health Information for Teens,
2nd Edition

Skin Health Information for Teens, 2nd
Edition

Sleep Information for Teens

Sports Injuries Information for Teens,
2nd Edition

Stress Information for Teens

Suicide Information for Teens, 2nd
Edition

Tobacco Information for Teens, 2nd
Edition

Blood and Circulatory Disorders

SOURCEBOOK

Third Edition

Health Reference Series

Third Edition

Blood and Circulatory Disorders

SOURCEBOOK

Basic Consumer Health Information about Blood and Circulatory System Disorders, Such as Anemia, Leukemia, Lymphoma, Rh Disease, Hemophilia, Thrombophilia, Other Bleeding and Clotting Deficiencies, and Artery, Vascular, and Venous Diseases, Including Facts about Blood Types, Blood Donation, Bone Marrow and Stem Cell Transplants, Tests and Medications, and Tips for Maintaining Circulatory Health

Along with a Glossary of Related Terms and a List of Resources for Additional Help and Information

Edited by
Sandra J. Judd

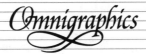

P.O. Box 31-1640, Detroit, MI 48231

Bibliographic Note
Because this page cannot legibly accommodate all the copyright notices, the Bibliographic Note portion of the Preface constitutes an extension of the copyright notice.

Edited by Sandra J. Judd

Health Reference Series

Karen Bellenir, *Managing Editor*
David A. Cooke, MD, FACP, *Medical Consultant*
Elizabeth Collins, *Research and Permissions Coordinator*
Cherry Edwards, *Permissions Assistant*
EdIndex, Services for Publishers, *Indexers*

* * *

Omnigraphics, Inc.
Matthew P. Barbour, *Senior Vice President*
Kevin M. Hayes, *Operations Manager*

* * *

Peter E. Ruffner, *Publisher*

Copyright © 2010 Omnigraphics, Inc.

ISBN 978-0-7808-1081-5

Library of Congress Cataloging-in-Publication Data

Blood and circulatory disorders sourcebook : basic consumer health information about blood and circulatory system disorders, such as anemia, leukemia, lymphoma, Rh disease, hemophilia, thrombophilia, other bleeding and clotting deficiencies, and artery, vascular, and venous diseases, including facts about blood types, blood donation, bone marrow and stem cell transplants, tests and medications, and tips for maintaining circulatory health; along with a glossary of related terms and a list of resources for additional help and information / edited by Sandra J. Judd. -- 3rd ed.
    p. cm.
  Includes bibliographical references and index.
  ISBN 978-0-7808-1081-5 (hardcover : alk. paper) 1. Blood--Diseases--Popular works. 2. Blood-vessels--Diseases--Popular works. I. Judd, Sandra J.
  RC636.B556 2010
  616.1'5--dc22
                                        2010013182

Table of Contents

Visit www.healthreferenceseries.com to view *A Contents Guide to the Health Reference Series*, a listing of more than 15,000 topics and the volumes in which they are covered.

Part II: Diagnosing and Treating Blood and Circulatory Disorders

Part III: Blood Disorders

Part IV: Bleeding and Clotting Disorders

Part VI: Additional Help and Information

Preface

About This Book

Blood plays many important roles in the human body. It carries oxygen and nutrients to the body's cells, helps fight infection, and works to heal wounds. When a disorder inhibits its ability to meet the body's needs or prevents blood from flowing or coagulating properly, a myriad of problems can result. According to the National Heart Lung and Blood Institute, nearly a quarter million deaths per year in the United States—approximately nine percent of all U.S. deaths—are attributable to blood diseases.

Blood and Circulatory Disorders Sourcebook, Third Edition offers facts about blood function and composition, the maintenance of a healthy circulatory system, and the types of concerns that arise when processes go awry. It discusses the diagnosis and treatment of many common blood cell disorders, bleeding disorders, and circulatory disorders, including anemia, hemochromatosis, leukemia, lymphoma, hemophilia, hypercoagulation, thrombophilia, atherosclerosis, blood pressure irregularities, coronary artery and heart disease, and peripheral vascular disease. Blood donation, cord blood banking, blood transfusions, and bone marrow and stem cell transplants are also discussed. The book concludes with a glossary of related terms and a list of resources for further help and information.

How to Use This Book

This book is divided into parts and chapters. Parts focus on broad areas of interest. Chapters are devoted to single topics within a part.

Part I: Understanding Blood and the Circulatory System explains the composition and types of blood and how it functions in the body. It describes blood donation and cord blood banking procedures, and it also discusses how aging affects the heart and blood vessels.

Part II: Diagnosing and Treating Blood and Circulatory Disorders provides information about medical tests commonly used to identify and monitor blood and circulatory disorders. It offers facts about many of the medications often used in the treatment of these disorders and discusses such procedures as blood transfusion and bone marrow transplants.

Part III: Blood Disorders describes ailments that affect the composition of the blood itself. These include anemia and other hemoglobin disorders, cancers of the blood, plasma cell disorders, and white blood cell disorders. Information about the causes of these disorders is provided, and treatment strategies are discussed.

Part IV: Bleeding and Clotting Disorders provides information about bleeding disorders resulting from insufficient clotting, such as hemophilia and von Willebrand disease, and those resulting from excess clotting, including deep vein thrombosis and pulmonary embolism. Methods of diagnosis and treatment options are included.

Part V: Circulatory Disorders describes disorders affecting the veins, arteries, and heart. It includes information about aneurysms, stroke, blood pressure irregularities, atherosclerosis, carotid artery disease, coronary artery disease, heart disease, peripheral vascular disease, and venous disorders such as thrombophlebitis and varicose and spider veins. Information about causes and diagnosis, as well as treatment options, is provided.

Part VI: Additional Help and Information includes a glossary of terms related to blood and circulatory disorders and a directory of resources offering additional help and support.

Bibliographic Note

This volume contains documents and excerpts from publications issued by the following U.S. government agencies: Agency for Healthcare Research and Quality; Centers for Disease Control and Prevention; National Cancer Institute; National Heart Lung and Blood Institute;

National Human Genome Research Institute; National Institute of Arthritis and Musculoskeletal and Skin Diseases; National Institute of Diabetes and Digestive and Kidney Diseases; National Institute on Aging; National Women's Health Information Center; NIH Clinical Center; NIH Senior Health; U.S. Food and Drug Administration; and Walter Reed Army Medical Center.

In addition, this volume contains copyrighted documents from the following organizations and individuals: A.D.A.M., Inc.; American Academy of Family Physicians; American Heart Association; American Partnership for Eosinophilic Disorders; American Pregnancy Association; American Red Cross; Arizona Department of Health Services; Cedars-Sinai Medical Center; Cincinnati Children's Hospital Medical Center; Cleveland Clinic; College of American Pathologists; Florida Blood Services; HowStuffWorks.com; International Myeloma Foundation (UK); Leukemia and Lymphoma Society; Merck and Co., Inc.; Damien Mosquera, M.D.; MyDR.com.au; National Anemia Action Council; National Hemophilia Foundation; Nemours Foundation; New Zealand Dermatological Society; St. Luke's Cataract and Laser Institute; Texas Department of State Health Services; UC Davis Vascular Center; University of Iowa Hospitals and Clinics; University of Rochester/Strong Health; Utah Department of Health; Vascular Disease Foundation; and Virtual Medical Centre.

Acknowledgements

Thanks go to the many organizations, agencies, and individuals who have contributed materials for this *Sourcebook* and to medical consultant Dr. David Cooke and document engineer Bruce Bellenir. Special thanks go to managing editor Karen Bellenir and permissions coordinator Liz Collins for their help and support.

About the Health Reference Series

The *Health Reference Series* is designed to provide basic medical information for patients, families, caregivers, and the general public. Each volume takes a particular topic and provides comprehensive coverage. This is especially important for people who may be dealing with a newly diagnosed disease or a chronic disorder in themselves or in a family member. People looking for preventive guidance, information about disease warning signs, medical statistics, and risk factors for health problems will also find answers to their questions in the *Health Reference Series*. The *Series*, however, is not intended to serve as a tool for diagnosing illness, in prescribing treatments, or as a substitute for the physician/patient relationship. All people concerned about medical symptoms or the possibility of disease are encouraged to seek professional care from an appropriate healthcare provider.

A Note about Spelling and Style

Health Reference Series editors use *Stedman's Medical Dictionary* as an authority for questions related to the spelling of medical terms and the *Chicago Manual of Style* for questions related to grammatical structures, punctuation, and other editorial concerns. Consistent adherence is not always possible, however, because the individual volumes within the *Series* include many documents from a wide variety of different producers and copyright holders, and the editor's primary goal is to present material from each source as accurately as is possible following the terms specified by each document's producer. This sometimes means that information in different chapters or sections may follow other guidelines and alternate spelling authorities. For example, occasionally a copyright holder may require that eponymous terms be shown in possessive forms (Crohn's disease *vs.* Crohn disease) or that British spelling norms be retained (leukaemia *vs.* leukemia).

Locating Information within the Health Reference Series

The *Health Reference Series* contains a wealth of information about a wide variety of medical topics. Ensuring easy access to all the fact sheets, research reports, in-depth discussions, and other material contained within the individual books of the series remains one of our highest priorities. As the *Series* continues to grow in size and scope, however, locating the precise information needed by a reader may become more challenging.

A *Contents Guide to the Health Reference Series* was developed to direct readers to the specific volumes that address their concerns. It presents an extensive list of diseases, treatments, and other topics of general interest compiled from the Tables of Contents and major index headings. To access *A Contents Guide to the Health Reference Series*, visit www.healthreferenceseries.com.

Medical Consultant

Medical consultation services are provided to the *Health Reference Series* editors by David A. Cooke, MD, FACP. Dr. Cooke is a graduate of Brandeis University, and he received his M.D. degree from the University of Michigan. He completed residency training at the University of Wisconsin Hospital and Clinics. He is board-certified in Internal Medicine. Dr. Cooke currently works as part of the University of Michigan Health System and practices in Ann Arbor, MI. In his free time, he enjoys writing, science fiction, and spending time with his family.

Our Advisory Board

We would like to thank the following board members for providing guidance to the development of this series:

Dr. Lynda Baker, Associate Professor of Library
and Information Science, Wayne State University,
Detroit, MI

Nancy Bulgarelli, William Beaumont Hospital Library,
Royal Oak, MI

Karen Imarisio, Bloomfield Township Public Library,
Bloomfield Township, MI

Karen Morgan, Mardigian Library,
University of Michigan-Dearborn, Dearborn, MI

Rosemary Orlando, St. Clair Shores Public Library,
St. Clair Shores, MI

Health Reference Series *Update Policy*

The inaugural book in the *Health Reference Series* was the first edition of *Cancer Sourcebook* published in 1989. Since then, the *Series* has been enthusiastically received by librarians and in the medical community. In order to maintain the standard of providing high-quality health information for the layperson the editorial staff at Omnigraphics felt it was necessary to implement a policy of updating volumes when warranted.

Medical researchers have been making tremendous strides, and it is the purpose of the *Health Reference Series* to stay current with the most recent advances. Each decision to update a volume is made on an individual basis. Some of the considerations include how much new information is available and the feedback we receive from people who use the books. If there is a topic you would like to see added to the update list, or an area of medical concern you feel has not been adequately addressed, please write to:

Editor
Health Reference Series
Omnigraphics, Inc.
P.O. Box 31-1640
Detroit, MI 48231
E-mail: editorial@omnigraphics.com

Part One

Understanding Blood and the Circulatory System

Chapter 1

Blood Function and Composition

Blood Facts

- Approximately 8 percent of an adult's body weight is made up of blood.

- Females have around 4 to 5 liters (8.5 to 10.5 pints), while males have around 5 to 6 liters (10.5 to 12.5 pints). This difference is mainly due to the differences in body size between men and women.

- Its mean temperature is 38 degrees Celsius (100.4 degrees Fahrenheit).

- It has a pH of 7.35 to 7.45, making it slightly basic (less than 7 is considered acidic).

- Whole blood is about 4.5 to 5.5 times as viscous as water, indicating that it is more resistant to flow than water. This viscosity is vital to the function of blood because if blood flows too easily or with too much resistance, it can strain the heart and lead to severe cardiovascular problems.

- Blood in the arteries is a brighter red than blood in the veins because of the higher levels of oxygen found in the arteries.

- An artificial substitute for human blood has not been found.

"Blood Types," © 2009 Virtual Medical Centre (www.virtualmedicalcentre.com). All rights reserved. Reprinted with permission.

Functions of Blood

Blood has three main functions: transport, protection, and regulation.

Transport

Blood transports the following substances:

- Gases, namely oxygen (O_2) and carbon dioxide (CO_2), between the lungs and rest of the body
- Nutrients from the digestive tract and storage sites to the rest of the body
- Waste products to be detoxified or removed by the liver and kidneys
- Hormones from the glands in which they are produced to their target cells
- Heat to the skin so as to help regulate body temperature

Protection

Blood has several roles in inflammation:

- Leukocytes, or white blood cells, destroy invading microorganisms and cancer cells
- Antibodies and other proteins destroy pathogenic substances
- Platelet factors initiate blood clotting and help minimize blood loss

Regulation

Blood helps regulate:

- pH by interacting with acids and bases;
- water balance by transferring water to and from tissues.

Composition of Blood

Blood is classified as a connective tissue and consists of two main components:

- Plasma, which is a clear extracellular fluid
- Formed elements, which are made up of the blood cells and platelets

The formed elements are so named because they are enclosed in a plasma membrane and have a definite structure and shape. All formed elements are cells except for the platelets, which are tiny fragments of bone marrow cells.

Formed elements are:

- erythrocytes, also known as red blood cells (RBCs);

- leukocytes, also known as white blood cells (WBCs);

- platelets.

Leukocytes are further classified into two subcategories: granulocytes, which consist of neutrophils, eosinophils, and basophils; and agranulocytes, which consist of lymphocytes and monocytes.

The formed elements can be separated from plasma by centrifuge, where a blood sample is spun for a few minutes in a tube to separate its components according to their densities. RBCs are denser than plasma, and so become packed into the bottom of the tube to make up 45 percent of total volume. This volume is known as the hematocrit. WBCs and platelets form a narrow cream-colored coat known as the buffy coat immediately above the RBCs. Finally, the plasma makes up the top of the tube, which is a pale yellow color and contains just under 55 percent of the total volume.

Blood Plasma

Blood plasma is a mixture of proteins, enzymes, nutrients, wastes, hormones, and gases. The specific composition and function of its components are as follows.

Proteins

These are the most abundant substance in plasma by weight and play a part in a variety of roles including clotting, defense, and transport. Collectively, they serve several functions:

- They are an important reserve supply of amino acids for cell nutrition. Cells called macrophages in the liver, gut, spleen, lungs, and lymphatic tissue can break down plasma proteins so as to release their amino acids. These amino acids are used by other cells to synthesize new products.

- Plasma proteins also serve as carriers for other molecules. Many types of small molecules bind to specific plasma proteins and are transported from the organs that absorb these proteins to other tissues for utilization. The proteins also help to keep the blood slightly basic at a stable pH. They do this by functioning as weak bases themselves to bind excess H+ ions. By doing so, they remove excess H+ from the blood, which keeps it slightly basic.

- The plasma proteins interact in specific ways to cause the blood to coagulate, which is part of the body's response to injury to the blood vessels (also known as vascular injury), and helps protect against the loss of blood and invasion by foreign microorganisms and viruses.

- Plasma proteins govern the distribution of water between the blood and tissue fluid by producing what is known as a colloid osmotic pressure.

There are three major categories of plasma proteins, and each individual type of protein has its own specific properties and functions in addition to their overall collective role:

- **Albumins:** These are the smallest and most abundant plasma proteins. Reductions in plasma albumin content can result in a loss of fluid from the blood and a gain of fluid in the interstitial space (space within the tissue), which may occur in nutritional, liver, and kidney disease. Albumin also helps many substances dissolve in the plasma by binding to them, hence playing an important role in plasma transport of substances such as drugs, hormones, and fatty acids.

- **Globulins:** These can be subdivided into three classes from smallest to largest in molecular weight into alpha, beta, and gamma globulins. The globulins include high-density lipoproteins (HDL), an alpha-1 globulin, and low-density lipoproteins (LDL), a beta-1 globulin. HDL functions in lipid transport, carrying fats to cells for use in energy metabolism, membrane reconstruction, and hormone function. HDLs also appear to prevent cholesterol from invading and settling in the walls of arteries. LDL carries cholesterol and fats to tissues for use in manufacturing steroid hormones and building cell membranes, but it also favors the deposition of cholesterol in arterial walls and thus appears to play a role in disease of the blood vessels and heart. HDL and LDL therefore play important parts in the regulation of cholesterol and hence have a large impact on cardiovascular disease.

- **Fibrinogen:** This is a soluble precursor of a sticky protein called fibrin, which forms the framework of blood clots. Fibrin plays a key role in coagulation of blood, which is discussed later in this chapter under "Platelets."

Amino Acids

These are formed from the breakdown of tissue proteins or from the digestion of digested proteins.

Nitrogenous Waste

Being toxic end products of the breakdown of substances in the body, these are usually cleared from the bloodstream and are excreted by the kidneys at a rate that balances their production.

Nutrients

Those absorbed by the digestive tract are transported in the blood plasma. These include glucose, amino acids, fats, cholesterol, phospholipids, vitamins, and minerals.

Gases

Some oxygen and carbon dioxide are transported by plasma. Plasma also contains a substantial amount of dissolved nitrogen.

Electrolytes

The most abundant of these are sodium ions, which account for more of the blood's osmolarity than any other solute.

Red Blood Cells

Red blood cells (RBCs), also known as erythrocytes, have two main functions:

- To pick up oxygen from the lungs and deliver it to tissues elsewhere

- To pick up carbon dioxide from other tissues and unload it in the lungs

An erythrocyte is a disc-shaped cell with a thick rim and a thin, sunken center. The plasma membrane of a mature RBC has glycoproteins and glycolipids that determine a person's blood type. On its inner surface are two proteins called spectrin and actin that give the membrane resilience and durability. This allows the RBCs to stretch, bend, and fold as they squeeze through small blood vessels, and to spring back to their original shape as they pass through larger vessels.

RBCs are incapable of aerobic respiration, preventing them from consuming the oxygen they transport because they lose nearly all their inner cellular components during maturation. The inner cellular components lost include their mitochondria, which normally provide energy to a cell, and their nucleus, which contains the genetic material of the cell and enable it to repair itself. The lack of a nucleus means that RBCs are unable to repair themselves. However, the resulting biconcave shape means that the cell has a greater ratio of surface area to volume, enabling O_2 and CO_2 to diffuse quickly to and from hemoglobin (Hb).

The cytoplasm of an RBC consists mainly of a 33-percent solution of Hb, which gives RBCs their red color. Hemoglobin carries most of the oxygen and some of the carbon dioxide transported by the blood.

Circulating erythrocytes live for about 120 days. As an RBC ages, its membrane grows increasingly fragile. Without key organelles such as a n ucleus or ribosomes, RBCs cannot repair themselves. Many RBCs die in the spleen, where they are trapped in narrow channels, broken up, and destroyed. Hemolysis refers to the rupture of RBCs, where hemoglobin is released, leaving empty plasma membranes, which are easily digested by cells known as macrophages in the liver and spleen. The Hb is then further broken down into its different components and either recycled in the body for further use or disposed of.

White Blood Cells

White blood cells (WBCs) are also known as leukocytes. They can be divided into granulocytes and agranulocytes. The former have cytoplasms that contain organelles that appear as colored granules through light microscopy, hence their name. Granulocytes consist of neutrophils, eosinophils, and basophils. In contrast, agranulocytes do not contain granules. They consist of lymphocytes and monocytes.

Granulocytes

Neutrophils: These contain very fine cytoplasmic granules that can be seen under a light microscope. Neutrophils are also called polymorphonuclear (PMN) because they have a variety of nuclear shapes.

They play roles in the destruction of bacteria and the release of chemicals that kill or inhibit the growth of bacteria.

Eosinophils: These have large granules and a prominent nucleus that is divided into two lobes. They function in the destruction of allergens and inflammatory chemicals, and release enzymes that disable parasites.

Basophils: They have a pale nucleus that is usually hidden by granules. They secrete histamine, which increases tissue blood flow via dilating the blood vessels, and also secrete heparin, which is an anticoagulant that promotes mobility of other WBCs by preventing clotting.

Agranulocytes

Lymphocytes: These are usually classified as small, medium, or large. Medium and large lymphocytes are generally seen mainly in fibrous connective tissue and only occasionally in the circulation bloodstream. Lymphocytes function in destroying cancer cells, cells infected by viruses, and foreign invading cells. In addition, they present antigens to activate other cells of the immune system. They also coordinate the actions of other immune cells, secrete antibodies, and serve in immune memory.

Monocytes: They are the largest of the formed elements. Their cytoplasm tends to be abundant and relatively clear. They function in differentiating into macrophages, which are large phagocytic cells, and digest pathogens, dead neutrophils, and the debris of dead cells. Like lymphocytes, they also present antigens to activate other immune cells.

Platelets

Platelets are small fragments of bone marrow cells and are therefore not really classified as cells themselves.

Platelets have the following functions:

- Secrete vasoconstrictors, which constrict blood vessels, causing vascular spasms in broken blood vessels
- Form temporary platelet plugs to stop bleeding
- Secrete procoagulants (clotting factors) to promote blood clotting
- Dissolve blood clots when they are no longer needed

- Digest and destroy bacteria

- Secrete chemicals that attract neutrophils and monocytes to sites of inflammation

- Secrete growth factors to maintain the linings of blood vessels

The first three functions listed above refer to important hemostatic mechanisms in which platelets play a role during bleeding: vascular spasms, platelet plug formation, and blood clotting (coagulation).

Vascular Spasm

This is a prompt constriction of the broken blood vessel and is the most immediate protection against blood loss. Injury stimulates pain receptors. Some of these receptors directly innervate nearby blood vessels and cause them to constrict. After a few minutes, other mechanisms take over. Injury to the smooth muscle of the blood vessel itself causes a longer-lasting vasoconstriction where platelets release a chemical vasoconstrictor called serotonin. This maintains vascular spasm long enough for the other hemostatic mechanisms to come into play.

Platelet Plug Formation

Under normal conditions, platelets do not usually adhere to the wall of undamaged blood vessels, since the vessel lining tends to be smooth and coated with a platelet repellent. When a vessel is broken, platelets put out long spiny extensions to adhere to the vessel wall as well as to other platelets. These extensions then contract and draw the walls of the vessel together. The mass of platelets formed is known as a platelet plug, and can reduce or stop minor bleeding.

Coagulation

This is the last and most effective defense against bleeding. During bleeding, it is important for the blood to clot quickly to minimize blood loss, but it is equally important for blood not to clot in undamaged vessels. Coagulation is a very complex process aimed at clotting the blood at appropriate amounts. The objective of coagulation is to convert plasma protein fibrinogen into fibrin, which is a sticky protein that adheres to the walls of a vessel. Blood cells and platelets become stuck to fibrin, and the resulting mass helps to seal the break in the blood vessel. The forming of fibrin is what makes coagulation so complicated, as it involved numerous chemical reactions and many coagulation factors.

Production of Blood

Hemopoiesis

Hemopoiesis is the production of the formed elements of blood. Hemopoietic tissues refer to the tissues that produce blood. The earliest hemopoietic tissue to develop is the yolk sac, which also functions in the transfer of yolk nutrients of the embryo. In the fetus, blood cells are produced by the bone marrow, liver, spleen, and thymus. This changes during and after birth. The liver stops producing blood cells around the time of birth, while the spleen stops producing them soon after birth but continues to produce lymphocytes for life. From infancy onward, all formed elements are produced in the red bone marrow. Lymphocytes are additionally produced in lymphoid tissues and organs widely distributed in the body, including the thymus, tonsils, lymph nodes, spleen, and patches of lymphoid tissues in the intestine.

Erythropoiesis

Erythropoiesis refers specifically to the production of erythrocytes or red blood cells (RBCs). These are formed through the following sequence of cell transformations:

The proerythroblast has receptors for the hormone erythropoietin (EPO). Once EPO receptors are in place, the cell is committed to exclusively producing RBCs. The erythroblasts then multiply and synthesize hemoglobin (Hb), which is a red oxygen transport protein. The nucleus from the erythroblasts is then discarded, giving rise to cells named reticulocytes. The overall transformation from hemocytoblast to reticulocytes involves a reduction in cell size, an increase in cell number, the synthesis

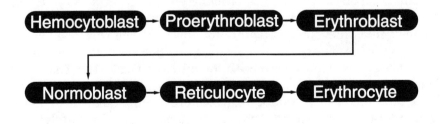

Figure 1.1. *Erythropoiesis*

of hemoglobin, and the loss of the cell nucleus. These reticulocytes leave the bone marrow and enter the bloodstream, where they mature into erythrocytes when their endoplasmic reticulum disappears.

Leukopoiesis

Leukopoiesis refers to the production of leukocytes (WBCs). It begins when some types of hemocytoblasts differentiate into three types of committed cells:

- B progenitors, which are destined to become B lymphocytes

- T progenitors, which become T lymphocytes

- Granulocyte-macrophage colony-forming units, which become granulocytes and monocytes

These cells have receptors for colony-stimulating factors (CSFs). Each CSF stimulates a different WBC type to develop in response to specific needs. Mature lymphocytes and macrophages secrete several types of CSFs in response to infections and other immune challenges. The red bone marrow stores granulocytes and monocytes until they are needed in the bloodstream. However, circulating leukocytes do not stay in the blood for very long. Granulocytes circulate for four to eight hours and then migrate into the tissues, where they live for another four to five days. Monocytes travel in the blood for ten to twenty hours, then migrate into the tissues and transform into a variety of macrophages, which can live as long as a few years. Lymphocytes are responsible for long-tern immunity and can survive from a few weeks to decades. They are continually recycled from blood to tissue fluid to lymph and finally back to the blood.

Thrombopoiesis

Thrombopoiesis refers to the production of platelets in the blood, because platelets used to be called thrombocytes. This starts when a hemocytoblast develops receptors for the hormone thrombopoietin, which is produced by the liver and kidneys. When these receptors are in place, the hemocytoblast becomes a committed cell called a megakaryoblast. This replicates its deoxyribonucleic acid (DNA), producing a large cell called a megakaryocyte, which breaks up into tiny fragments that enter the bloodstream. About 25 to 40 percent of the platelets are stored in the spleen and released as needed. The remainder circulate freely in the blood and live for about ten days.

Aging Changes in the Blood

The properties of blood change as we grow older. It is thought that these changes might contribute to the increased incidence of clot formation and atherosclerosis in older people. Some of the most prominent findings on these changes include:

- rise in fibrinogen;
- rise in blood viscosity;
- rise in plasma viscosity;
- increased red blood cell rigidity;
- increased formation of fibrin degradation products;
- earlier activation of the coagulation system.

The increased level of plasma fibrinogen is thought to be due to either its rapid production or slower degradation. As age progresses, fibrinogen and plasma viscosity tend to be positively correlated, with the rise in plasma viscosity being largely attributed to the rise in fibrinogen.

The viscosity of blood depends on factors such as shear rate, hematocrit, red cell deformability, plasma viscosity, and red cell aggregation. Although there are many factors involved, hyperviscosity syndrome can be generated by a rise in only one factor. A state of hyperviscosity causes sluggish blood flow and reduced oxygen supply to the tissue.

An age-dependent increase in various coagulation factors, a positive correlation with fibrinogen, and a negative correlation with plasma albumin has also been found. Both platelet and red cell aggregation increase with age, with red cell aggregation appearing to be the primary factor responsible for a rise in blood viscosity at low shear rates.

The decrease in red cell deformability (increase in rigidity) refers to its ability to deform under flow forces. Less deformable cells offer more resistance to flow in the microcirculation, which influences the delivery of oxygen to the tissues. Studies have found that older people have less fluid membranes in their red cells.

Blood H+ has also been found to be positively correlated with age, making the blood slightly more acidic as we age. This results in a swelling of the cell, making the red cells less deformable. This sets up a cycle for further increase in blood viscosity and worsening of blood flow parameters.

Since aging causes a reduction in total body water, blood volume decreases due to less fluid being present in the bloodstream. The number of red blood cells, and the corresponding hemoglobin and hematocrit levels, are reduced, which contributes to fatigue in the individual. Most of the white blood cells stay at their original levels, although there is a decrease in lymphocyte number and ability to fight off bacteria, leading to a reduced ability to resist infection.

Overall, the rise in fibrinogen is the most common and significant change in blood during aging because it contributes to a rise in plasma viscosity, red blood cell aggregation, and a rise in blood viscosity at low shear rates. Increased age is associated with a state of hypercoagulation of blood, making older people more susceptible to clot formation and atherosclerosis.

References

Ajmani RS, Rifkind JM. Hemorheological changes during human aging. *Gerontology* 1998; 44 (2): 111–20.

Coagulation cascade [online]. 2003 [cited 2007 Sep 9]. Available from: URL: http://labtestsonline.org/understanding/analytes/coag_cascade/coagulation_cascade.html

Marieb EN. *Human anatomy & physiology*. 4th ed. Menlo Park, Calif.: Benjamin/Cummings; 1998.

Saladin KS. *Anatomy and physiology—the unity of form and function*. 3rd ed. New York: McGraw-Hill; 2004.

Sherwood L. *Human physiology—from cells to systems*. 5th ed. Belmont, Calif: Brooks/Cole; 2004.

Chapter 2

Blood Types

Chapter Contents

Section 2.1

Introduction to Blood Types

All cells, including those that make up blood, have a combination of substances known as antigens on their surfaces that is inherited. Antigens function to enable our immune system to distinguish the body's own cells from foreign invaders. When invaders are recognized, they are destroyed by antibodies, which are also produced by the immune system. In blood typing, antigens on the surfaces of red blood cells (RBCs) are also known as agglutinogens and the antibodies that react against them are also called agglutinins. Antibodies in the blood are found in the plasma.

The ABO Blood Group

The ABO blood groups are made up of four types of blood—A, B, AB, and O. An individual's ABO blood type is determined by the hereditary presence or absence of the antigens A and B on the surfaces of RBCs. Antibodies of the ABO group appear in the plasma two to eight months after birth mainly in response to the bacteria that inhabit the intestines. However, antibodies cross-react with RBC antigens that are different to those present on the individual's own RBCs. This cross-reaction can be fatal and therefore has great significance in blood transfusions.

Identifying ABO Blood Types

People with type A blood have the antigen A on the surface of their RBCs, while people with type B blood have the B antigen. Individuals with type AB blood have both A and B antigens, whereas people with type O blood have no antigens present (there is no antigen O). The antibody that reacts against antigen A is called anti-A, and is found in the plasma of people who do not possess antigen A on their own RBCs—that is, people with type O or type B blood. The antibody that reacts against antigen B is called anti-B and is present in those who do not possess antigen B in their RBCs—people with type O or type A blood.

Importance of ABO Blood Groups in Transfusions

An antibody can attach to several RBCs at once and bind them together. Agglutination is the clumping of RBCs bound together by antibodies. In giving transfusions, it is very important that the donor's RBCs not agglutinate as they enter the recipient's bloodstream. For example, if type B blood (with B antigens) were transfused into a type A recipient (with anti-B antibodies), the recipient's anti-B antibodies would immediately agglutinate the donor's RBCs, causing a transfusion reaction where the agglutinated RBCs block small vessels and release their hemoglobin (Hb) over the next few hours to days. This free Hb can block the kidney tubules and cause death from kidney failure within a day or so. Therefore, a person with type A (anti-B) blood cannot receive B or AB blood, a person with type B (anti-A) blood cannot receive A or AB blood, and a person with type O (anti-A and anti-B) blood cannot receive A, B, or AB blood. Type AB blood is sometimes called the universal recipient because it lacks both anti-A and anti-B antibodies so it will not agglutinate donor RBCs of any ABO type. Type O may sometimes be called the universal donor, because since there is no "anti-O" antibody, recipients of any ABO type may receive type O blood.

The Rhesus Blood Group

The Rhesus or Rh blood group is named after the rhesus monkeys in which they were first discovered. Individuals either belong to the Rh-positive (Rh+) or Rh-negative (Rh-) Rhesus blood group. People with the Rh+ blood group have D antigens on the surface of their red blood cells, while Rh- individuals do not.

In contrast to the ABO group, anti-D antibodies that react against D antigens are not usually present in the blood under normal conditions. They only form in Rh- individuals who are exposed to Rh+ blood. If an Rh- receives an Rh+ transfusion, the recipient produces anti-D antibodies. Since anti-D does not form instantaneously, there is little danger in the first mismatched transfusion. However, because the recipient will now start producing anti-D, a subsequent Rh+ transfusion could agglutinate the donor's RBCs.

Implications of Rhesus Blood Groups during Pregnancy

A related condition can occur when an Rh- woman is pregnant with an Rh+ fetus. The first pregnancy is generally uneventful since anti-D does not form right away, so that even if the mother is exposed to Rh+

fetal blood via miscarriage or placental tearing at the time of birth, there is no danger to her first Rh+ child. However, she does begin to produce anti-D antibodies upon her first exposure to Rh+ fetal blood, although this does not occur instantaneously. If she becomes pregnant again with an Rh+ fetus, her anti-D antibodies can pass through the placenta and agglutinate the fetal RBCs. Agglutinated RBCs hemolyze (release their Hb), and the baby is born with a severe anemia called hemolytic disease of the newborn (HDN), which may kill the infant or leave it brain damaged.

HDN is relatively easy to prevent, while very difficult to treat. An Rh- mother is at risk of having an Rh+ baby if the baby's father is Rh+. As a result, it is now common to give immunoglobulin at twenty-eight to thirty-two weeks gestation and at birth to any pregnancy involving an Rh- mother and an Rh+ father. Immunoglobulin binds fetal RBC antigens so that they cannot stimulate the mother's immune system to produce anti-D, hence preventing HDN.

Reference

Saladin KS. *Anatomy and physiology—the unity of form and function*. 3rd ed. New York: McGraw-Hill; 2004.

Sherwood L. *Human physiology—from cells to systems*. 5th ed. Belmont, Calif: Brooks/Cole; 2004.

Section 2.2

Blood Types in the United States

All human blood may look alike but when it is tested using special agents, differences become apparent. The main red blood cell groups are A, B, AB, and O. The letters stand for the presence or absence of two antigens (chemical substances that can be targeted by one's immune system) labeled A and B:

- Group A blood has only the A antigen on red cells (and B antibody in the plasma).

- Group B blood has the only the B antigen on red cells (and A antibody in the plasma).

- Group AB blood has both antigens on red cells (but neither A nor B antibody in the plasma).

- Group O blood has neither antigen on red cells (but both A and B antibodies are in the plasma).

You can't donate red blood cells to just anyone and you can't receive blood from just anyone—blood groups need to be matched. Figure 2.1 shows how the blood groups match.

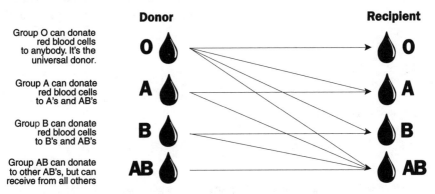

Figure 2.1. *Donor and Recipient Blood Group Matching*

Blood groups further classified as Rh-positive or Rh-negative are called blood types. Blood is Rh-positive if the blood antigen called the "Rh factor" is present and it is Rh-negative if the "Rh factor" antigen is absent.

The most common blood type is O+. Not all racial and ethnic groups have the same mix of these blood types. Hispanic people, for example, have a relatively high number of O's, while Asian people have a relatively high number of B's. The mix of the different blood types in the U.S. population is shown in Table 2.1.

Table 2.1. Blood Types in the U.S. Population

	White	African American	Hispanic	Asian
O +	37%	47%	53%	39%
O -	8%	4%	4%	1%
A +	33%	24%	29%	27%
A -	7%	2%	2%	0.5%
B +	9%	18%	9%	25%
B -	2%	1%	1%	0.4%
AB +	3%	4%	2%	7%
AB -	1%	0.3%	0.2%	0.1%

Some patients require a closer blood match than that provided by the ABO +/- blood typing. For example, sometimes if the donor and recipient are from the same racial or ethnic background, the chance of a reaction can be reduced. That's why an African American blood donation may be the best hope for the needs of patients with sickle cell disease, 98 percent of whom are of African American descent.

Blood Type Inheritance

It's inherited . . .

Like eye color, blood type is passed genetically from parents to children. Whether your blood type is A, B, AB, or O is based on the blood types of your mother and father.

Table 2.2. Blood Type Inheritance

Parent 1	AB	AB	AB	AB	B	A	A	O	O	O
Parent 2	AB	B	A	O	B	B	A	B	A	O
Possible blood type of child										
O					X	X	X	X	X	X
A		X	X	X	X		X	X		X	
B		X	X	X	X	X	X		X	
AB		X	X	X		X				

Note: Testing difficulties can cause exceptions to the above patterns. ABO blood typing is not sufficient to prove or disprove paternity or maternity.

Chapter 3

Donating and Preserving Blood

Chapter Contents

Section 3.1

Frequently Asked Questions about Blood Donation

Who can donate blood?

Anyone who is least sixteen years old, weighs at least 110 pounds, and enjoys generally good health.

What does "generally good health" mean?

You should not have cold, flu, or sore throat symptoms, and your blood's iron level should be adequate. There is no upper age limit, and even prescription medications do not necessarily disqualify you.

Are there any restrictions?

You should not donate blood if you are pregnant (or have been in the past six weeks), had hepatitis since age ten, had major surgery within the past year, or participated in activities that put you at risk for human immunodeficiency virus (HIV)/acquired immunodeficiency syndrome (AIDS).

How long does it take to donate blood?

Blood collection takes ten minutes or less, but we will also collect information, conduct a mini-physical (including a blood pressure test), and provide light refreshment. Allow about an hour for the entire process (two hours for platelet collection.) You will not even have to change your diet before donating.

Is donating blood safe?

Donating blood is a safe process. Needles and bags used to collect blood are used only once and then discarded, making spread of infection to the donor not possible.

Can I give if I have been turned down before?

Most reasons for which donors are turned away from donating blood are temporary, not permanent. For example, one common reason for a deferral is low iron level in the blood, but iron levels fluctuate daily and are affected by what you eat. A "mini-physical" is given to all potential donors to ensure they are healthy enough to donate.

How often can one give blood?

Regulations in the United States allow people to donate whole blood once every 56 days. The waiting period between donations can be different for other blood components. For example, donating only platelets in a process called apheresis requires only a 3-day wait before a person can give again. Donating two units of red blood cells through a similar process doubles the waiting period to 112 days.

Are the health history questions and my test results confidential?

Yes. The health history will be conducted by a trained professional in an individual booth arranged to preserve confidentiality. Your answers will be kept confidential, except where required by law. If your blood tests positive to any of the administered standard tests, you will receive confidential notification.

How much blood is taken—won't it make me weak?

A blood donation equals approximately one pint of blood. The average adult body has ten to twelve pints. The vast majority of people will not feel any different because of the donation. A very small percentage may experience temporary dizziness, but some rest and fluids will help you feel better quickly. Your body will replace the lost fluid within twenty-four hours.

How can I ensure a pleasant donation experience?

You'll want a good night's sleep the night before, and a good breakfast or lunch before your donation. Drink fluids like juice, milk, or soda ahead of time. Take your normal medications as prescribed. Ensure you have adequate iron level by making iron-rich foods part of your daily diet. These include red meat, poultry, fish, green leafy vegetables, iron-fortified cereals, nuts, raisins, and prunes. During your donation, relax. After your donation, have some juice and cookies. Then you can go about your daily activities, but avoid heavy lifting or strenuous exercise for the remainder of the day.

Should I give blood now or wait until I am called?

Under normal circumstances eligible donors are encouraged to donate as often as possible. During emergency circumstances please listen to media reports in your area and donate as requested.

Section 3.2

Tips for a Good Donation Experience

Before Donating

- Have a good breakfast or lunch.
- Drink extra water and fluids to replace the volume you will donate (avoid tea, coffee, or other beverages with caffeine).
- Eat iron-rich foods—red meat, fish, poultry or liver, beans, iron-fortified cereals, raisins and prunes.
- Avoid fatty foods, such as hamburgers, fries, or ice cream before donating. Tests for infections done on all donated blood can be affected by fatty materials—lipids—that appear in your blood for several hours after eating fatty foods. When this occurs and required testing cannot be performed, the blood may need to be discarded.

During the Donation

- Wear clothing with sleeves that can be raised above the elbow.
- Show the staff any "good veins" that have been used successfully in the past to draw blood.

- Relax.
- Take the time to enjoy a snack and a drink in the refreshments area immediately after donating.

After Donation

- Rehydrate by drinking plenty of fluids over the next twenty-four to forty-eight hours.
- Avoid strenuous physical activity or heavy lifting for about five hours after donation.
- If you feel lightheaded, lie down, preferably with feet elevated, until the feeling passes.
- In rare cases when bleeding occurs after removing the bandage, apply pressure to the site and raise your arm for three to five minutes; if bleeding or bruising occurs under the skin, apply a cold pack to the area periodically during the first twenty-four hours.
- If for any reason something doesn't feel right, call the American Red Cross toll-free number provided to you after your donation.

Section 3.3

Apheresis

Reprinted from "Blood Donation," Walter Reed Army Medical Center. The text of this document is available online at http://www.wramc.army.mil/SUPPORT/VOLUNTEER/Pages/donation.aspx; accessed April 20, 2009.

What is apheresis?

Apheresis is a special kind of blood donation that allows whole blood to be withdrawn from a donor and separated into its component parts, with all but the needed component being returned to the donor The needed blood component, such as platelets, is then made immediately available to the patient.

Why is blood separated?

Whole blood is made of several components, including red blood cells, white blood cells, platelets, and plasma. Each component has a special use. Apheresis procedures are used to collect platelets, plasma, and white blood cells. Each unit of whole blood contains only two tablespoons (30 ml) of platelet concentrate. Six to ten regular whole-blood donations would be required to supply enough platelets for one patient. However, one apheresis donation from a single donor can provide sufficient platelets for one transfusion.

Who needs apheresis?

Patients with cancer or leukemia, and transplant patients with blood disorders, such as aplastic anemia, benefit from apheresis blood products. Many times during chemotherapy and radiation treatment both cancer cells and healthy cells are destroyed, so patients need transfusions to prevent bleeding or to fight infection.

Who can be an apheresis donor?

Requirements for apheresis donors are similar to those for whole blood donations. Apheresis donors must:

- meet specific age requirements;
- meet a minimum weight requirement;
- be willing to give one to two hours of time per donation;
- not have taken aspirin or products containing aspirin, ibuprofen, or other anti-inflammatory medications for seventy-two hours.

Are platelet donations safe?

Yes. Each donation is closely supervised by trained staff who observe the donor throughout process. The donation does not significantly decrease the number of platelets in the donor's body and the donated platelets are quickly replaced. Donors experience no bleeding problems. It is impossible to get acquired immunodeficiency syndrome (AIDS) or any viral disease by donating platelets. The needles, tubing, and collection bags in the machine are sterile and discarded after each donation.

How does apheresis work?

Blood is drawn from the donor's arm and sent through sterile tubing into a centrifuge located in a cell-separator machine. The machine spins the blood to separate the platelets from the other components. The platelets are collected and the remaining components are returned to the donor in the other arm. The cell separator is a closed, sterile system utilizing disposable needles and plastic tubing that is used only once and then disposed of safely.

How long does it take?

Platelet donation takes about one to two hours. Donors are welcome to watch television or read during the process. You already spend about an hour donating whole blood. Why not take a little extra time to donate platelets? It's worth it!

Section 3.4

Cord Blood Banking

"Umbilical Cord Blood," © 2007 Arizona Department of Health Services
(www.azdhs.gov). Reprinted with permission.

What is cord blood?

After your baby is born, the umbilical cord is clamped and cut. The blood remains in the placenta and umbilical cord. In the past this blood, commonly called cord blood, was usually thrown away. We now know cord blood contains stem cells that can be used to help people with certain serious diseases. Now, families have three options available: discard the blood, donate it to a public cord bank, or retain it in a family cord blood bank. Cord blood that has been collected for storage at either a public cord blood bank or family cord blood bank is frozen and can be used when needed to help treat many serious diseases.

It is important to discuss questions regarding cord blood banking options with your health care provider as soon as possible during your pregnancy.

How can cord blood help?

The stem cells in cord blood are very important because they make many different types of cells in the body, including blood cells that carry oxygen, fight disease, and help stop bleeding. The stem cells in cord blood are primitive or undeveloped and can be transplanted in people to treat a number of life-threatening diseases. If needed, blood-forming cord blood stem cells can sometimes be used in autologous transplants (when a person receives his or her own umbilical cord blood) or more commonly, allogeneic transplants (when a person receives umbilical cord blood donated from someone else). A cord blood transplant does not need to be as perfectly matched to the person who receives it as in most other types of transplants. Because cord blood stem cells are more primitive, they have a lower rate of complications than with other stem cell transplants such as in bone marrow.

What disease can cord blood be used for?

There are more than sixty diseases that can now be helped through cord blood transplantation. These diseases include malignant and non-malignant conditions, such as blood cancers, rare inherited disorders of metabolism, immune diseases, and more. Treatment of these diseases using umbilical cord blood is not experimental. Cord blood transplantation has already helped thousands of people. There is ongoing research to find more diseases that can be helped by cord blood. While the research is still in the experimental stages, scientists are hopeful that one day cord blood transplantation will help in many heart, bone, liver, and brain diseases, even diseases like heart attack and stroke.

How is cord blood collected? Is it safe?

Collecting cord blood is completely safe for babies and mothers. It will not affect your baby's health or your birth experience because the blood is collected after your baby is born. The blood remaining in the umbilical cord is drained into a special collection bag and sent to the public or family cord blood bank you selected.

If you would like your baby's cord blood to be collected and stored for future use, you must make arrangements with either a public or family cord blood bank before the baby is born. When you contact a cord blood bank, they will send you information about cord blood collection and storage, forms to fill out, and a kit to take the hospital for your baby's birth.

What are the ways cord blood can be stored? What is the right decision for my family?

Types of cord blood banks: Cord blood can be donated to a public cord blood bank for use by someone in need or stored at a family cord blood bank for your baby's or family's use. Donating your baby's cord blood or storing it for private use is a personal decision that you must make for yourself after discussion with your healthcare provider and after performing your own research. If you have a family member with leukemia or another disease that may be treatable by stem cell transplant, you should talk to their healthcare provider about the advisability of family cord blood banking, which would typically be performed under these circumstances without cost.

Public cord blood banks: Public cord blood banks save and use cord blood for transplants to help people with one of the treatable diseases or for scientific research to learn more about the possible uses of cord blood. Transplants are anonymous and no information about you or your baby is given to the person receiving the cord blood. Donated cord blood becomes the property of the public cord blood bank. Before being accepted for donation, you will need to complete a health questionnaire to screen for genetic disorders and infectious diseases.

Family cord blood banks: There are many family cord blood banks available for families who wish to save their baby's cord blood for potential future use. Using family cord blood banks, the family controls the use of the cord blood. Studies show there are fewer graft versus host disease complications and better survival rates when cord blood from a related source is transplanted. However, there is no guarantee that the saved cord blood will be able to be used in all situations. When making a decision about family cord blood banks, it is important to ask what the total cost is, how experienced the company is in cord blood banking, how experienced the company is in cord blood transplantation, if the company is financially sound, and what would happen if the company went out of business.

How much does it cost to donate or bank cord blood?

Donating cord blood to a public cord blood bank does not usually cost you any money. Ask your healthcare provider if there will be any charge to collect the blood. Family banking of cord blood for the baby's or family's future use usually costs between $1,000 and $2,000 at the time of the baby's birth. There will also be an annual storage fee of approximately $100 to $150.

Chapter 4

Maintaining a Healthy Circulatory System

Keeping Your Arteries Healthy

The well-being of your arteries depends on a healthy endothelium, the inner lining of your blood vessels.

"Endothelial cells are the prima donnas within the blood vessels. They control almost every activity that occurs in the vessels, and they're fundamentally altered with age," says Dr. Edward Lakatta, M.D., chief of the Laboratory of Cardiovascular Science at the National Institutes of Health. "People who maintain a healthy endothelium as they get older and those who make an effort to do things that promote the repair of injured endothelium can reduce the risk of heart attacks and strokes caused by atherosclerosis or hypertension."

Although scientists still have much to learn about the endothelium and what can be done to keep it healthy, a number of studies suggest that certain modifiable risk factors can have an important impact on the cardiovascular system. For instance, regular moderate exercise, such as running, walking, or swimming can reduce body fat, increase lean muscle mass, decrease blood pressure, increase high-density lipoprotein (HDL) cholesterol (the "good" cholesterol) levels, and lessen the extent of arterial stiffening. All of these exercise-induced changes can have a positive influence on endothelial cells.

In addition, scientists have long known that tobacco smoke contains numerous toxic compounds, such as carbon monoxide, that promote

Excerpted from "Blood Vessels and Aging: The Rest of the Journey," National Institute on Aging, National Institutes of Health, October 16, 2008.

endothelial cell damage. Smoking also increases blood pressure and heart rate. Free radicals in smoke slash the amount of nitric oxide available in the blood stream. Nitric oxide, as you may recall, is a signaling molecule that helps keep arteries pliable. Because nicotine causes narrowing of blood vessels, less oxygen is transported to the heart. If you smoke, blood platelets become stickier and are more apt to form clots in your arteries.

High blood pressure—hypertension—causes blood vessels to thicken, diminishes production of nitric oxide, promotes blood clotting, and contributes to the development of atherosclerotic plaques in the arteries. Blood pressure is considered high when systolic pressure exceeds 140 mmHg and when diastolic blood pressure is higher than 90 mmHg.

Excessive weight increases the risk of high blood pressure and can increase the likelihood that you'll have high blood triglycerides and low HDL cholesterol, Dr. Lakatta says. Being overweight can also increase the probability you'll develop insulin resistance, a precursor of diabetes.

Diabetes, a disease in which the body does not produce or properly use insulin, becomes more common as we age. In fact, nearly half of all cases are diagnosed after age fifty-five. Atherosclerosis develops earlier and is more aggressive in people who have diabetes. In part, this occurs because diabetes causes the endothelium to produce excessive amounts of superoxide anion, a free radical that destroys nitric oxide. People age sixty-five and older who have diabetes are nearly four times more likely than those who don't to develop peripheral vascular disease, a condition that clogs the arteries that carry blood to the legs or arms. And cardiovascular diseases and stroke are leading causes of diabetes-related deaths. If you suspect you have or are at risk for diabetes, check with your doctor. Symptoms include increased thirst, increased hunger, fatigue, increased urination—especially at night, unexplained weight loss, blurred vision, and slow healing of wounds and sores.

Exercise: Your Heart's Best Friend

Scientists have long known that regular exercise causes certain changes in the hearts of younger people: Resting heart rate is lower, heart mass is higher, and stroke volume is higher than in their sedentary counterparts. These differences make the heart a better pump. Evidence now suggests these changes occur even when exercise training begins later in life, at age sixty or seventy, for instance. In other words, you don't lose the ability to become better physically conditioned. In addition, several studies have shown that exercise not only helps reduce debilitating symptoms such as breathlessness and fatigue in people who have heart failure, it also prolongs life.

Exercise training may be effective because it appears to improve the function of virtually every cell in the cardiovascular system. Animal studies, for instance, suggest that regular aerobic workouts help heart muscle cells remove calcium from their inner fluid at a faster rate after a contraction. This improved calcium cycling allows the heart to relax more and fill with more blood between beats.

Exercise also improves blood vessel elasticity and endothelial function, in part, by blocking the production of damaging free radicals and maintaining the production of nitric oxide, an important signaling molecule that helps protect the inner layer of the arteries. Together, these changes can slow the progression of atherosclerosis and other age-related cardiovascular conditions.

Metabolic Syndrome Increases Arterial Stiffness

Many older Americans have high blood pressure or high blood sugar or just a bit too much fat on the belly. While each of these conditions alone is bad enough, having all of these conditions at once—a cluster called metabolic syndrome—magnifies the risk of developing heart disease and stroke. And National Institute on Aging (NIA) scientists may have discovered a reason why: Metabolic syndrome appears to accelerate stiffening and thickening of the arteries.

Metabolic syndrome—also known as syndrome X or insulin resistance syndrome—may affect as many as forty-seven million Americans, according to the Centers for Disease Control and Prevention (CDC). After age fifty, a person has a better than one in three chance of developing this group of medical conditions characterized by insulin resistance and the presence of obesity, abdominal fat, high blood sugar and triglycerides, low HDL (good) blood cholesterol, and high blood pressure.

To determine the effects of metabolic syndrome on aging arteries, NIA researchers studied 471 participants—average age fifty-nine— in the Baltimore Longitudinal Study of Aging (BLSA). None of these participants had any detectable signs of cardiovascular disease when initially examined. But those who had three or more conditions associated with metabolic syndrome developed stiffer and thicker arteries at earlier ages than those who didn't have the syndrome.

"It's as if the metabolic syndrome makes your blood vessels older," says Angelo Scuteri, M.D., Ph.D., an investigator at the NIA's Laboratory of Cardiovascular Science. "If you have metabolic syndrome, when you are forty your arteries look like they are fifty-five or sixty."

Researchers have also found that stress reduction techniques, such as taking a walk, practicing yoga, or deep breathing are important to cardiovascular health. Emotional stress triggers the release of adrenaline from the adrenal gland and noradrenaline from the nerve endings in your heart and blood vessels. These hormones make the heart beat faster and adversely affect blood vessels. Under stress, an older person's blood pressure rises more rapidly and stays higher longer than a younger person's because the older person's blood vessels are stiffer and have lost much of their elasticity.

Healthy Foods, Healthy Arteries: Is There a Connection?

What you eat can help keep your heart and arteries healthy—or lead to excessive weight, high blood pressure, and high blood cholesterol—three key factors that increase the risk of developing cardiovascular disease, according to the National Heart, Lung, and Blood Institute. Based on the best available scientific evidence, the American Heart Association (AHA) recommends a diet that includes a variety of fruits, vegetables, and grains, while limiting consumption of saturated fat and sodium.

Fruits and vegetables have lots of antioxidants such as vitamin C and vitamin A that neutralize free radicals and may prevent oxidation in the arteries, dietary experts say. Fruits and vegetables also contain plenty of soluble fiber, a substance that has been shown to reduce blood cholesterol levels, which is healthy for the endothelium.

Breads, cereals, and other grain foods, which provide complex carbohydrates, vitamins, minerals, and fiber, are associated with a decreased risk of cardiovascular disease, according to the AHA Dietary Guidelines. However, some studies suggest eating less sugar, bread, and other simple and complex carbohydrates can lower blood insulin levels and decrease body fat and weight—three factors that are linked to an increased risk of heart disease and stroke. In recent years, a number of dietary recommendations based on these findings have become popular and are currently catching the public's awareness. While contentious, these are important issues and long-term studies are required to determine the risks and benefits of such diets, Dr. Lakatta says.

Saturated fats are usually solid at room temperature. These fats are primarily found in animal foods like meat, poultry, and dairy products like butter. Saturated fats tend to raise levels of "bad" low-density lipoprotein (LDL) and increase the risk of atherosclerosis. In fact, within two hours of eating a high saturated fat meal, endothelial cells don't work as well. Such meals can cause a temporary 50 percent dip in endothelial function, even in healthy young people who have no risk factors for atherosclerosis, Dr. Lakatta says.

In addition to saturated fats, some scientists are concerned about trans-fatty acids—unsaturated fats that have been artificially solidified by food manufacturers in a process called hydrogenation to make products like margarine and vegetable shortenings. These scientists suspect that trans-fatty acids, which are often described as hydrogenated or partially hydrogenated fats on many food labels, are more damaging to the heart and arteries than saturated fats.

But researchers have found other types of fats may be beneficial. Monounsaturated fats, found mainly in plant foods such as peanuts and olives, help lower LDL cholesterol. Like polyunsaturated fats, monounsaturated fats are usually liquid at room temperature. Polyunsaturated fats, found in fish, nuts, and dark leafy vegetables, have been getting a lot of attention from scientists in the past few years. They've concluded that one type of polyunsaturated fat—omega-3 fatty acid—found in fish may promote several things that improve endothelial function, including increasing nitric oxide production, slashing the production of free radicals and other substances that cause inflammation, and boosting HDL cholesterol levels. Fish such as salmon, herring, and mackerel are good sources of omega-3s.

Control over the condition of our arteries may also lie in how much salt we consume. In cultures where little sodium (in the form of salt) is consumed, blood pressures do not rise with age. Cultural differences have also been found in arterial stiffness. One study compared rural and urban populations in China. The urban population consumed much higher levels of sodium than the rural groups. And they had stiffer arteries. Other researchers found that sodium appears to accelerate age-associated stiffening of arteries. In particular, sodium promotes thickening of aging arterial walls, reduces the amount of nitric oxide available to endothelial cells, and promotes the formation of oxygen free radicals. But shifting to a low-sodium diet, research suggests, can begin to diminish arterial stiffness in as little as two weeks.

Most of the sodium in your diet comes from processed foods. The remaining is added at the table and while cooking. Scientists who study this issue suggest limiting the amount of sodium that you consume from all these sources to no more than 1,500 milligrams (mg) each day (an average American adult consumes about 3,300 milligrams daily). They recommend reading food labels carefully and buying foods that say "reduced sodium," "low in sodium," "sodium free," or "no salt added." Some dietitians suggest seasoning foods with herbs and spices like oregano, onion powder, or garlic instead of sodium.

Scientists suspect the more lifestyle changes, including diet and exercise, you can incorporate into your life, the better off your arteries will be, because these interventions work independently as well as in unison to promote the vitality of endothelial cells and contribute to reducing the risk of cardiovascular disease.

Chapter 5

How Aging Affects the Heart and Blood Vessels

Some changes in the heart and blood vessels normally occur with age, but many others are modifiable factors that, if not treated, can lead to heart disease.

Background

The heart has two sides. The right side pumps blood to the lungs to receive oxygen and get rid of carbon dioxide. The left side pumps oxygen-rich blood to the body.

Blood flows out of the heart through arteries, which branch out and get smaller and smaller as they go into the tissues. In the tissues, they become tiny capillaries.

Capillaries are where the blood gives up oxygen and nutrients to the tissues, and receives carbon dioxide and wastes back from the tissues. Then, the vessels begin to collect together into larger and larger veins, which return blood to the heart.

Aging causes changes in the heart and in the blood vessels. Heart and blood vessel diseases are some of the most common disorders in the elderly.

Excerpted from "Aging Changes in the Heart and Blood Vessels," © 2009 A.D.A.M., Inc. Reprinted with permission.

Aging Changes

Heart

- The heart has a natural pacemaker system that controls the heartbeat. Some of the pathways of this system may develop fibrous tissue and fat deposits. The natural pacemaker (the sino-atrial [SA] node) loses some of its cells. These changes may result in a slightly slower heart rate.

- A slight increase in the size of the heart, especially the left ventricle, is not uncommon. The heart wall thickens, so the amount of blood that the chamber can hold may actually decrease despite the increased overall heart size. The heart may fill more slowly.

- Heart changes cause the electrocardiogram (ECG) of a normal, healthy, older person to be slightly different than the ECG of a healthy younger adult. Abnormal rhythms (arrhythmias) such as atrial fibrillation are common in older people. They may be caused by heart disease.

- Normal changes in the heart include deposits of the "aging pigment," lipofuscin. The heart muscle cells degenerate slightly. The valves inside the heart, which control the direction of blood flow, thicken and become stiffer. A heart murmur caused by valve stiffness is fairly common in the elderly.

Blood Vessels

- Receptors, called baroreceptors, monitor the blood pressure and make changes to help maintain a fairly constant blood pressure when a person changes positions or activities. The baroreceptors become less sensitive with aging. This may explain why many older people have orthostatic hypotension, a condition in which the blood pressure falls when a person goes from lying or sitting to standing. This causes dizziness because there is less blood flow to the brain.

- The capillary walls thicken slightly. This may cause a slightly slower rate of exchange of nutrients and wastes.

- The main artery from the heart (aorta) becomes thicker, stiffer, and less flexible. This is probably related to changes in the connective tissue of the blood vessel wall. This makes the blood pressure higher and makes the heart work harder, which may lead to hypertrophy (thickening of the heart muscle). The other arteries also thicken and stiffen. In general, most elderly people experience a moderate increase in blood pressure.

Blood

- The blood itself changes slightly with age. Normal aging causes a reduction in total body water. As part of this, there is less fluid in the bloodstream, so blood volume decreases.

- The number of red blood cells (and correspondingly, the hemoglobin and hematocrit levels) are reduced. This contributes to fatigue. Most of the white blood cells stay at the same levels, although certain white blood cells important to immunity (lymphocytes) decrease in number and ability to fight off bacteria. This reduces the ability to resist infection.

Effect of Changes

Under normal circumstances, the heart continues to adequately supply all parts of the body. However, an aging heart may be slightly less able to tolerate increased workloads, because changes reduce this extra pumping ability (reserve heart function).

Some of the things that can increase heart workload include illness, infections, emotional stress, injuries, extreme physical exertion, and certain medications.

Common Problems

- Angina (chest pain caused by temporarily reduced blood flow to the heart muscle), shortness of breath with exertion, and heart attack can result from coronary artery disease.

- Abnormal heart rhythms (arrhythmias) of various types can occur.

- Anemia may occur, possibly related to malnutrition, chronic infections, blood loss from the gastrointestinal tract, or as a complication of other diseases or medications.

- Arteriosclerosis (hardening of the arteries) is very common. Fatty plaque deposits inside the blood vessels cause them to narrow and can totally block blood vessels.

- Congestive heart failure is also very common in the elderly. In people older than seventy-five, congestive heart failure occurs ten times more often than in younger adults.

- Coronary artery disease is fairly common. It is often a result of arteriosclerosis.

- Heart and blood vessel diseases are fairly common in older people. Common disorders include high blood pressure and orthostatic hypotension.

- Transient ischemic attacks (TIA) or strokes can occur if blood flow to the brain is disrupted.

- Valve diseases are fairly common. Aortic stenosis, or narrowing of the aortic valve, is the most common valve disease in the elderly.

Other problems with the heart and blood vessels include the following:

- Blood clots

  - Deep vein thrombosis

  - Thrombophlebitis

- Peripheral vascular disease, resulting in claudication (intermittent pain in the legs when walking)

- Varicose veins

Prevention

You can help your circulatory system (heart and blood vessels). Heart disease risk factors that you have some control over include high blood pressure, cholesterol levels, diabetes, obesity, and smoking. Here are some things you can do help maintain your circulatory system:

- Eat a heart-healthy diet with reduced amounts of saturated fat and cholesterol, and control your weight. Follow your health care provider's recommendations for treatment of high blood pressure, high cholesterol, or diabetes. Minimize or stop smoking.

- Exercise may help prevent obesity and helps people with diabetes control their blood sugar.

- Exercise may help you maintain your maximum abilities as much as possible and reduces stress.

- Have regular check-ups for your heart:

  - Have your blood pressure checked every year. If you have diabetes, heart disease, kidney problems, or certain other conditions, your blood pressure may need to be monitored more closely.

- If your cholesterol level is normal, have it rechecked every three to five years. If you have diabetes, heart disease, kidney problems, or certain other conditions, your cholesterol may need to be monitored more closely.

- Moderate exercise is one of the best things you can do to keep your heart, and the rest of your body, healthy. Consult with your health care provider before beginning a new exercise program. Exercise moderately and within your capabilities, but do it regularly.

- People who exercise usually have less body fat and smoke less than people who do not exercise. They also tend to have fewer blood pressure problems and less heart disease.

References

Schwartz JB, Zipes DP. Cardiovascular Disease in the Elderly. In: Libby P, Bonow RO, Mann DL, Zipes DP, eds. *Braunwald's Heart Disease: A Textbook of Cardiovascular Medicine*. 8th ed. Philadelphia, Pa; Saunders Elsevier; 2007: chap 75.

Part Two

Diagnosing and Treating Blood and Circulatory Disorders

Chapter 6

Blood Tests

Chapter Contents

45

Section 6.1

Blood Typing

Alternative Names

Cross matching; Rh typing; ABO blood typing

Definition

Blood typing is a method to tell what specific type of blood you have. What type you have depends on whether or not there are certain proteins, called antigens, on your red blood cells.

Blood is often grouped according to the ABO blood typing system. This method breaks blood types down into four categories:

- Type A
- Type B
- Type AB
- Type O

Your blood type (or blood group) depends on the types that are been passed down to you from your parents.

How the Test Is Performed

Blood is drawn from a vein, usually from the inside of the elbow or the back of the hand. The puncture site is cleaned with a germ-killing product. An elastic band is placed around the upper arm to apply pressure, which causes the vein to swell with blood.

A needle is inserted into the vein, and the blood is collected into a tube. During the procedure, the elastic band is removed to restore circulation. Once the blood has been collected, the needle is removed, and a Band-Aid or gauze is applied.

In infants or young children, the area is cleansed with antiseptic and punctured with a sharp needle or a lancet. The blood may be collected in a pipette (small glass tube), on a slide, onto a test strip, or into a small container. A bandage may be applied if there is any bleeding.

The test to determine your blood group is called ABO typing. Your blood sample is mixed with antibodies against type A and B blood, and the sample is checked to see whether or not the blood cells stick together (agglutinate). If blood cells stick together, it means the blood reacted with one of the antibodies.

The second step is called back typing. The liquid part of your blood without cells (serum) is mixed with blood that is known to be type A and Type B. Persons with Type A blood have anti-B antibodies, and those with Type B blood have anti-A antibodies. Type O blood contains both types of antibodies. These two steps can accurately determine your blood type.

Blood typing is also done to tell whether or not you have a substance called Rh factor on the surface of your red blood cells If you have this substance, you are considered Rh+ (positive). Those without it are considered Rh- (negative). Rh typing uses a method similar to ABO typing.

How to Prepare for the Test

No special preparation is necessary for this test.

How the Test Will Feel

Some people have discomfort when the needle is inserted. Others may only feel a tiny prick or stinging sensation. Afterward, there may be some throbbing or a bruise may develop.

Why the Test Is Performed

This test is done to determine a person's blood type. Health care providers need to know your blood type when you get a blood transfusion or transplant, because not all blood types are compatible with each other. For example:

- If you have type A blood, you can only receive types A and O blood.

- If you have type B blood, you can you can only receive types B and O blood.

- If you have type AB blood, you can only receive types A, B, AB, and O blood.

- If you have type O blood, you can you can only receive type O blood.

Type O blood can be given to anyone with any blood type. That is why people with type O blood are called universal donors.

Blood typing is especially important during pregnancy. If the mother is found to be Rh-, the father should also be tested. If the father has Rh+ blood, the mother needs to receive a treatment to help prevent the development of substances that may harm the unborn baby.

If you are Rh+, you can receive Rh+ or Rh- blood. If you are Rh-, you can only receive Rh- blood.

Normal Results

If your blood cells stick together when mixed with:

- anti-A serum, you have type A blood;

- anti-B serum, you have type B blood;

- both anti-A and anti-B serums, you have type AB blood.

If your blood cells do not stick together when anti-A and B is added, you have type O blood.

Back Typing

- If your blood clumps together when B cells are added to your sample, you have type A blood.

- If your blood clumps together when A cells are added to your sample, you have type B blood.

- If your blood clumps together when both types of cells are added to your sample, you have type O blood.

Lack of blood cells sticking together when your sample is mixed with both types of blood indicates you have type AB blood.

Rh Typing

- If your blood cells stick together when mixed with anti-Rh serum, you have type Rh-positive blood.

- If your blood does not clot when mixed with anti-Rh serum, you have type Rh-negative blood.

Risks

Risks associated with taking blood may include:

- fainting or feeling light-headed;
- multiple punctures to locate veins;
- excessive bleeding;
- hematoma (blood accumulating under the skin);
- infection (a slight risk any time the skin is broken).

Considerations

There are many antigens besides the major ones (A, B, and Rh). Many minor ones are not routinely detected during blood typing. If they are not detected, you may still have a reaction when receiving certain types of blood, even if the A, B, and Rh antigens are matched.

A process called cross-matching followed by a Coombs test can help detect these minor antigens.

References

Goodnough LT. Transfusion medicine. In: Goldman L, Ausiello D, eds. Cecil *Medicine*. 23rd ed. Philadelphia, Pa: Saunders Elsevier; 2007: chap 183.

Section 6.2

Complete Blood Count

"Full Blood Count (FBC)," reviewed August 2009, reproduced with permission from myDr.com.au. Copyright CMPMedica Australia 2000–2009. Subject to myDr's disclaimer.

The full blood count (FBC), sometimes referred to as a full blood examination or complete blood count, is one of the most commonly performed blood tests, as it can tell us so much about the status of our health. It is important for diagnosing conditions in which the number of blood cells is abnormally high or abnormally low, or the cells themselves are abnormal.

A full blood count measures the status of a number of different features of the blood, including:

- the amount of hemoglobin in the blood;
- the number of red blood cells (red cell count);
- the percentage of blood cells as a proportion of the total blood volume (hematocrit or packed cell volume);
- the volume of red blood cells (mean cell volume);
- the average amount of hemoglobin in the red blood cells (known as mean cell hemoglobin);
- the number of white blood cells (white cell count);
- the percentages of the different types of white blood cells (leukocyte differential count); and
- the number of platelets.

The following provides an explanation of the various components that are measured, and helps to demystify some of the jargon you may hear in relation to this blood test.

Hemoglobin (Hb)

Hemoglobin is an iron-containing compound found in the red blood cells, which transports oxygen around the body. Measuring the concentration of hemoglobin in the blood can help diagnose anemia, a condition caused by a deficiency of hemoglobin. Anemia can arise due to:

- too few red blood cells;
- inadequate iron intake;
- inadequate folate or vitamin B_{12} intake;
- microscopic bleeding or other blood loss;
- blood cell destruction;
- a chronic illness; or
- a defect in the hemoglobin molecule itself.

This measurement may also detect abnormally high concentrations of hemoglobin. This may occur in people with chronic lung disease, as an adaptation to high altitudes, or because of an abnormal increase in red cell production by the bone marrow (polycythemia vera).

The normal hemoglobin level for adult males is 130–70 g/L, and 120–50 g/L for adult females.

Red Cell Count (RCC)

Red cell count is an estimation of the number of red blood cells per liter of blood.

Abnormally low numbers of red blood cells may indicate anemia as a result of blood loss, bone marrow failure, malnutrition such as iron deficiency, overhydration, or mechanical damage to red blood cells.

Abnormally high numbers of red blood cells may indicate congenital heart disease, some lung diseases, dehydration, kidney disease, or polycythemia vera.

The normal red cell count for adult males is 4.5–5.5 x 10^{12}/L, and 3.8–4.8 x 10^{12}/L for adult females.

Packed Cell Volume (PCV) or Hematocrit (Hct)

Hematocrit is a measure of the percentage of red blood cells to the total blood volume.

A low hematocrit may indicate anemia, blood loss, bone marrow failure, leukemia, multiple myeloma, nutritional deficiency, overhydration, or rheumatoid arthritis.

A high hematocrit may indicate dehydration (for example, due to burns or diarrhea), eclampsia (a serious condition that can occur during pregnancy), or polycythemia vera.

The normal hematocrit range for adult males is 40–50 percent, and 36–46 percent for adult females.

Mean Cell Volume or Mean Corpuscular Volume (MCV)

Mean cell volume is an estimate of the volume of red blood cells. It is useful for determining the type of anemia a person might have.

A low MCV may indicate iron deficiency, chronic disease, pregnancy, anemia due to blood cell destruction, or bone marrow disorders.

A high MCV may indicate anemia due to nutritional deficiencies, bone marrow abnormalities, liver disease, alcoholism, chronic lung disease, or therapy with certain medications.

The normal MCV range for adults is 83–101 fL.

Mean Cell Hemoglobin (MCH) and Mean Cell Hemoglobin Concentration (MCHC)

These measures, also known as mean corpuscular hemoglobin and mean corpuscular hemoglobin concentration, are further guides to the investigation of anemia.

The MCH is the hemoglobin content of the average red cell. The MCHC is the average hemoglobin concentration in a given volume of packed red cells.

The MCH may be low in types of anemia where the red blood cells are abnormally small, or high in other types of anemia where the red blood cells are enlarged (for example, as a result of folic acid or vitamin B_{12} deficiency).

The MCHC is low in iron deficiency, blood loss, pregnancy, and anemias caused by chronic disease.

The normal MCH range for adults is 27–32 pg, and the normal MCHC range is 315–345 g/L.

White Cell (Leukocyte) Count

White cell count estimates the total number of white blood cells per liter of blood.

An abnormal high or low white cell count can indicate many possible medical conditions and a leukocyte differential count, which provides numbers of the different types of white cells, is usually needed to help make any diagnosis.

Abnormally low numbers of white blood cells may indicate liver or spleen disorders, bone marrow disorders, or exposure to radiation or toxic substances.

Abnormally high levels of white blood cells may indicate infection, tissue damage, leukemia, or inflammatory diseases.

The normal white cell count for adults is 4.0–10.0 x 10^9/L.

Leukocyte (White Cell) Differential Count

Leukocyte differential count provides an estimate of the numbers of the five main types of white blood cells. These are: neutrophils; monocytes; lymphocytes; eosinophils; and basophils.

Each of the five types has a specific role in the body.

Neutrophils and monocytes protect the body against bacteria and eat up small particles of foreign matter.

Lymphocytes are involved in the immune process, producing antibodies against foreign organisms, protecting against viruses, and fighting cancer.

Eosinophils kill parasites and are involved in allergic responses. High numbers of eosinophils may be associated with worm infections or exposure to substances that cause allergic reactions.

Basophils also take part in allergic responses and increased basophil production may be associated with bone marrow disorders or viral infection.

The normal ranges for the number of the different types of white cells in adults are:

- Neutrophils: 2.0–7.0 x 10^9/L

- Eosinophils: 0.02–0.5 x 10^9/L

- Basophils: 0.05–0.1 x 10^9/L

- Monocytes: 0.2–1.0 x 10^9/L

- Lymphocytes: 1.0–3.0 x 10^9/L

Platelet Count

Platelet count is an estimation of the number of platelets per liter of blood. Abnormally low numbers of platelets is known as thrombocytopenia, while an abnormally high level of platelets is known as thrombocytosis.

Platelet counts are often used to monitor medications such as heparin, which may cause low numbers of platelets, as well as medications that can have toxic effects on bone marrow. They may also be used to help diagnose problems associated with abnormal bleeding or bruising.

The normal platelet count for adults is 150–400 x 10^9/L.

A Note on Differing Laboratory Values

The ranges for what is considered normal given here are typical figures. However, different laboratories may use slightly different ranges, depending on how they perform the measurements. Ask your doctor if you are unsure about your results.

The material provided by CMPMedica Australia Pty Ltd is intended for Australian residents only, is of a general nature, and is provided for information purposes only. The material is not a substitute for independent professional medical advice from a qualified healthcare professional. It is not intended to be used by anyone to diagnose, treat, cure, or prevent any disease or medical condition. No person should act in reliance solely on a statement contained in the material provided, and at all times should obtain specific advice from a qualified healthcare professional.

Section 6.3

Fibrinogen Test

"Fibrinogen," © 2009 A.D.A.M., Inc. Reprinted with permission.

Alternative Names

Serum fibrinogen; plasma fibrinogen; factor I; hypofibrinogenemia test

Definition

Fibrinogen is a protein produced by the liver. This protein helps stop bleeding by helping blood clots to form. A blood test can be done to tell how much fibrinogen you have in the blood.

How the Test Is Performed

Blood is typically drawn from a vein, usually from the inside of the elbow or the back of the hand. The site is cleaned with germ-killing medicine (antiseptic). The healthcare provider wraps an elastic band around the upper arm to apply pressure to the area and make the vein swell with blood.

Next, the healthcare provider gently inserts a needle into the vein. The blood collects into an airtight vial or tube attached to the needle. The elastic band is removed from your arm.

Once the blood has been collected, the needle is removed, and the puncture site is covered to stop any bleeding.

In infants or young children, a sharp tool called a lancet may be used to puncture the skin and make it bleed. The blood collects into a small glass tube called a pipette, or onto a slide or test strip. A bandage may be placed over the area if there is any bleeding.

How to Prepare for the Test

There is no special preparation needed.

How the Test Will Feel

When the needle is inserted to draw blood, some people feel moderate pain, while others feel only a prick or stinging sensation. Afterward, there may be some throbbing.

Why the Test Is Performed

Your doctor may order this test if you have problems with blood clotting, particularly if you have excessive bleeding.

Normal Results

The normal range is 200–400 milligrams per deciliter (mg/dL).

Note: Normal value ranges may vary slightly among different laboratories. Talk to your doctor about the meaning of your specific test results.

What Abnormal Results Mean

Abnormal results may be due to:

- excessive fibrinogen use (as in disseminated intravascular coagulation);
- fibrinolysis;
- hemorrhage;
- lack of fibrinogen production (acquired or from birth).

Additional conditions under which the test may be performed:

- hemophilia A;
- hemophilia B;
- placenta abruption.

Risks

There is very little risk involved with having your blood taken. Veins and arteries vary in size from one patient to another and from one side of the body to the other. Taking blood from some people may be more difficult than from others.

Other risks associated with having blood drawn are slight but may include:

- excessive bleeding;
- fainting or feeling light-headed;
- hematoma (blood accumulating under the skin);
- infection (a slight risk any time the skin is broken).

Note: This test is most often performed on people who have bleeding disorders. The risk of excessive bleeding is slightly greater in such people than for those who do not have bleeding problems.

References

Kessler C. Hemorrhagic disorders: Coagulation factor deficiencies. In: Goldman L, Ausiello D, eds. *Cecil Medicine*. 23rd ed. Philadelphia, Pa: Saunders Elsevier; 2007: chap 180.

Section 6.4

Reticulocyte Count

"Reticulocyte Count," © 2009 A.D.A.M., Inc. Reprinted with permission.

A reticulocyte count measures the percentage of reticulocytes (slightly immature red blood cells) in blood.

How the Test Is Performed

Blood is typically drawn from a vein, usually from the inside of the elbow or the back of the hand. The site is cleaned with germ-killing medicine (antiseptic). The healthcare provider wraps an elastic band around the upper arm to apply pressure to the area and make the vein swell with blood.

Next, the healthcare provider gently inserts a needle into the vein. The blood collects into an airtight vial or tube attached to the needle. The elastic band is removed from your arm.

Once the blood has been collected, the needle is removed, and the puncture site is covered to stop any bleeding.

In infants or young children, a sharp tool called a lancet may be used to puncture the skin and make it bleed. The blood collects into a small glass tube called a pipette, or onto a slide or test strip. A bandage may be placed over the area if there is any bleeding.

The blood sample is sent to a laboratory. A special stain is used to identify the reticulocytes.

How to Prepare for the Test

No special preparation is necessary.

How the Test Will Feel

When the needle is inserted to draw blood, some people feel moderate pain, while others feel only a prick or stinging sensation. Afterward, there may be some throbbing.

Why the Test Is Performed

The test is done to determine if red blood cells are being created in the bone marrow at an appropriate rate. The number of reticulocytes in the blood is a sign of how quickly they are being produced and released by the bone marrow.

Normal Results

The normal range depends on the level of hemoglobin, and the range is higher if there has been bleeding or red cell destruction.

What Abnormal Results Mean

A higher-than-normal percentage of reticulocytes may indicate:

* bleeding;
* erythroblastosis fetalis;
* hemolytic anemia;
* kidney disease with increased erythropoietin production.

A lower-than-normal percentage of reticulocytes may indicate:

* bone marrow failure (for example, from toxicity, tumor, or infection);
* cirrhosis of the liver;
* folate deficiency;
* iron deficiency;
* kidney disease with decreased erythropoietin production;
* radiation therapy;
* vitamin B-12 deficiency.

Additional conditions under which the test may be performed:

* anemia of chronic disease;
* congenital spherocytic anemia;
* drug-induced immune hemolytic anemia;
* hemolytic anemia due to glucose-6-phosphate dehydrogenase (G6PD) deficiency
* idiopathic aplastic anemia;

- idiopathic autoimmune hemolytic anemia;

- immune hemolytic anemia;

- pernicious anemia;

- secondary aplastic anemia.

Risks

There is very little risk involved with having your blood taken. Veins and arteries vary in size from one patient to another and from one side of the body to the other. Taking blood from some people may be more difficult than from others.

Other risks associated with having blood drawn are slight but may include:

- excessive bleeding;

- fainting or feeling lightheaded;

- hematoma (blood accumulating under the skin);

- infection (a slight risk any time the skin is broken).

Considerations

The reticulocyte count may be increased during pregnancy.

References

Zuckerman K. Approach to the anemias. In: Goldman L, Ausiello D, eds. *Cecil Medicine*. 23rd ed. Philadelphia, Pa: Saunders Elsevier; 2007: chap 162.

Chapter 7

Bone Marrow Tests

What Are Bone Marrow Tests?

Bone marrow tests are used to check whether your bone marrow is healthy. These tests also show whether your bone marrow is making normal amounts of blood cells.

Bone marrow is the sponge-like tissue inside the bones. It contains stem cells that develop into the three types of blood cells that the body needs:

- Red blood cells carry oxygen through the body.

- White blood cells fight infection.

- Platelets stop bleeding.

Another type of stem cell, called an embryonic stem cell, can develop into any type of cell in the body. These cells aren't found in bone marrow.

Overview

The two bone marrow tests are aspiration and biopsy.

Bone marrow aspiration usually is done first. For this test, your doctor removes a small amount of fluid bone marrow through a needle. He or she may have some idea of what the problem is, and the sample gives him or her useful information about the cells in the marrow.

Excerpted from "Bone Marrow Tests," National Heart Lung and Blood Institute, National Institutes of Health, September 2007.

A bone marrow biopsy is a follow-up test. It's done when an aspiration doesn't give needed information. Or, it's done when the doctor wants to examine the bone marrow structure itself. For a bone marrow biopsy, your doctor removes a small amount of bone marrow tissue through a larger needle.

Who Needs Bone Marrow Tests?

You may need bone marrow tests if your doctor suspects that you have a blood or bone marrow disease or condition. These diseases and conditions include the following:

- **Myelodysplastic syndrome:** This is a group of diseases in which your bone marrow doesn't make enough normal blood cells.

- **Neutropenia:** This is a condition in which you have a lower than normal number of white blood cells in your blood.

- **Anemia:** This is a condition in which you have a lower than normal number of red blood cells, or the red blood cells don't have enough of an iron-rich protein that carries oxygen from the lungs to the rest of the body. Bone marrow tests also are used to diagnose aplastic anemia. This is a rare and serious condition in which bone marrow stops making enough new blood cells.

- **Myelofibrosis:** This is a serious bone marrow disorder that disrupts normal production of blood cells and leads to severe anemia.

- **Thrombocytopenia:** This group of conditions occurs when your body doesn't make enough platelets and your blood doesn't clot as it should.

- **Essential thrombocythemia:** This is a disease in which your bone marrow makes too many blood cells, especially platelets.

- **Leukemia:** This is a cancer of the white blood cells. Types of leukemia include acute and chronic leukemias and multiple myeloma.

You also may need bone marrow tests if you have other types of cancer. These may include breast cancer that has spread to the bone or Hodgkin and non-Hodgkin lymphomas (which are cancers of a particular type of white blood cell).

Bone marrow tests help show what stage the cancer is in. That is, the tests help doctors know how serious the cancer is and how much it has spread in the body.

Bone marrow tests also can show what's causing a fever. The tests may be used for people who have diseases in which their immune systems aren't working properly. They're also used for patients who may have uncommon bacterial infections.

What to Expect During Bone Marrow Tests

Bone marrow aspiration and biopsy take about twenty minutes each. Before the test(s), the doctor or nurse will tell you what will happen. Your breathing, heart rate, and pain will be monitored throughout the test.

These tests are generally done on the pelvic bone. Part of this bone is accessible in most people on the lower back. If your doctor uses that part of the pelvic bone, you will lie on your stomach for the test. Aspiration also can be done on the breastbone.

The area on your body where the doctor will insert the needle is cleaned and draped with a cloth. Your doctor sees only the site where the needle is inserted. He or she numbs the skin at the site and then makes a small incision (cut). This makes it easier to insert the needle into the bone. Stitches may be needed to close the cut after the test.

For bone marrow aspiration, your doctor inserts the needle into the marrow and removes a small amount of fluid bone marrow. You may feel a brief, sharp pain. The fluid that's removed from the bone marrow is taken to a lab and studied under a microscope.

If your doctor decides to do a bone marrow biopsy, it's done after the aspiration. For the biopsy, your doctor uses a needle to remove a small amount of the bone marrow tissue. Thin sections of this tissue are studied under a microscope.

During both tests, it's important for you to remain still and as relaxed as possible.

What to Expect After Bone Marrow Tests

After the bone marrow test(s), the nurse holds a bandage on the site where the needle was inserted until the bleeding stops. Then he or she puts a smaller bandage on the site. Most people can go home the same day.

After twenty-four hours, you can take off the bandage. Call your doctor if you develop a fever, have a lot of pain, or see redness, swelling, or discharge at the site. These are signs of infection.

Expect mild discomfort for about a week. Your doctor may tell you to take an over-the-counter pain medicine.

What Do Bone Marrow Tests Show?

Bone marrow tests show whether your bone marrow is making enough healthy blood cells. If it's not, the results can tell your doctor which cells are unhealthy and why.

Your doctor combines information from your bone marrow test with information from a physical exam, blood tests, and other tests such as imaging scans and x-rays. This information helps your doctor diagnose your condition and plan how to treat it.

What Are the Risks of Bone Marrow Tests?

Bleeding and infection are the two most common risks of bone marrow tests, but they're rare.

To prevent bleeding from the site where the needle was inserted, don't do any heavy lifting or vigorous exercise for a few days.

To prevent infection, don't shower or bathe for the first day. After twenty-four hours, you can take off the bandage. Call your doctor if you develop a fever, have a lot of pain, or see redness, swelling, or discharge at the site. These are signs of infection.

Expect mild discomfort for about a week. Your doctor may tell you to take an over-the-counter pain medicine.

Bone marrow tests are safe for most people. In some cases, these tests aren't safe for people with certain bleeding disorders (like hemophilia). Your doctor can tell you whether bone marrow tests are safe for you.

Chapter 8

Bleeding and Clotting Tests

Chapter Contents

Section 8.1

Bleeding Time

Bleeding time is a blood test that looks at how fast small blood vessels close to stop you from bleeding.

How the Test Is Performed

A blood pressure cuff inflates around your upper arm. While the cuff is on your arm, the healthcare provider makes two small cuts on the lower arm. They are just deep enough to cause a tiny amount of bleeding.

The blood pressure cuff is immediately deflated. Blotting paper is touched to the cuts every thirty seconds until the bleeding stops. The healthcare provider records the time it takes for the cuts to stop bleeding.

How to Prepare for the Test

Certain medications may change the test results. Always tell your doctor what medications you are taking, even over-the-counter drugs. Drugs that may increase bleeding times include dextran, nonsteroidal anti-inflammatory drugs (NSAIDs), and salicylates (including aspirin).

Your doctor may tell you to stop taking certain medicines a few days before the test. Never stop taking medicine without first talking to your doctor.

How the Test Will Feel

The tiny cuts are very shallow. Most people say it feels like a skin scratch.

Why the Test Is Performed

This test helps diagnose bleeding problems.

Normal Results

Bleeding normally stops within one to nine minutes. However, values may vary from lab to lab.

What Abnormal Results Mean

Longer-than-normal bleeding time may be due to:

- blood vessel defect;
- platelet aggregation defect;
- thrombocytopenia (low platelet count).

Additional conditions under which the test may be performed:

- acquired platelet function defect;
- congenital platelet function defects;
- primary thrombocythemia;
- von Willebrand disease.

Risks

There is a very slight risk of infection where the skin is broken. Excessive bleeding is rare.

References

Schafer A. Hemorrhagic disorders: Approach to the patient with bleeding and thrombosis. In: Goldman L, Ausiello D, eds. *Cecil Medicine.* 23rd ed. Philadelphia, Pa: Saunders Elsevier; 2007: chap 178.

Section 8.2

Partial Thromboplastin Time

What It Is

A partial thromboplastin time (PTT) test measures how long it takes for a clot to form in a blood sample. A clot is a thick lump of blood that the body produces to seal leaks, wounds, cuts, and scratches and prevent excessive bleeding.

The blood's ability to clot involves platelets (also called thrombocytes) and proteins called clotting factors. Platelets are oval-shaped cells made in the bone marrow. Most clotting factors are made in the liver.

When a blood vessel breaks, platelets are first to the area to help seal off the leak and temporarily stop or slow the bleeding. But for the clot to become strong and stable, the action of clotting factors is required.

The body's twelve clotting factors are numbered using the Roman numerals I through XII (thromboplastin is factor III). They work together in a specialized sequence, almost like pieces of a puzzle. When the last piece is in place, the clot develops—but if even one piece is missing or defective, the clot can't form.

The PTT test is used to evaluate the ability of a person's blood to clot. If it takes an abnormally long time for the blood to clot, it can indicate a problem with one or more of several different clotting factors. This may be a sign of:

- a missing, deficient, or defective clotting factor or factors;

- liver disease (because many clotting factors are made in the liver);

- treatment with heparin, a blood-thinning medication.

Why It's Done

Doctors may order the PTT test as part of an evaluation for a bleeding disorder such as hemophilia or von Willebrand disease. Symptoms of a bleeding disorder can include easy bruising, nosebleeds that won't stop, excessive bleeding after dental procedures, heavy menstrual periods, blood in the urine, or swollen or painful joints. Even in the absence of symptoms, doctors may use the test to ensure that clotting ability is normal before a patient undergoes a major procedure such as surgery.

The PTT test is especially useful in monitoring the effects of the blood-thinning medication heparin. Blood thinners are frequently given to prevent clots in patients who've had a heart attack or stroke, or who have an artificial heart valve. Because dosing is critical—enough medication must be given to prevent dangerous clots, but not so much so as to cause excessive bleeding—close monitoring is necessary. In many cases, the PTT test is performed with a prothrombin time (PT) test to give doctors a more complete picture of clotting factor function.

Preparation

No special preparations are needed for this test. If you take blood-thinning medication, antihistamines, or aspirin, you should tell the doctor because these can affect test results.

On the day of the test, it may help to wear a short-sleeve shirt to allow easier access for the technician who will be drawing the blood.

The Procedure

A health professional will clean the skin surface with antiseptic and place an elastic band (tourniquet) around the upper arm to apply pressure and cause the veins to swell with blood. Then a needle is inserted into a vein (usually in the arm inside of the elbow or on the back of the hand) and blood is withdrawn and collected in a vial or syringe.

After the procedure, the elastic band is removed. Once the blood has been collected, the needle is removed and the area is covered with cotton or a bandage to stop the bleeding. Collecting the blood for the test will only take a few minutes.

What to Expect

Collecting a sample of blood is only temporarily uncomfortable and can feel like a quick pinprick. Afterward, there may be some mild bruising, which should go away in a day or so.

Getting the Results

Partial thromboplastin time is measured in seconds. PTT test results are compared with the average clotting time of healthy people. The time is longer in people who take blood thinners.

Risks

The PTT test is considered a safe procedure. However, as with many medical tests, some problems can occur with having blood drawn:

- fainting or feeling lightheaded;

- hematoma (blood accumulating under the skin causing a lump or bruise);

- pain associated with multiple punctures to locate a vein.

Helping Your Child

Having a blood test is relatively painless. Still, many children are afraid of needles. Explaining the test in terms your child can understand might help ease some of the fear.

Allow your child to ask the technician any questions he or she might have. Tell your child to try to relax and stay still during the procedure, as tensing muscles and moving can make it harder and more painful to draw blood. It also may help if your child looks away when the needle is being inserted into the skin.

Chapter 9

Tests Used in the Assessment of Vascular Disease

History and Examination

The initial assessment of a patient is the most important part of the management of any patient. It is at this assessment that a mutual trust should develop between surgeon and patient. The assessment needs to be tailored to the presenting problem, but should be detailed enough to understand the full situation of each individual. Patients deserve a period of undistracted thought, concentrated on their particular problem. This is absolutely crucial in subsequent management, when often extremely important decisions are being made which can affect the subsequent life and limb of the patient.

The first part of the assessment of any patient, with any problem, is taking a detailed medical history and performing a physical examination. The time taken to do this initial assessment will depend on the presenting problem.

History

Arterial. When a patient develops symptoms of pain in the leg due to arterial disease there are certain typical features. The pain is typically brought on by exercise and relieved by rest (claudication). Sometimes these features are not clear-cut and close questioning by your vascular surgeon will be required to try to decide if your symptoms could be related to vascular disease. Sometimes it is more clear-cut that arterial disease is present. The presence of gangrene or severe, unremitting pain in the foot at rest, are good indicators of more severe vascular disease.

Pain that is intermittently present in the foot or leg and occurs with exercise, but is also present at rest is frequently not related to arterial disease. Other common causes are arthritis or nerve problems (neuropathy).

If you are seeing your surgeon because of a previous stroke or ministroke then your surgeon will want more detail on that stroke and exactly how it affected you.

Aneurysms do not often cause symptoms, but your surgeon will often ask about back and abdominal pain, which can be a sign of impending trouble.

General vascular history includes asking about previous heart attacks and angina, current medication, and general fitness particularly with regard to respiratory problems. This is important because many older people with arterial disease have serious co-existing disease, which may influence future decisions about treatment.

Venous. For patients with varicose veins or chronic venous insufficiency, your surgeon will want to know how long varicose veins have been present. The symptoms caused by your varicose veins will be important. It is important that the aching and discomfort in the legs is due to the veins, if you are to have surgery to your veins. Sometimes leg discomfort can be due to arthritis in the knees even when varicose veins are present. It is important to clarify the exact nature of the symptoms at an early stage so the true benefits of treatment can be assessed. Previous history of deep venous thrombosis, leg ulcers, and broken bones in the leg can be important.

In patients with leg ulcers it is important to know how long they have been present and how they started. A previous history of leg ulcers can be important.

Lymphatic. The duration of swelling in the leg(s) and problems it has caused are important. Infection is the commonest problem. Any previous surgery and/or radiotherapy to the limb is important. Surgery in the armpit or groin may be particularly important in patients with lymphedema.

Examination

Examination mainly comprises looking (inspection) and feeling (palpation). Tapping (percussion) and listening (auscultation) are also examination tools that can be helpful, but less so in vascular disease.

A full arterial examination can involve examining the hands or fingers for signs of smoking and raised cholesterol in the blood. The pulses in the arms will be compared and blood pressure measured in both arms. Raised cholesterol can also cause a white ring to appear around the iris (arcus). In the neck turbulent blood flow can produce a sound (bruit) that can be heard with a stethoscope. A bruit, however, is not a reliable indicator of underlying vascular disease in the carotid arteries in the neck.

In the abdomen an aneurysm can sometimes be felt, although this can vary enormously depending on the size of the patient and feeling is a poor way to detect an aneurysm or assess its size.

In the legs the appearance of the skin of the leg and foot may be helpful. The temperature of the skin and the presence of pulses in the leg and foot should be assessed.

The health of the skin is important in lymphedema. It can frequently become thickened and scaly.

In venous disease the shape and color of the leg are important. The distribution and size of varicose veins are recorded. The major venous junctions at the groin and behind the knee will be examined.

Blood Tests

No blood test can be used to diagnose arterial or venous disease, but blood tests may assist in providing extra information. For instance the blood sugar level can determine if undiagnosed diabetes is present. The cholesterol level can be monitored and kidney function assessed. The full blood count will tell the surgeon whether you are anemic or occasionally if there are too many blood cells present (polycythemia).

Less commonly performed tests may be important in certain circumstances. Tests that assess the presence of a tendency to form blood clots (thrombophilia) and homocysteine levels can be useful because treatments are available to help these problems. In microvascular disease a vasculitic screen to assess the presence of destructive antibodies causing blood vessel inflammation (vasculitis) is used.

Hand-Held Doppler

The hand-held Doppler is an instrument that detects blood flow. It can be a very useful tool in assessing how good the blood flow is to the foot or hand. It is a painless test and very similar to taking blood pressure using a stethoscope. It is particularly useful for assessment of arterial disease but can also be used for venous problems. It is also commonly used to listen to the heartbeat of a baby in the womb and is completely harmless.

Using the Doppler, the blood pressure can be measured in the arm and the leg to assess whether any differences are present. Usually the blood pressure in the arm and the leg are the same and in these circumstances the ankle-brachial index (ABI) will be close to 1.0. If there is arterial disease in the leg then the blood pressure may be lower in the leg than in the arm and the ABI will be less than 1.0, for example 0.5.

Doppler measurements can also be performed before and after exercise. The leg pressure will decrease further in patients after exercise if there is atherosclerosis present.

Listening to the type of sound produced by the arterial flow is also useful. In normal patients the arterial signal has three phases (triphasic), but in the presence of arterial disease this signal becomes monophasic (one phase). Interpretation of the sounds is of particular benefit in patients when there is difficulty in measuring the pressures, such as in some patients with diabetes and renal failure.

The ABI and hand-held Doppler give the surgeon a more objective assessment of the severity of the arterial problem. It does not indicate to the surgeon whether treatment is required and is only complementary to the findings from the history and examination.

Duplex Ultrasound

Ultrasound scanning has become one of the most important investigations used in the assessment of vascular disease. This is because it provides accurate information on the flow of blood in the arteries and veins, but it is painless and risk free. Ultrasound has been used safely for years to assess babies in the womb.

Color flow ultrasound provides accurate information on most arteries. It can assess the flow of blood and whether there is any impairment of flow caused by hardening of the arteries. It is commonly used to assess aortic aneurysms, carotid arteries, and the arteries to the legs. It is especially useful in the assessment of venous disease as it can identify the sites in the veins leading to reflux (reverse flow).

Ultrasound requires a skilled operator to produce the most accurate information.

Angiogram

An angiogram (digital subtraction angiogram) produces a road map of the blood vessels. It is a good way of examining the anatomy of the blood vessels and tells the surgeon which blood vessels are open and which are diseased, narrowed (stenosed), or blocked. Angiography is the most commonly used method of assessing the arteries before surgery.

It has one major disadvantage compared with the other techniques because it requires the placement of a needle in the artery. This can be uncomfortable, but it is the only method of assessment, which can also be used to treat arterial disease by angioplasty.

Magnetic Resonance Angiography

Magnetic resonance angiography (MRI and MRA) is one of the newer techniques. It is a technically complicated imaging method which relies on powerful magnets to align water molecules in the body tissues. It is a painless and fairly rapid form of assessment especially on the latest machines, but is noisy and some patients feel hemmed in or claustrophobic by the procedure.

It can be used to assess almost any artery in the body but has been found particularly useful in the assessment of carotid artery disease. It is also good for assessing the renal (kidney) arteries. It does not require puncture of an artery and consequently is only useful in the diagnosis of disease and cannot be used to treat arterial problems.

MRA is becoming an increasingly popular imaging technique for blood vessels.

CT (Computed Tomography) Angiography

This test uses x-rays to produce horizontal cross-sectional images through the body which are then reconstructed using computers to produce longitudinal and three-dimensional (3-D) images. The advantage of CT is that it does not require a puncture of an artery. If an angioplasty is required then this must be performed separately using conventional angiography.

CT angiography is also becoming more popular as sixty-four-slice CT scanners become more prevalent. In the right hands CT angiography is probably as accurate as conventional angiography. Newer imaging suites are able to combine cross-sectional CT images with angiography in three dimensions.

Chapter 10

Commonly Used Medications for Cardiovascular Health

Chapter Contents

Section 10.1

Facts about Using Aspirin

Reprinted from "Aspirin for Reducing Your Risk of Heart Attack and Stroke:
Know the Facts," U.S. Food and Drug Administration, April 30, 2009.

You can walk into any pharmacy, grocery, or convenience store and
buy aspirin without a prescription. The Drug Facts label on medication products will help you choose aspirin for relieving headache, pain,
swelling, or fever. The Drug Facts label also gives directions that will
help you use the aspirin so that it is safe and effective.

But what about using aspirin for a different use, time period, or in
a manner that is not listed on the label? For example, using aspirin to
lower the risk of heart attack and clot-related strokes. In these cases,
the labeling information is not there to help you with how to choose
and how to use the medicine safely. Since you don't have the labeling
directions to help you, you need the medical knowledge of your doctor,
nurse practitioner, or other health professional.

You can increase the chance of getting the good effects and decrease
the chance of getting the bad effects of any medicine by choosing and
using it wisely. When it comes to using aspirin to lower the risk of heart
attack and stroke, choosing and using wisely means knowing the facts
and working with your health professional.

Fact: Daily Use of Aspirin Is Not Right for Everyone

Aspirin has been shown to be helpful when used daily to lower the
risk of heart attack, clot-related strokes, and other blood flow problems.
Many medical professionals prescribe aspirin for these uses. There may
be a benefit to daily aspirin use for you if you have some kind of heart
or blood vessel disease, or if you have evidence of poor blood flow to
the brain. However, the risks of long-term aspirin use may be greater
than the benefits if there are no signs of, or risk factors for, heart or
blood vessel disease.

Every prescription and over-the-counter medicine has benefits and
risks—even such a common and familiar medicine as aspirin. Aspirin
use can result in serious side effects, such as stomach bleeding, bleeding

in the brain, kidney failure, and some kinds of strokes. No medicine is completely safe. By carefully reviewing many different factors, your health professional can help you make the best choice for you.

When you don't have the labeling directions to guide you, you need the medical knowledge of your doctor, nurse practitioner, or other health professional.

Fact: Daily Aspirin Can Be Safest When Prescribed by a Medical Health Professional

Before deciding if daily aspirin use is right for you, your health professional will need to consider the following things:

- Your medical history and the history of your family members
- Your use of other medicines, including prescription and over-the-counter
- Your use of other products, such as dietary supplements, including vitamins and herbals
- Your allergies or sensitivities, and anything that affects your ability to use the medicine
- What you have to gain, or the benefits, from the use of the medicine
- Other options and their risks and benefits
- What side effects you may experience
- What dose, and what directions for use are best for you
- How to know when the medicine is working or not working for this use

Make sure to tell your health professional all the medicines (prescription and over-the-counter) and dietary supplements, including vitamins and herbals, that you use—even if only occasionally.

Fact: Aspirin Is a Drug

If you are at risk for heart attack or stroke your doctor may prescribe aspirin to increase blood flow to the heart and brain. But any drug—including aspirin—can have harmful side effects, especially when mixed with other products. In fact, the chance of side effects increases with each new product you use.

New products include prescription and other over-the-counter medicines, dietary supplements (including vitamins and herbals), and sometimes foods and beverages. For instance, people who already use a prescribed medication to thin the blood should not use aspirin unless recommended by a health professional. There are also dietary supplements known to thin the blood. Using aspirin with alcohol or with another product that also contains aspirin, such as a cough-sinus drug, can increase the chance of side effects.

Your health professional will consider your current state of health. Some medical conditions, such as pregnancy, uncontrolled high blood pressure, bleeding disorders, asthma, peptic (stomach) ulcers, and liver and kidney disease, could make aspirin a bad choice for you.

Make sure that all your health professionals are aware that you are using aspirin to reduce your risk of heart attack and clot-related strokes.

Fact: Once Your Doctor Decides That Daily Use of Aspirin Is for You, Safe Use Depends on Following Your Doctor's Directions

There are no directions on the label for using aspirin to reduce the risk of heart attack or clot-related stroke. You may rely on your health professional to provide the correct information on dose and directions for use. Using aspirin correctly gives you the best chance of getting the greatest benefits with the fewest unwanted side effects. Discuss with your health professional the different forms of aspirin products that might be best suited for you.

Aspirin has been shown to lower the risk of heart attack and stroke, but not all over-the-counter pain and fever reducers do that. Even though the directions on the aspirin label do not apply to this use of aspirin, you still need to read the label to confirm that the product you buy and use contains aspirin at the correct dose. Check the Drug Facts label for "active ingredients: aspirin" or "acetylsalicylic acid" at the dose that your health professional has prescribed.

Remember, if you are using aspirin every day for weeks, months, or years to prevent a heart attack, stroke, or for any use not listed on the label—without the guidance from your health professional—you could be doing your body more harm than good.

Section 10.2

Anticoagulants and Antiplatelet Agents

"What Are Anticoagulants and Antiplatelet Agents?" reprinted with permission. © 2007 American Heart Association, Inc. (www.americanheart.org).

What are anticoagulants and antiplatelet agents?

Anticoagulants and antiplatelet agents are medicines that reduce blood clotting in an artery, a vein, or the heart. Clots can block the blood flow to your heart muscle and cause a heart attack. They can also block blood flow to your brain, causing a stroke.

What should I know about anticoagulants?

Anticoagulants are drugs that are given to prevent your blood from clotting or prevent existing clots from getting larger. They can keep harmful clots from forming in your heart, veins, or arteries. Clots can block blood flow and cause a heart attack or stroke.

Common names for anticoagulants are "warfarin" and "heparin."

You must take anticoagulants just the way your doctor tells you.

Regular blood tests tell your doctor how the anticoagulants are working.

You must tell other doctors and dentists that you're taking anticoagulants.

Never take aspirin with anticoagulants unless your doctor tells you to.

Ask your doctor before taking anything else—such as vitamins, cold medicine, sleeping pills, or antibiotics. These can make anticoagulants stronger or weaker, which can be dangerous.

Tell your family how you take them and carry an emergency medical identification (ID) card.

Could anticoagulants cause problems?

If you do as your doctor tells you, there probably won't be problems. But you must tell your doctor right away if:

- your urine turns red or dark brown;
- your stools turn red, dark brown, or black;
- you bleed more than normal when you have your period;
- your gums bleed;
- you have a very bad headache or stomach pain that doesn't go away;
- you get sick or feel weak, faint, or dizzy;
- you think you're pregnant;
- you often find bruises or blood blisters;
- you have an accident of any kind.

What should I know about antiplatelet agents?

These drugs, such as aspirin, keep blood clots from forming. Many doctors now prescribe aspirin to heart patients for this reason.

Aspirin can save your life if you have heart problems. You don't need a prescription to get it, but it's just as important as any other medicine your doctor tells you to take. You must use it just as you're told.

Aspirin:

- helps keep blood from clotting;
- has been shown to reduce the risk of a heart attack, stroke, or transient ischemic attack (TIA);
- should not be taken with anticoagulants unless your doctor tells you to;
- must be used as your doctor orders—most often in small doses every day or every other day if you already have cardiovascular disease (CVD) or are at high risk for CVD;
- might not be taken while you're having surgery.

Do I need to wear an emergency medical ID?

Yes, always carry it in your purse or wallet. It needs to include:

- the name of the drug you're taking;
- your name, phone number, and address;
- the name, address, and phone number of your doctor.

How can I learn more?

Talk to your doctor, nurse, or other healthcare professionals. If you have heart disease or have had a stroke, members of your family also may be at higher risk. It's very important for them to make changes now to lower their risk.

Call 800-AHA-USA1 (800-242-8721) or visit americanheart.org to learn more about heart disease.

For more information on stroke, call 888-4-STROKE (888-478-7653) or visit StrokeAssociation.org.

The American Heart Association has many other fact sheets and educational booklets to help you make healthier choices to reduce your risk, manage disease, or care for a loved one. Knowledge is power, so learn and live!

Section 10.3

Using Coumadin Safely

Excerpted from "Your Guide to Coumadin®/Warfarin Therapy," Agency for Healthcare Research and Quality, AHRQ Publication No. 08-0028-A, August 2008.

What Coumadin®/Warfarin Is and What It Does for You

If your blood is too thick and forms clots, you could be at risk for heart attack, stroke, and other serious medical problems. Coumadin®/warfarin is a medicine that helps prevent blood clots. The drug is an anticoagulant. "Anti" means against and "coagulant" means to thicken into a gel or solid. Sometimes this drug is called a blood thinner. Think of syrup being poured—it is sticky and thick and flows slowly. Coumadin®/warfarin helps your blood flow easier and not clot.

Some people are more likely to get blood clots. Talk to your doctor to find out if you are at risk.

Coumadin®/warfarin will do the following:

• Keep your blood from making clots

• Help your blood flow more easily

How to Take Coumadin®/Warfarin

Always take your pills as directed. You must take the pills only on the days your doctor tells you to. The amount of Coumadin®/warfarin each person needs is different. The dose is based on a blood test called the international normalized ratio (INR). The amount of medication you take may change, based on the blood test. It needs to be taken at the same time, usually in the evening.

Coumadin®/warfarin can be taken with other medications. Never skip a dose, and never take a double dose. If you miss a dose, take it as soon as you remember.

If you don't remember until the next day, please call your doctor for instructions. If this happens on a weekend or holiday, skip the missed dose and start again the next day. Mark the missing dose in a diary. A daily pillbox will help you keep track of your dose.

Checklist:

- Go for blood tests as directed.

- Never skip a dose.

- Never take a double dose.

- Take Coumadin®/warfarin at the same time as directed by your doctor.

Blood Tests

The doctor decides how much Coumadin®/warfarin you need by testing your blood. The test measures how fast your blood is clotting and lets the doctor know if your dosage should change. If your blood test is too high, you might be at risk for bleeding problems. If it is too low, you might be at risk for forming clots. Your doctor has decided on a range on the blood test that is right for you.

Regulating your blood with Coumadin®/warfarin is like balancing a scale. If you take too much you will increase bleeding; if you take too little, your blood will clot. Getting your blood within the target range is getting it balanced.

When you first start taking Coumadin®/warfarin you may have your blood checked often. Once the blood test is in the target range and the correct dose is reached, this test is done less often. Because your dose is based on the INR blood test, it is very important that you get your blood tested on the date and at the time that you are told.

Illness can affect your INR blood test and your Coumadin®/warfarin dose. If you become sick with a fever, the flu, or an infection, call your doctor. Also call if you have diarrhea and vomiting lasting more than one day.

Possible Side Effects

Side effects with Coumadin®/warfarin may happen. Side effects may include bleeding. To lower the risk of bleeding, your blood Coumadin®/warfarin level will be kept within a range that is right for you. Even when your INR blood test is in range, you might see a little bleeding like bruises on your body or slight gum bleeding when you brush your teeth. Some people may experience hair loss or skin rashes, but this is rare. If you notice something wrong that you feel may be caused by your medication, call your doctor.

Slight bleeding—you may notice from time to time:

- Gum bleeding while brushing teeth
- Occasional nosebleed
- Easy bruising
- Bleeding after a minor cut that stops within a few minutes
- Menstrual bleeding that is a little heavier than normal

Major bleeding—call your doctor, or go to the hospital emergency room if you have any of the following:

- Red-, dark-, coffee-, or cola-colored urine
- Bowel movements that are red or look like tar
- Bleeding from the gums or nose that does not stop quickly
- Vomit that is coffee-colored or bright red
- Anything red in color that you cough up
- Severe pain, such as a headache or stomachache
- Sudden appearance of bruises for no reason
- Menstrual bleeding that is much heavier than normal
- A cut that will not stop bleeding within ten minutes
- A serious fall or hit on the head
- Dizziness or weakness

Stay Safe While Taking Coumadin®/Warfarin

You will need to be careful using objects, such as knives and scissors, that could make you bleed. You will need to avoid some activities and sports that could cause injury. For example, it is not a good idea to take up risky sports while you are on Coumadin®/warfarin. This does not mean you cannot do the things that you enjoy. If you like to work in the yard, be sure to wear sturdy shoes and gloves. Activities that would be safe for you include swimming and walking.

It is very important to know that you can be bleeding and not see any blood. For example, you could fall and hit your head, and bleeding could occur under your skull. Or, you could fall and hurt your arm and notice a large purple bruise. This would be bleeding under the skin. Call your doctor or go to the hospital immediately if you have taken a bad fall, even if you are not bleeding.

Talk to your doctor about wearing a medical alert bracelet or necklace. If you are badly injured and unable to speak, the bracelet would tell healthcare workers that you are on Coumadin®/warfarin.

To prevent injury indoors:

- Be very careful using knives and scissors.

- Use an electric razor.

- Use a soft toothbrush.

- Use waxed dental floss.

- Do not use toothpicks.

- Wear shoes or nonskid slippers in the house.

- Take care trimming your toenails.

- Do not trim corns or calluses yourself.

To prevent injury outdoors:

- Always wear shoes.

- Wear gloves when using sharp tools.

- Avoid activities and sports that can easily hurt you.

- Wear gardening gloves when doing yard work.

Use of Other Medications

When Coumadin®/warfarin is taken with other medicines it can change the way other medicines work. Other medicines can also change the way Coumadin®/warfarin works. It is very important to talk with your doctor about all of the other medicines that you are taking, including over-the-counter medicines, antibiotics, vitamins, or herbal products.

Any product containing aspirin may lessen the blood's ability to form clots and may harm you when you take Coumadin®/warfarin. If you take a daily aspirin, talk with your doctor about what dose is right for you.

Other medicines you get over the counter may have aspirin in them. All medications must be approved by your doctor, including medicines you have taken before you started Coumadin®/warfarin. Following is a list of some common medications that should be approved by your doctor:

- Pain relievers, such as the following:
  - Excedrin®
  - Acetaminophen (Tylenol®)
  - Naproxen (Aleve®)
  - Ibuprofen (Advil®, Motrin®, Nuprin®, Midol®, Pamprin HB®)

- Stomach remedies, such as the following:
  - Cimetidine (Tagamet HB®)
  - Bismuth subsalicylate (Pepto Bismol®)
  - Laxatives and stool softeners
  - Alka-Seltzer®

- Herbal products, such as the following:
  - Garlic
  - Green tea
  - Ginkgo

- Vitamins

Check the Coumadin®/warfarin you are taking. Does the medicine seem different from what your doctor wrote on the prescription or look different from what you expected? Does your refill look different than what you used before? Is the color the same as what you were previously given? If something seems different, ask the pharmacist to double-check it. Most errors are first found by patients.

Check Your Medicine

Always tell your doctor about all the medicines you are taking. Tell your doctor when you start taking new medicine and when you stop. Bring a list of current medications, over-the-counter drugs—such as aspirin—and any vitamins and herbal products you take.

Diet for Coumadin®/Warfarin Users

The foods you eat can affect how well Coumadin®/warfarin works for you. High amounts of vitamin K might work against Coumadin®/warfarin. Talk to your doctor about the amount of vitamin K that is right for you.

These foods contain vitamin K:

- Fruits and vegetables, such as:
  - Kiwi
  - Cabbage
  - Asparagus
  - Lettuce
  - Kale
  - Blueberries
  - Brussels sprouts
  - Cauliflower
  - Spinach
  - Endive
  - Broccoli
  - Green onions
  - Peas
  - Parsley
  - Turnip, collard, and mustard greens

- Meats, such as:
  - Beef liver
  - Pork liver
- Other:
  - Mayonnaise
  - Soybean oil
  - Cashews
  - Margarine
  - Vitamins
  - Canola oil
  - Soybeans

Keep Your Diet the Same

Do not make any major changes in your diet or start a weight loss plan without calling your doctor.

Call your doctor if you are unable to eat for several days, for whatever reason. Also call if you have stomach problems, vomiting, or diarrhea that lasts more than one day. These problems could affect your Coumadin®/warfarin dosage.

Limit alcohol. Alcohol can affect your Coumadin®/warfarin dosage but it does not mean you must avoid all alcohol. Serious problems can occur with alcohol and Coumadin®/warfarin when you drink more than two drinks a day or when you change your usual pattern. Binge drinking is not good for you. Be careful on special occasions or holidays, and drink only what you usually would on any regular day of the week.

Share Information with Your Other Doctors

Because you are on Coumadin®/warfarin you will be seen regularly by the doctor who ordered your medication. You may also see other doctors regularly to keep yourself healthy. When you see other doctors, it is very important that you tell them you are taking Coumadin®/warfarin. You should also tell your dentist and the person who cleans your teeth. If another doctor orders a new medication for you, please call the doctor who ordered your Coumadin®/warfarin so it can be noted in your file.

Chapter 11

Commonly Used Medications for Anemia

Chapter Contents

Section 11.1

Iron Supplements

"A Patient's Guide to Oral Iron Supplements," © 2008 National Anemia
Action Council (NAAC), reprinted with permission. For more information,
including NAAC's Online Resources for Patients, visit www.anemia.org.

If you are diagnosed with iron-deficiency anemia, your doctor may
recommend that you increase your iron intake. Eating an iron-rich diet
and taking a multivitamin with iron may be a useful way to prevent
iron-deficiency anemia, but it is usually not enough to treat anemia
once it has developed. Your doctor will probably recommend that you
take an iron supplement. The goal of this anemia treatment is to eliminate any symptoms you may be experiencing and boost your levels of
stored iron and hemoglobin.

Dr. William Ershler, M.D., a hematologist at the National Institutes
of Health, feels that it is extremely important for you and your doctor
to determine why you have iron-deficiency anemia as well as treat the
symptoms. Iron-deficiency anemia may be an early sign of another
disease. Finding the cause of your anemia may catch a potentially
serious disease before it gets worse.

If your doctor wants you to take an iron supplement, you and your
doctor will need to find the supplement that is best for you. Iron supplements usually do not need a prescription, and are commonly sold in
drugstores and supermarkets. There are a large number of iron preparations available with different amounts of iron, different iron salts,
complexes, combinations, and dosing regimens. After reading about
the different types of iron, browse the shelves of your local drugstore
to see all the iron products available to you.

Types of Iron Supplements

There are two general types of iron supplements which contain either the ferrous or ferric form of iron. Ferrous iron is the best-absorbed
form of iron supplements. Most available iron pills contain ferrous
iron. There are three types of ferrous iron supplements commonly
found: ferrous sulfate, ferrous fumarate, and ferrous gluconate. While

all three come in a 325 mg tablet size, each one contains a different amount of the form of iron used by your body, called "elemental iron." When choosing an iron supplement, it is important to remember to look at the amount of "elemental iron" in each tablet, instead of the size of the tablet.[1]

Adults will usually require a dose of 60–200 mg of elemental iron daily, depending on the severity of the anemia.[2] Since the amount of iron absorbed decreases as doses get larger, most people should take their daily iron supplement in two or three equally spaced doses. For adults who are not pregnant, the Centers for Disease Control and Prevention (CDC) generally recommends taking 50–60 mg of oral elemental iron (the approximate amount of elemental iron in one 325 mg tablet of ferrous sulfate) twice daily for three months for the treatment of iron-deficiency anemia.[3] However, your doctor will individually evaluate your condition and prescribe the amount of iron you need.

Iron supplements are available in regular tablets and capsules, liquid, drops, and coated or extended-release tablets and capsules. Regular tablets and capsules are the best-absorbed iron pill and are usually the most economical. Liquid and drop iron supplements are necessary for young children and people with problems swallowing pills, but may temporarily stain your teeth. Iron from coated or delayed-release preparations may have fewer side effects, but is not as well absorbed and not usually recommended. If your doctor recommends an iron supplement, consider the type of iron and pill, as well as the cost.[4]

Controlling the Side Effects

All iron supplements will cause your stool to become dark in color, but some people may also experience side effects which make it hard to follow recommended dosages. An upset stomach and constipation are the most common side effects of iron. If iron makes you constipated, consider taking a stool softener. Here are some tips to help you take your iron more comfortably and effectively:

- Iron supplements can upset your stomach. Starting with half the recommended dose and gradually increasing to the full dose will help minimize these side effects.

- Iron supplements are absorbed better if taken an hour before meals. However your doctor may tell you to take your iron with food to reduce an upset stomach.

- If iron makes you constipated, consider taking a stool softener such as docusate sodium along with your iron. Many products are available with this ingredient. Your pharmacist can help you choose the product that is best for you.

- Milk, caffeine, antacids, and calcium supplements can decrease iron absorption and should not be taken at the same time as iron supplements.

- You can get the most benefit from iron pills if you take them with vitamin C or drink orange juice. Vitamin C increases the absorption of iron.[1]

Dr. Ershler states, "Some patients will not be able to take an oral iron supplement, no matter how hard they try. If you are one of these patients who cannot take an iron supplement by mouth, your doctor may recommend an iron injection. Iron injections are a safe and effective alternative when iron tablets do not work or cannot be tolerated."

If you think you have anemia, please contact your doctor. Do not try to treat yourself or take iron pills without talking to your doctor. Taking too much iron over a period of time can be dangerous. It is important to keep iron pills out of the reach of children.

References

1. National Institute of Health. Office of Dietary Supplements. Dietary Supplement Fact Sheet: Iron.

2. Medline Plus. Drugs and Supplements: Iron.

3. Centers for Disease Control and Prevention. CDC Recommendations to prevent and control iron deficiency in the United States. *MMWR Recomm Rep* 1998;47:1–29.

4. Fishbane S, Mittal SK, Maesaka JK. Beneficial effects of iron therapy in renal failure patients on hemodialysis. *Kidney Int Suppl*. 1999 Mar;69:S67–70.

Section 11.2

Erythropoiesis-Stimulating Agents

"ESA Drugs Treat Anemia by Stimulating Red Blood Cell Production,"
© 2009 National Anemia Action Council (NAAC), reprinted with permission. For more information, including NAAC's Online Resources for Patients, visit www.anemia.org.

Medications that increase the production of red blood cells, called erythropoiesis-stimulating agents (ESAs), are one of the most common drugs used to treat anemia. ESAs stimulate your body's natural process for making more red blood cells. They can be given alone or in combination with some other treatments for the underlying cause of anemia. Before the mid-1980s there were no effective therapies to increase the production of red blood cells. People with severe anemia were treated with blood transfusions, which can cause infections, allergic reactions, and other immunologic effects.[1] In 1989, the first ESA drug was approved for use, revolutionizing the treatment of anemia. Today, blood transfusions are usually reserved for life-threatening situations and ESAs have become a common treatment for anemia.

While ESAs are a common anemia therapy, they are not the only available treatment. Many different conditions can cause anemia, including poor nutrition, bleeding, pregnancy, kidney disease, and other chronic diseases. Knowing how to treat anemia depends largely on what is causing you to have fewer red blood cells—measured as hemoglobin level. Some treatments can include iron, B_{12}, or folic acid supplements; treating the underlying disease; or increasing the number of healthy red blood cells with ESAs or a blood transfusion.

The Roles of Natural Erythropoietin and ESAs

If you have anemia your blood isn't able to carry and distribute enough oxygen to different tissues and organs. As a result, you may feel tired or have other symptoms depending on the severity of anemia. People with severe anemia may feel tired or fatigued or experience shortness of breath, which can cause problems carrying out routine activities. Erythropoietin is a natural substance made by certain kidney cells. These kidney cells are very sensitive to the amount of oxygen in your blood. When these cells determine that your oxygen level is low, they release more erythropoietin. The erythropoietin then signals your bone marrow to make more red blood cells in order to carry more oxygen throughout the body.[2]

Sometimes the kidneys cannot make enough erythropoietin. If this is the case, your doctor may prescribe an ESA. Synthetic ESA drugs act like the natural erythropoietin, and are given to help the body produce more red blood cells and raise hemoglobin levels. Currently there are two ESA drugs available in the United States to treat anemia: erythropoietin alfa, which is also referred to by the brand names Epogen®[3] and Procrit®[4], and darbepoetin alfa, which is also referred to by the brand name Aranesp®.[5]

What Types of Patients Receive ESAs?

ESAs are approved by the Food and Drug Administration (FDA) to treat anemia which has been caused by cancer chemotherapy treatment, kidney failure, or a drug used to treat acquired immunodeficiency syndrome (AIDS). Erythropoietin has also been approved for use to increase the red blood cell count in anemic patients who are scheduled to have surgery. This can decrease the need for blood transfusions following surgery. Though not yet approved by the Food and Drug Administration (FDA), ESAs have also been shown to be of benefit in managing anemia in elderly people,[6] in people with inflammatory bowel disease,[7] and in people with rheumatoid arthritis.[8]

How Synthetic ESA Drugs Work

Erythropoietin is a natural substance made in your body by the kidneys. Sometimes the kidneys cannot produce enough erythropoietin to make the red blood cells you need. If this is the case, your doctor may prescribe an erythropoiesis-stimulating agent (ESA). Synthetic ESA drugs act like the natural erythropoietin, and can be given to increase red blood cells.

How Are ESAs Administered?

ESAs are given by injection, either subcutaneously (under the skin) or intravenously (through an IV). They can be given in many dosing schedules, ranging from several times a week to once a month, depending on the drug chosen, the dose needed, and the reason you are receiving it.[3-5] It may take several weeks to raise your hemoglobin level and relieve some of your symptoms. This is because your body must make new red blood cells to replace those that were lost. It normally takes about five to seven days to make a healthy red blood cell.[9]

Monitoring Your Body's Response to ESAs

It is important to note that not everyone responds to ESAs and your hemoglobin levels may not go up. It is estimated that as many as 5 to 10 percent of patients have a decreased response, or no response, to ESA treatment. Some of the reasons for this lack of response include iron deficiency, blood loss, infection, or inflammation. Sometimes correcting these problems will help your body to better respond to ESA drugs.[10]

ESAs stimulate your bone marrow to make more red blood cells. Having more red blood cells raises your hemoglobin level. If your hemoglobin level stays too high or if your hemoglobin goes up too quickly, this may lead to health problems.[11] Recently, the FDA has changed the instructions for ESA drugs, in order to make sure that hemoglobin levels stay below 12 g/dL.[12] A recent study has shown that patients who need high doses of ESAs to maintain their hemoglobin levels may have a greater risk of cardiovascular problems and death.[13]

Your doctor will monitor your red blood cell counts on a regular basis if you are taking ESAs. All medicines may cause side effects, but many people have no, or minor, side effects. Occasionally, these medications may affect your heart function or may increase your chance of developing a blood clot, or after prolonged use, cause your red blood cell count to decrease. Let your doctor know immediately if you have chest pain, shortness of breath, or leg swelling and pain.[11]

Treating Anemia

The first step to treating anemia is to determine its cause. Once the cause is determined, your doctor can decide on the best treatment to correct the anemia. Many kinds of anemia can be alleviated by treating the underlying disease or problem. Several medications, including ESAs, are available to help correct anemia. ESAs have been administered successfully to millions of patients worldwide and are the standard of care for anemia treatment. ESAs may be the best treatment for you, but always discuss all treatment options thoroughly with your doctor. Communicate symptoms before, during, and following any type of treatment, especially ESA treatment.

References

1. Henry DH. Supplemental Iron: A Key to Optimizing the Response of Cancer-Related Anemia to rHuEPO? *Oncologist.* 1998;3(4):275–78.

2. Beaulieu NJ. Erythropoietin. In: *Gale Encyclopedia of Cancer* available at Healthline. Detroit, MI: The Gale Group Inc; 2002. Accessed: March 3, 2009.

3. Epogen Product Package Insert. August 2008. Accessed: March 3, 2009.

4. Procrit Product Package Insert. August 2008. Accessed: March 3, 2009.

5. Aranesp Product Package Insert. August 2008. Accessed: March 3, 2009.

6. Trovarelli T, Kahn B, Vernon S. Transfusion-free surgery is a treatment plan for all patients. *AORN J.* 1998 Nov;68(5):773–88.

7. Gasché C, Dejaco C, Waldhoer T, Tillinger W, Reinisch W, Fueger GF, Gangl A, Lochs H. Intravenous iron and erythropoietin for anemia associated with Crohn disease. A randomized, controlled trial. *Ann Intern Med.* 1997 May 15;126(10):782–87.

8. Murphy EA, Bell AL, Wojtulewski J, Brzeski M, Madhok R, Capell HA. Study of erythropoietin in treatment of anaemia in patients with rheumatoid arthritis. *BMJ.* 1994 Nov 19;309(6965):1337–78.

9. van Iperen CE, Kraaijenhagen RJ, Biesma DH, Beguin Y, Marx JJ, van de Wiel A. Iron metabolism and erythropoiesis after surgery. *Br J Surg.* 1998 Jan;85(1):41–45.

10. Wei M, Bargman JM, Oreopoulos DG. Factors related to erythropoietin hypo-responsiveness in patients on chronic peritoneal dialysis. *Int Urol Nephrol.* 2007;39(3):935–40.

11. Procrit Medication Guide. August 2008. Accessed: March 3, 2009.

12. U.S. Food and Drug Administration. Information for Healthcare Professionals. Erythropoiesis Stimulating Agents (ESAs). Accessed: March 3, 2009.

13. Bohlius J, Brillant C, Clarke M et al. Recombinant Human Erythropoiesis Stimulating Agents in Cancer Patients: Individual Patient Data Meta-Analysis on Behalf of the EPO IPD Meta-Analysis Collaborative Group. *ASH Annual Meeting Abstracts* 2008;112:LBA-6.

Chapter 12

Blood Transfusion

What Is a Blood Transfusion?

A blood transfusion is a safe, common procedure in which blood is given to you through an intravenous (IV) line in one of your blood vessels. Blood transfusions are done to replace blood lost during surgery or a serious injury. A transfusion also may be done if your body can't make blood properly because of an illness.

During a blood transfusion, a small needle is used to insert an IV line into one of your blood vessels. Through this line, you receive healthy blood. The procedure usually takes one to four hours, depending on how much blood you need.

Blood transfusions are very common. Each year, almost five million Americans need a blood transfusion. Most blood transfusions go well. Mild complications can occur. Very rarely, serious problems develop.

Important Information about Blood

The heart pumps blood through a network of arteries and veins throughout the body. Blood has many vital jobs. It carries oxygen and other nutrients to your body's organs and tissues. Having a healthy supply of blood is important to your overall health.

Blood is made up of various parts, including red blood cells, white blood cells, platelets, and plasma. Blood is transfused either as whole blood (with all its parts) or, more often, as individual parts.

Excerpted from "Blood Transfusion," National Heart Lung and Blood Institute, National Institutes of Health, September 2007.

Blood Types

Every person has one of the following blood types: A, B, AB, or O. Also, every person's blood is either Rh-positive or Rh-negative. So, if you have type A blood, it's either A positive or A negative.

The blood used in a transfusion must work with your blood type. If it doesn't, antibodies (proteins) in your blood attack the new blood and make you sick.

Type O blood is safe for almost everyone. About 40 percent of the population has type O blood. People with this blood type are called universal donors. Type O blood is used for emergencies when there's no time to test a person's blood type.

People with type AB blood are called universal recipients. This means they can get any type of blood.

If you have Rh-positive blood, you can get Rh-positive or Rh-negative blood. But if you have Rh-negative blood, you should get only Rh-negative blood. Rh-negative blood is used for emergencies when there's no time to test a person's Rh type.

Blood Banks

Blood banks collect, test, and store blood. They carefully screen all donated blood for possible infectious agents, such as viruses that could make you sick.

Blood bank staff also screen each blood donation to find out whether it's A, B, AB, or O and whether it's Rh-positive or Rh-negative. Getting a blood type that doesn't work with your own blood type will make you very sick. That's why blood banks are very careful when they test the blood.

To prepare blood for a transfusion, some blood banks remove white blood cells. This process is called white cell or leukocyte reduction. Although rare, some people are allergic to white blood cells in donated blood. Removing these cells makes allergic reactions less likely.

Not all transfusions use blood donated from a stranger. If you're going to have surgery, you may need a blood transfusion because of blood loss during the operation. If it's surgery that you're able to schedule months in advance, your doctor may ask whether you would like to use your own blood, rather than donated blood.

If you choose to use your own blood, you will need to have blood drawn a few times prior to the surgery. A blood bank will store your blood for your use.

Alternatives to Blood Transfusions

Researchers are trying to find ways to make blood. There is currently no man-made alternative to human blood. However, researchers have developed medicines that may help do the job of some blood parts.

For example, some patients with kidney problems can now take a medicine called erythropoietin that helps their bodies make more red blood cells. This means they may need fewer blood transfusions.

Surgeons try to reduce the amount of blood lost during surgery so that fewer patients need blood transfusions. Sometimes they can collect and reuse the blood for the patient.

Types of Blood Transfusions

Blood is transfused either as whole blood (with all its parts) or, more often, as individual parts. The type of blood transfusion you need depends on your situation.

For example, if you have an illness that stops your body from properly making a part of your blood, you may need only that part to treat the illness.

Red Blood Cell Transfusions

Red blood cells are the most commonly transfused part of the blood. These cells carry oxygen from the lungs to your body's organs and tissues. They also help your body get rid of carbon dioxide and other waste products. You may need a transfusion of red blood cells if you've lost blood due to an injury or surgery.

You also may need this type of transfusion if you have severe anemia due to disease or blood loss. Anemia is a condition in which your blood has a lower than normal number of red blood cells, or the red blood cells don't have enough hemoglobin. Hemoglobin—an iron-rich protein that gives blood its red color—carries oxygen from the lungs to the rest of the body.

Platelets and Clotting Factor Transfusions

Platelets and clotting factors help stop bleeding, including internal bleeding that you can't see. Some illnesses may cause your body to not make enough platelets or other clotting factors. You may need regular transfusions of these parts of your blood to stay healthy.

For example, if you have hemophilia A, you may need a special clotting factor to replace the clotting factor you're lacking. Hemophilia is a rare, inherited bleeding disorder in which your blood doesn't clot normally.

If you have hemophilia, you may bleed for a longer time than others after an injury or accident. You also may bleed internally, especially in the joints (knees, ankles, and elbows).

Plasma Transfusions

Plasma is the liquid part of your blood. It's mainly water, but also contains proteins, clotting factors, hormones, vitamins, cholesterol, sugar, sodium, potassium, calcium, and more.

If you have been badly burned or have liver failure or a severe infection, you may need a plasma transfusion.

Who Needs a Blood Transfusion?

Blood transfusions are very common. Each year, almost five million Americans need blood transfusions. This procedure is used for people of all ages.

Many people who have surgery need blood transfusions because they lose blood during the operation. For example, about one-third of all heart surgery patients have a transfusion.

Some people who have serious injuries—such as from car wrecks, war, or natural disasters—need blood transfusions to replace blood lost during the injury.

Some people need blood or parts of the blood because of illnesses. You may need a blood transfusion if you have any of the following:

- A severe infection or liver disease that stops your body from properly making blood or some parts of blood.

- An illness that causes anemia, such as kidney disease or cancer. Medicines or radiation used to treat a medical condition also can cause anemia. There are many different types of anemia, including aplastic, Fanconi, hemolytic, iron-deficiency, and sickle cell anemias and thalassemia.

- A bleeding disorder, such as hemophilia or thrombocytopenia.

What To Expect Before a Blood Transfusion

Before a blood transfusion, a technician tests your blood to find out what blood type you have (that is, A, B, AB, or O and Rh positive or Rh negative). He or she pricks your finger with a needle to get a few drops of blood or draws blood from one of your veins.

The blood type used in your transfusion must work with your blood type. If it doesn't, antibodies (proteins) in your blood attack the new blood and make you sick.

Some patients have allergic reactions even when the blood given does work with their own blood type. To prevent this, your doctor may prescribe a medicine to stop allergic reactions.

If you have allergies or have had an allergic reaction during a past transfusion, your doctor will make every effort to make sure you're safe.

Most patients don't need to change their diet or activities before or after a blood transfusion. Your doctor will let you know whether you need to make any lifestyle changes prior to the procedure.

What to Expect during a Blood Transfusion

Blood transfusions take place in either a doctor's office or a hospital. Sometimes they're done at the patient's home, but this is less common.

A needle is used to insert an intravenous (IV) line into one of your blood vessels. Through this line, you receive healthy blood. The procedure usually takes one to four hours. The time depends on how much blood you need and what part of the blood you receive.

During the blood transfusion, a nurse carefully watches you, especially for the first fifteen minutes. This is when reactions are most likely to occur. The nurse continues to watch you during the rest of the procedure as well.

What to Expect after a Blood Transfusion

After a blood transfusion, your vital signs are checked (such as your temperature, blood pressure, and heart rate). The intravenous line (IV) is taken out. You may have some bruising or soreness for a few days at the site where the IV was inserted.

You may need blood tests that show how your body is reacting to the transfusion.

Your doctor will let you know about signs and symptoms to watch for and report.

What Are the Risks of a Blood Transfusion?

Most blood transfusions go very smoothly. However, mild problems and, very rarely, serious problems can occur.

Allergic Reaction

Some people have allergic reactions to the blood given during transfusions. This can happen even when the blood given is the right blood type.

Allergic reactions can be mild or severe. Symptoms can include the following:

- Anxiety

- Chest and/or back pain

- Trouble breathing

- Fever, chills, flushing, and clammy skin

- A high pulse or low blood pressure

- Nausea (feeling sick to the stomach)

A transfusion is stopped at the first signs of an allergic reaction. The healthcare team determines how mild or severe the reaction is, what treatments are needed, and if the transfusion can safely be restarted.

Viruses and Infectious Diseases

Some infectious agents, such as human immunodeficiency virus (HIV), can survive in blood and infect the person receiving the blood transfusion. To keep blood safe, blood banks carefully screen donated blood.

There is a risk of catching a virus from a blood transfusion, but it's very low:

- **HIV:** Your risk of getting HIV from a blood transfusion is lower than your risk of getting killed by lightning. Only about 1 in 2 million donations may carry HIV and transmit HIV if given to a patient.

- **Hepatitis B and C:** The risk of having a donation that carries hepatitis B is about 1 in 205,000. The risk for hepatitis C is 1 in 2 million. If you receive blood during a transfusion that contains hepatitis, you will likely develop the virus.

- **Variant Creutzfeldt-Jakob disease (vCJD):** Variant CJD is the human version of mad cow disease. It's a very rare, yet fatal brain disorder. There is a possible risk of getting vCJD from a blood transfusion, although the risk is very low. Because of this, people who may have been exposed to vCJD aren't eligible blood donors.

Fever

You may get a sudden fever during or within a day of your blood transfusion. This is usually your body's normal response to white blood cells in the donated blood. Over-the-counter fever medicine will usually treat the fever.

Some blood banks remove white blood cells from whole blood or different parts of the blood. This makes it less likely that you will have a reaction after the transfusion.

Iron Overload

Getting many blood transfusions can cause too much iron to build up in your blood (iron overload). People with a blood disorder like thalassemia, which requires multiple transfusions, are at risk of iron overload. Iron overload can damage your liver, heart, and other parts of your body.

If you have iron overload, you may need iron chelation therapy. For this therapy, medicine is given through an injection or as a pill to remove the extra iron from your body.

Lung Injury

Although it's unlikely, blood transfusions can damage your lungs, making it difficult to breathe. This usually occurs within about six hours of the procedure. Most patients recover. However, 5 to 25 percent of patients who develop lung injuries die from the injury. These people usually were very ill before the transfusion.

Doctors aren't completely sure why blood transfusions damage the lungs. Antibodies (proteins)—which are more likely to be found in the plasma of women who have been pregnant—may disrupt the normal way that lung cells work. Because of this risk, hospitals are starting to use men and women's plasma differently.

Acute Immune Hemolytic Reaction

Acute immune hemolytic reaction is very serious, but also very rare. It occurs if the blood type you get during a transfusion doesn't match or work with your blood type. Your body attacks the new red blood cells, which then produce substances that harm your kidneys.

The symptoms include chills, fever, nausea, pain in the chest or back, and dark urine. The doctor will stop the transfusion at the first sign of this reaction.

Delayed Hemolytic Reaction

This is a much slower version of acute immune hemolytic reaction. Your body destroys red blood cells so slowly that the problem can go unnoticed until your red blood cell level is very low.

Both the acute and delayed hemolytic reactions are most common in patients who have had a previous transfusion.

Graft-Versus-Host Disease

Graft-versus-host disease (GVHD) is when white blood cells in the new blood attack your tissues. GVHD is usually fatal. People who have weakened immune systems are the most likely to get GVHD.

Symptoms start within a month of the blood transfusion. They include fever, rash, and diarrhea. To protect against GVHD, patients with weakened immune systems should receive blood that has been treated so the white blood cells can't cause GVHD.

Chapter 13

Bone Marrow and Stem Cell Transplants

What Is a Blood and Marrow Stem Cell Transplant?

A blood and marrow stem cell transplant replaces a person's abnormal or faulty stem cells with healthy ones from another person (a donor). This procedure allows the recipient to get new stem cells that work properly.

Stem cells are found in bone marrow—a sponge-like tissue inside the bones. Stem cells develop into the three types of blood cells that the body needs:

- Red blood cells carry oxygen through the body.

- White blood cells fight infection.

- Platelets help blood clot.

Small numbers of stem cells also are found in the blood and in the umbilical cord (the cord that connects a fetus to its mother's placenta).

Another type of stem cell, called an embryonic stem cell, can develop into any type of cell in the body. These cells aren't found in bone marrow.

Excerpted from "Blood and Marrow Stem Cell Transplant," National Heart Lung and Blood Institute, National Institutes of Health, September 2007.

Overview

Doctors use stem cell transplants to treat people who have the following illnesses:

- Certain types of cancer, such as leukemia. The high doses of chemotherapy and radiation used to treat some cancers can severely damage or destroy bone marrow. A transplant replaces the stem cells that the treatment destroyed.

- Severe blood diseases, such as thalassemia, aplastic anemia, and sickle cell anemia. In these diseases, the body doesn't make enough red blood cells or they don't work properly.

- Certain immune-deficiency diseases that prevent the body from making some kinds of white blood cells. Without these cells, a person can develop life-threatening infections. A transplant provides stem cells that replace the missing white blood cells.

Types of Transplants

Two main types of stem cell transplants are autologous and allogenic.

For an autologous transplant, a person's own stem cells are collected and stored for use later on. This works best when a person still has enough healthy stem cells even though he or she is sick. For a person with cancer, doctors also make sure that cancer cells are removed or destroyed from the collected cells.

For an allogenic transplant, a person gets stem cells from a donor. The donor can be a relative (like a brother or sister) or an unrelated person. A person also may get stem cells from umbilical cord blood donated by an unrelated person.

To prevent problems, the donor's stem cells should match the recipient's as closely as possible. Donors and recipients are matched through a blood test called human leukocyte antigen (HLA) tissue typing.

Collection Process

Stem cells used in transplants are collected from donors in several ways. They can be collected:

- Through a type of blood donation called apheresis. A needle is placed in the donor's arm to draw blood. Then, his or her blood is passed through a machine that removes the stem cells from the blood. The rest of the blood is returned to the donor.

- Directly from a donor's pelvis. This procedure isn't used very much anymore because it must be done in a hospital using local or general anesthesia. A hollow needle is inserted repeatedly into the pelvis, and marrow is sucked out of the bone.

- From an umbilical cord and placenta. Blood containing stems cells may be collected from an umbilical cord and placenta after a baby is born. The blood is frozen and stored at a cord blood bank for future use.

Outlook

Stem cell transplants have serious risks. Some complications are life threatening. For some people, however, a stem cell transplant is the best hope for a cure or a longer life.

Who Needs a Blood and Marrow Stem Cell Transplant?

You may need a blood and marrow stem cell transplant if you have a disease or condition that prevents your body from making enough healthy blood cells.

These diseases and conditions include the following:

- Some types of cancer, such as leukemia, lymphoma, myeloma, and breast cancer

- Severe blood diseases, such as thalassemia, aplastic anemia, and sickle cell anemia

- Immune-deficiency diseases, such as severe combined immunodeficiency syndrome, congenital neutropenia, and chronic granulomatous disease

When deciding whether you need a stem cell transplant, your doctors will consider the following things:

- The type of disease you have and how severe it is

- Your age and overall health

- Other possible treatment options

Your doctors also will order tests to make sure you're healthy enough to have the procedure. They also want to find out whether you have any medical problems that could cause complications after the transplant.

What to Expect Before a Blood and Marrow Stem Cell Transplant

Finding a Donor

If you're going to receive stem cells from another person, your doctors will want to find a donor whose stem cells match yours as closely as possible.

A close match can reduce the risk that your immune system will attack the donor cells. It also reduces the risk that cells from the donor's marrow or blood will attack your body.

HLA Tissue Typing

People having transplants are matched with donors through a test called HLA tissue typing. HLAs are proteins found on the surface of white blood cells. Your immune system uses HLAs to tell which cells belong to you and which don't.

Because HLA markers are inherited, an identical twin is the best donor match. Brothers or sisters also can be good matches. However, many people don't have a good match within their families.

If no matching donor is found in your family, the search widens to include people outside the family. Millions of volunteer donors are registered with the National Marrow Donor Program. Your doctors will look for the following:

- Donors who are an HLA match but not a family member
- Family members who aren't exact HLA matches
- Unrelated donors who aren't exact HLA matches
- Umbilical cord blood that's an HLA match

People who provide their own stem cells for use later don't need to go through HLA matching.

Medical Tests and Exams

You also will need other medical tests and exams before a stem cell transplant. Your doctors will want to make sure you're healthy enough to have a transplant. They also want to find out whether you have any medical problems that could cause complications after the transplant.

Blood Tests

Blood tests are used to check for human immunodeficiency virus (HIV), herpes, pregnancy, and other conditions. These tests help doctors learn about your overall health.

Chest X-ray and Lung Function Tests

A chest x-ray provides a picture of your heart and lungs. It can show whether the heart is enlarged or whether the lungs have extra blood flow or extra fluid.

Lung function tests tell doctors whether you have any lung infection or disease. They also show how well your blood is able to carry oxygen through your body.

Computed Tomography Scan, Skeletal X-ray, or Bone Scan

These tests provide detailed images of your body. They're used to see whether you have any tumors in your bones that might cause a problem for a transplant.

Dental Exam

A complete dental exam is used to check for problems that might cause an infection after your transplant.

Heart Tests

Heart tests, including EKG (electrocardiogram) and echocardiography, are used to find any conditions that might get worse after the transplant.

An EKG detects and records the electrical activity of your heart. Echocardiography uses sound waves to create a moving picture of your heart. The picture shows how well your heart is working and its size and shape.

Bone Marrow Biopsy

A bone marrow biopsy helps show whether your bone marrow is making enough healthy blood cells. If you're being treated for a blood cancer, this test shows whether your cancer is inactive.

What to Expect During a Blood and Marrow Stem Cell Transplant

A blood and marrow stem cell transplant has three parts: preparation, transplant, and recovery in the hospital.

Preparation

You will check in to the hospital a few days before the transplant. Using a simple surgical procedure, doctors will place a tube in a large vein in your chest. This tube is called a central venous catheter, or a central line. It allows easy access to your bloodstream.

Doctors use the central line to give you fluids, medicines, and blood products and to collect blood samples. The tube will stay in place for at least six months after your transplant.

To prepare your body for the transplant, your doctors will give you high doses of chemotherapy and possibly radiation. This treatment destroys the stem cells in your bone marrow that aren't working properly. It also suppresses your body's immune system so that it won't attack the new stem cells after the transplant.

The high doses of chemotherapy and radiation can cause side effects, including nausea (feeling sick to your stomach), vomiting, diarrhea, and tiredness. Medicines can help with these symptoms.

In older patients or those who aren't very strong, doctors may choose "reduced-intensity" treatment. This involves lower doses of chemotherapy or radiation.

Because your immune system is very weak after this treatment, you can easily get an infection. As a result, you will stay in a hospital room that has special features that keep the room as clean as possible.

Doctors, nurses, and visitors also have to wash their hands carefully and follow other procedures to make sure you don't get an infection. For example, they may wear a face mask while in contact with you.

Preparation before a transplant may take up to ten days. The time depends on your medical situation, general health, and whether you need chemotherapy or chemotherapy and radiation.

Transplant

During the transplant, which is like a blood transfusion, you get donated stem cells through your central line. Once the stem cells are in your body, they travel to your bone marrow and begin making new red blood cells, white blood cells, and platelets.

You're awake during the transplant. You may get medicine to help you stay calm and relaxed. Doctors and nurses will check your blood pressure, breathing, and pulse, and watch for signs of fever or chills. Side effects of the transplant can include headache or nausea—but you may not have side effects.

The transplant takes an hour or more. This includes the time to set up the procedure, the transplant itself, and time to check you afterward.

Recovery in the Hospital

You will stay in the hospital for weeks or even months after your stem cell transplant. In the first few days after the procedure, your blood cell levels will continue to go down. This is because of the chemotherapy or radiation you got before the transplant.

Your doctors will test your blood seven to ten days after the transplant to see whether new blood cells have begun to grow. They will check your blood counts every day to track your progress.

You will stay in the hospital until your immune system recovers and doctors are sure that your transplant was successful. During your time in the hospital, your doctors and nurses will carefully watch you for side effects from chemotherapy and radiation, infection, and graft-versus-host disease (GVHD) and graft failure.

Side Effects from Chemotherapy or Radiation

The chemotherapy and possible radiation you get before the transplant have side effects. These side effects begin to appear a few days after the transplant. Some of these side effects are painful or uncomfortable; others are very serious. They include the following:

- Painful sores in the mouth.

- Nausea, diarrhea, and intestinal cramps.

- Skin rashes.

- Hair loss.

- Liver damage. This occurs in about 10 percent of people who go through the transplant preparation.

- Interstitial pneumonia. This is a kind of pneumonia that affects certain tissues in the lungs. It affects about 5 percent of people who go through the transplant preparation.

Doctors use mouth rinses, medicines, and other treatments to treat these side effects. Some go away on their own once your blood cells begin to grow and your immune system recovers.

Infection

You can easily get an infection after the transplant because your immune system is weak. Some infections are serious. Infections can be caused by any of the following:

- Bacteria, such as those in your mouth or around your central line

- Viruses, such as herpes or cytomegalovirus

- Fungus or yeast, such as candida

To prevent infections, you will stay in a single room. The air will be filtered to keep germs out. Doctors, nurses, and others who visit you will wear face masks and wash their hands very carefully. Your doctor may have you take medicine to fight infections even if you don't already have an infection.

You also can take other steps to prevent infections:

- Bathe or shower daily.

- Carefully clean your teeth and gums.

- Keep the area clean where your central line enters your body.

- Avoid foods, such as raw fruits and vegetables, that may have harmful bacteria.

Graft-Versus-Host Disease and Graft Failure

Donated stem cells can attack your body. This is called graft-versus-host disease (GVHD). Your immune system also can attack the donated stem cells. This is called graft failure. These events can be minor or life threatening. They can happen soon after transplant or can develop slowly over months.

What to Expect After a Blood and Marrow Stem Cell Transplant

You will stay in the hospital for weeks or even months after your blood and marrow stem cell transplant. Your doctors want to be sure that you're healthy and strong enough to go home.

They want to make sure:

- your bone marrow is making enough healthy blood cells;

- you have no severe complications;

- you feel well and your mouth sores and diarrhea have improved or gone away;

- your appetite has improved;

- you have no fever or vomiting.

During the first weeks and months after you leave the hospital, you will make frequent trips to an outpatient clinic. This allows your doctors to track your progress. These visits will happen less often over time.

Staff at the clinic will teach you and your caregiver how to care for your central line, how to watch for and prevent infections, and other ways to care for you. They also will tell you who to call and what to do in case of emergency.

Recovery from a stem cell transplant can be slow. It takes six to twelve months to recover normal blood cell levels and immune function. During this time, it's important for you to take steps to reduce risk of infection, get plenty of rest, and follow your doctors' instructions about medicines and checkups.

What Are the Risks of a Blood and Marrow Stem Cell Transplant?

The main risks of a blood and marrow stem cell transplant are infection, graft-versus-host disease (GVHD), and graft failure.

Infection

You can easily get an infection after the transplant because your immune system is weak. The risk for infection decreases as your immune system recovers.

You can take steps to prevent infections, such as washing your hands and staying away from crowds. Doctors use medicines to prevent and treat infections.

Graft-Versus-Host Disease

GVHD is a common complication if you receive stem cells from a donor. In GVHD, the new stem cells attack your body.

Acute GVHD occurs within ninety to one hundred days after the transplant. Chronic GVHD begins more than ninety to one hundred days after the transplant or goes beyond ninety days after the transplant.

GVHD can be minor or life threatening. Signs and symptoms include the following:

- A rash that starts on the palms and soles of your feet and spreads to your mid-section. Over time, the rash may cover your entire body. Skin can blister or peel if the rash is very bad.

- Nausea (feeling sick to your stomach), vomiting, loss of appetite, abdominal cramps, and diarrhea. Doctors determine how bad GVHD is based on the severity of diarrhea.

- Jaundice (yellowing of the skin and eyes) and abdominal pain, which indicate liver damage.

Medicines are used to treat GVHD. Acute GVHD is treated with glucocorticoids, such as methyl prednisone, prednisone in combination with cyclosporine, antithymocyte globulin, or monoclonal antibodies.

Chronic GVHD is treated with steroids—usually cyclosporine and prednisone on alternating days.

Older people, people who have had acute GVHD before, and people who received stem cells from mismatched or unrelated donors are more likely to develop GVHD.

Doctors can reduce your chances of getting GVHD by doing the following:

- Closely matching your stem cells to your donor's through HLA tissue typing.

- Using medicines to suppress your immune system.

- Removing T cells from donor cells. T cells attack your body in GVHD.

- Using umbilical cord blood as the source of donor cells.

Graft Failure

Graft failure occurs when your immune system rejects the new stem cells. It also can occur if not enough stem cells are used, the new stem cells are damaged during storage, or your bone marrow is damaged after the transplant.

Graft failure is more likely in people who receive less preparation for their transplants. People who get stem cells from a poorly matched donor also are more likely to have graft failure.

Other Risks

Complications from chemotherapy and radiation treatment (used to prepare for a transplant) can occur long after a transplant. These complications include infertility, cataracts, new cancers, and damage to the liver, kidneys, lungs, or heart.

Chapter 14

Chelation Therapy: A Controversial Treatment Approach

For more than thirty years, people with fatty buildups of plaque in their arteries (atherosclerosis) may have heard about a "miracle cure" called chelation (pronounced "ke-LA'shun") therapy. But you may not know that the American Heart Association and other medical and scientific groups have spoken out against this treatment.

This answers the most frequently asked questions about chelation therapy. It also gives the American Heart Association's position on this procedure, as well as those of other highly regarded scientific organizations.

What's atherosclerosis?

Atherosclerosis is also called "hardening of the arteries." It occurs when the inner walls of the arteries become lined with deposits of fat, cholesterol, and other substances, including calcium. This fatty buildup usually starts early in life and gradually gets worse over many years. That's why middle-aged and older people are more likely to have the disease.

As plaque builds up, the arteries become hard and constricted. They lose their ability to expand and contract as blood flows through them and they get narrower. These changes make it harder for blood to flow through them, so the heart must work harder to pump blood throughout the body.

"Questions and Answers about Chelation Therapy," reprinted with permission. © 2009 American Heart Association, Inc. (www.americanheart.org).

If this plaque ruptures or a blood clot blocks a narrowed artery, a heart attack, stroke, or other serious medical problem can result. A heart attack happens when an artery bringing blood to the heart muscle is blocked. A stroke occurs when an artery to the brain is blocked.

What's chelation therapy?

Chelation therapy is administering a man-made amino acid called EDTA into the veins. (EDTA is an abbreviation for ethylenediamine tetra-acetic acid. It's marketed under several names, including edetate, disodium, Endrate, and sodium versenate.) EDTA is most often used in cases of heavy metal poisoning (lead or mercury). That's because it can latch onto or bind these metals, creating a compound that can be excreted in the urine.

Besides binding heavy metals, EDTA also "chelates" (naturally seeks out and binds) calcium, one of the components of atherosclerotic plaque. In the early 1960s, this led to speculation that EDTA could remove calcium deposits from buildups in arteries. The idea was that once the calcium was removed by regular treatments of EDTA, the remaining elements in the plaque would break up and the plaque would clear away. The narrowed arteries would be restored to their former state.

Based upon this thinking, chelation therapy has been proposed to treat existing atherosclerosis and to prevent it from forming.

After carefully reviewing all the available scientific literature on this subject, the American Heart Association has concluded that the benefits claimed for this form of therapy aren't scientifically proven. That's why we don't recommend this type of treatment.

How long does chelation therapy last and how much does it cost?

A single chelation treatment usually lasts from two to four hours and costs between $50 and $100. In the first month, patients usually receive from five to thirty treatments (with thirty being most common). Patients often are advised to continue preventive treatment once a month.

Patients must pay for this treatment themselves. EDTA isn't a medically accepted procedure for atherosclerosis, so insurance companies and Medicare won't reimburse for it.

Is there any proof that chelation therapy works?

Supporters of chelation therapy rely on the testimonies of people who've had it done. Many people claim that their lives were saved and their health improved because of chelation therapy.

But these aren't the only claims. Supporters also claim that chelation therapy significantly improves blood flow through previously narrowed blood vessels in some patients. Another claim is that chelation therapy has restored lost bodily function and reduced pain in some cases.

The American Heart Association can't say why some people feel better after having chelation therapy. And we don't deny that some people actually may feel better after treatment. So what's the problem?

The problem is, we question whether these patients feel better because of chelation therapy. It's possible they feel better because of something else.

For example, chelation therapists usually require their patients to make lifestyle changes. This can include quitting smoking, losing weight, eating more fruits and vegetables, avoiding foods high in saturated fats, and exercising regularly. These are healthy changes for anyone to make, and patients make them at the same time that they're undergoing chelation therapy. That's what clouds the issue. Research has shown that these lifestyle changes improve patients' quality of life and sense of well-being. In fact, we have advocated these lifestyle changes for many years.

The American Heart Association believes that these lifestyle changes are probably why the condition of some patients improves. We believe they don't feel better because of chelation therapy with EDTA, but because of better, healthier habits that they adopt.

Patients also may feel better for psychological reasons. Sometimes a sick person's symptoms disappear for no apparent reason, due to a placebo effect. This could be why some patients report that they feel better after they've spent $3,000 to $5,000 for chelation therapy.

Can chelation therapy be dangerous?

EDTA isn't totally safe as a drug. There's a real danger of kidney failure (renal tubular necrosis). EDTA can also cause bone marrow depression, shock, low blood pressure (hypotension), convulsions, disturbances of regular heart rhythm (cardiac arrhythmias), allergic-type reactions, and respiratory arrest.

In fact, a number of deaths in the United States have been linked with chelation therapy. Also, some people are on dialysis because of kidney failure caused, at least in part, by chelation therapy.

The American Heart Association is concerned that some people who rely on this therapy may delay undergoing proven therapies like drugs or surgery until it's too late. This is the added danger of relying on an unproven "miracle cure."

Clearly, people who choose chelation therapy are risking more than money.

What kind of scientific experiment or study is needed to validate (or invalidate) chelation therapy?

The best way to study chelation therapy would be to conduct a two-part study.

Step one would be a study that proves EDTA can remove calcium from arterial plaque (and that the plaque dissolves). The study should also show that this occurs without dangerous side effects.

Step two would be properly controlled clinical trials in a large population. This would only be done if EDTA had been proven successful in reducing arterial plaque without dangerous side effects.

What's a properly controlled clinical trial?

A properly controlled clinical trial meets these criteria:

- The patients or subjects receiving the treatment formally agree to participate, based upon reliable information given to them by the scientists conducting the trial. The patients would be told of the known risks involved and the possible (but unproven) benefits. Participants would have to give their "informed consent" to participate.

- The treatments are free to the patients or subjects.

- The trial is closely monitored and reviewed by 1) knowledgeable scientists who aren't involved in the trial, 2) representatives of the lay community, 3) representatives of the religious community, 4) statisticians, and 5) other interested persons.

- The trial is "double blind." This means that neither the patient nor the physician giving the treatment knows whether the patient is getting EDTA or a neutral control substance (placebo). Other precautions to ensure objectivity are 1) that the physician giving the treatment can't be the person who records the results and 2) the person observing the results can't know which substance a person under observation received.

Any study that doesn't follow this methodology will produce results open to question because the process lacks scientific safeguards. Accordingly, the results wouldn't be scientifically valid. To the knowledge of the American Heart Association, no study of chelation therapy that rigorously follows accepted scientific methodology has ever been completed.

Why hasn't the American Heart Association funded a project to research this question?

A scientifically valid trial would be very expensive. Also, according to qualified scientists who are familiar with research in heart disease, there's only a very small chance that chelation therapy will work.

Have scientists ever done a study on chelation therapy?

In the 1960s scientists started a small-scale study involving thirty patients. However, after two patients died and the others showed no signs of improvement, it was stopped.

Also, a recent study of chelation therapy, using currently approved scientific methodology, was done on people with intermittent claudication. (This is peripheral artery disease [fatty buildups] in leg arteries.) This study found that EDTA chelation therapy was no more effective than a placebo (sugar pill).

Finally, a recent study entitled "Chelation therapy for ischemic heart disease" was published in the *Journal of the American Medical Association* (*JAMA* 2002;287:481–86). The authors followed eighty-four patients for twenty-seven weeks. All of the patients had coronary artery disease. One-half of the patients received intravenous chelation therapy during the study period and the other one-half received intravenous placebo (fluid with no drug). Neither the physicians nor the patients knew whether they were receiving chelation or placebo. Patients were given exercise tests to see how long they could exercise before their electrocardiogram (ECG) showed changes indicating ischemia. They also answered quality-of-life questionnaires. At the end of the twenty-seven weeks, the patients who received chelation were no better than the patients who received placebo. The authors concluded that "Based on exercise time to ischemia, exercise capacity and quality-of-life measurements, there is no evidence to support a beneficial effect of chelation therapy in patients with ischemic heart disease, stable angina, and a positive treadmill test for ischemia."

Thus, there's still no scientific evidence that demonstrates any benefit from chelation therapy.

What's the American Heart Association's position?

We have a task force that examines the medical support for new and unestablished therapies, of which chelation is one. The report of the task force was adopted by the American Heart Association as our official policy statement on chelation therapy. This report states: "The

American Heart Association's Clinical Science Committee has reviewed the available literature on the use of chelation (EDTA) in the treatment of arteriosclerotic heart or blood vessel disease and finds no scientific evidence to demonstrate any benefit of this form of therapy. Furthermore, employment of this form of unproven treatment may deprive patients of the well-established benefits attendant to the many other valuable methods of treating these diseases."

What do other authorities say about this treatment?

Food and Drug Administration: "In the absence of evidence of safety and effectiveness, the use of this treatment for atherosclerosis is investigational. To date, no physician or sponsor has filed a plan or protocol to study its (EDTA's) use in such treatment. No party has ever provided us with an organized submission attempting to show that it is an effective therapy in atherosclerosis; instead, we have been handed unorganized data without any attempt to describe a formal study. Under the circumstances, we have had no choice but to attempt to prevent improper promotion of the drug and to point out its unproven status."

American College of Physicians: "Chelation therapy with EDTA has been used in the treatment and prevention of atherosclerosis. Because of the risk of severe renal (kidney) toxicity and lack of objective evidence suggesting therapeutic benefit from EDTA therapy . . . such therapy should be regarded as investigational and (should be) conducted under carefully controlled conditions in an academic institution by experienced investigators."

National Heart, Lung, and Blood Institute, National Institutes of Health: "There is no reason to expect benefit from chelation in the management of arteriosclerosis. More importantly, there has been no scientific evidence of such benefit—and there is scientific evidence of no benefit."

American Medical Association: The American Medical Association believes that chelation therapy for atherosclerosis is an experimental process without proven efficacy. They have also reaffirmed their 1984 House of Delegates Resolution stating: "there is no scientific documentation that the use of chelation therapy is effective in the treatment of cardiovascular disease, atherosclerosis, rheumatoid arthritis, and cancer . . . if chelation therapy is to be considered a useful medical treatment for anything other than heavy metal poisoning, hypercalcemia, or digitalis toxicity, it is the responsibility of its proponents to (a) conduct properly controlled scientific studies, (b) adhere to Food and Drug Administration (FDA) guidelines for the investigation of drugs, and (c) disseminate results of scientific studies in the usually accepted channels."

American College of Cardiology: "There is insufficient scientific evidence to justify the application of chelation therapy for atherosclerosis on a clinical basis. At the present time, therefore, chelation therapy should be applied only under an investigational protocol."

Isn't it true that practicing physicians and medical organizations oppose chelation therapy because widespread use of this procedure would mean a loss of income to cardiovascular specialists, particularly surgeons?

No. Organized medicine opposes chelation therapy because it's an unproven procedure and it involves extreme risks to patients who receive it.

The truth is that physicians who treat cardiovascular diseases could significantly increase their income if chelation therapy was a scientifically proven treatment procedure. Many people have atherosclerosis, but only a relatively small percentage develop problems severe enough to require surgery. If chelation were scientifically proven, EDTA could be administered to everyone who had atherosclerosis. Surgery can be done on only one patient at a time. With chelation, the number of patients who can be treated is limited only by the amount of room in the practitioner's office.

Are any new scientific studies of chelation therapy under way?

In August 2002, the National Center for Complementary and Alternative Medicine (NCCAM) and the National Heart, Lung, and Blood Institute (NHLBI), which are both components of the National Institutes of Health (NIH), announced that they have launched the Trial to Assess Chelation Therapy (TACT). This will be the first large-scale, multicenter study to find out if EDTA chelation therapy is safe and effective for people with coronary heart disease. This placebo-controlled, double-blind study will involve 2,372 participants age fifty years and older who've had a heart attack. They will be representative of the U.S. population. TACT will be more than twenty times larger than any prior study of chelation therapy—large enough to show if chelation therapy has mild or moderate benefits.

This study is being done because there is a public health need to conduct a large, well-designed clinical trial to find out if chelation therapy is safe and effective for treating people with coronary heart disease.

The trial will take place at about one hundred research sites across the United States and will test EDTA chelation therapy by using the most widely practiced means of administering it. Participants will begin being recruited in March 2003; patients will receive thirty weekly intravenous treatments, then ten more treatments given bimonthly, over a twenty-eight-month period. They will also receive high doses of vitamins, which are also often given with chelation therapy. (The effect of such vitamin doses will also be examined in the trial.) Once recruitment begins, the study will take about five years to complete.

Part Three

Blood Disorders

Chapter 15

Anemia

Chapter Contents

Section 15.1

Anemia: An Overview

Excerpted from "Anemia: Frequently Asked Questions,"
National Women's Health Information Center, May 13, 2008.

What is anemia?

Anemia occurs when you have less than the normal number of red blood cells in your blood or when the red blood cells in your blood don't have enough hemoglobin. Hemoglobin is a protein. It gives the red color to your blood. Its main job is to carry oxygen from your lungs to all parts of your body. If you have anemia, your blood does not carry enough oxygen to all the parts of your body. Without oxygen, your organs and tissues cannot work as well as they should. More than three million people in the United States have anemia. Women and people with chronic diseases are at the greatest risk for anemia.

What are the types and causes of anemia?

Anemia happens when:

- the body loses too much blood (such as with heavy periods, certain diseases, and trauma);

- the body has problems making red blood cells;

- red blood cells break down or die faster than the body can replace them with new ones; or

- more than one of these problems happen at the same time.

There are many types of anemia, all with different causes.

Iron-deficiency anemia (IDA). IDA is the most common type of anemia. IDA happens when you don't have enough iron in your body. You need iron to make hemoglobin. People with this type of anemia are sometimes said to have "iron-poor blood" or "tired blood."

A person can have a low iron level because of blood loss. In women, iron and red blood cells are lost when bleeding occurs from very heavy and long periods, as well as from childbirth. Women also can lose iron and red blood cells from uterine fibroids, which can bleed slowly. Other ways iron and red blood cells can be lost include the following:

- Ulcers, colon polyps, or colon cancer

- Regular use of aspirin and other drugs for pain

- Infections

- Severe injury

- Surgery

Eating foods low in iron also can cause IDA. Meat, poultry, fish, eggs, dairy products, or iron-fortified foods are the best sources of iron found in food. Pregnancy can cause IDA if a woman doesn't consume enough iron for both her and her unborn baby.

Some people have enough iron in their blood, but have problems absorbing it because of diseases, such as Crohn disease and celiac disease, or drugs they are taking.

Vitamin-deficiency anemia (or megaloblastic anemia). Low levels of vitamin B_{12} or folate are the most common causes of this type of anemia.

Vitamin B_{12} deficiency anemia (or pernicious anemia) happens due to a lack of vitamin B_{12} in the body. Your body needs vitamin B_{12} to make red blood cells and to keep your nervous system working normally. This type of anemia occurs most often in people whose bodies are not able to absorb vitamin B_{12} from food because of an autoimmune disorder. It also can happen because of intestinal problems.

You also can get this type of anemia if the foods you eat don't have enough vitamin B_{12}. Vitamin B_{12} is found in foods that come from animals. Fortified breakfast cereals also have vitamin B_{12}. Folic acid supplements (pills) can treat this type of anemia. But folic acid cannot treat nerve damage caused by a lack of vitamin B_{12}.

With this type of anemia, your doctor may not realize that you're not getting enough vitamin B_{12}. Not getting enough vitamin B_{12} can cause numbness in your legs and feet, problems walking, memory loss, and problems seeing. The treatment depends on the cause. But you may need to get vitamin B_{12} shots or take special vitamin B_{12} pills.

Folate, also called folic acid, is also needed to make red blood cells. Folate-deficiency anemia can occur if you don't consume enough folate or if you have problems absorbing vitamins. It also may occur during the third trimester of pregnancy, when a woman's body needs extra folate. Folate is a B vitamin found in foods such as leafy green vegetables, fruits, and dried beans and peas. Folic acid is found in fortified breads, pastas, and cereals.

Anemias caused by underlying diseases. Some diseases can hurt the body's ability to make red blood cells. For example, anemia is common in people with kidney disease. Their kidneys can't make enough of the hormones that signal the body to make red blood cells. Plus, iron is lost in dialysis (what some people with kidney disease must have to take out waste from the blood).

Anemias caused by inherited blood disease. If you have a blood disease in your family, you are at greater risk to also have this disease. Sickle cell anemia and thalassemia are two examples of this type of anemia.

The red blood cells of people with sickle cell disease are hard and have a curved edge. These cells can get stuck in the small blood vessels, blocking the flow of blood to the organs and limbs. The body destroys sickle red cells quickly but it can't make new red blood cells fast enough. These factors cause anemia.

People with thalassemia make less hemoglobin and fewer red blood cells than normal. This leads to mild or severe anemia. One severe form of this condition is Cooley anemia.

Aplastic anemia. This is a rare blood disorder in which the body stops making enough new blood cells. All blood cells—red cells, white cells, and platelets—are affected. Low levels of red blood cells leads to anemia. With low levels of white blood cells, the body is less able to fight infections. With too few platelets, the blood can't clot normally. This type of anemia can be caused by many things:

- Cancer treatments (radiation or chemotherapy)

- Exposure to toxic chemicals (like those used in some insecticides, paint, and household cleaners)

- Some drugs (like those that treat rheumatoid arthritis)

- Autoimmune diseases (like lupus)

- Viral infections

- Family diseases passed on by genes, such as Fanconi anemia

What are the signs of anemia?

Anemia takes some time to develop. In the beginning, you may not have any signs or they may be mild. But as it gets worse, you may have these symptoms:

- Fatigue (very common)

- Weakness (very common)

- Dizziness

- Headache

- Numbness or coldness in your hands and feet

- Low body temperature

- Pale skin

- Rapid or irregular heartbeat

- Shortness of breath

- Chest pain

- Irritability

- Not doing well at work or in school

All of these signs and symptoms can occur because your heart has to work harder to pump more oxygen-rich blood through the body.

How do I find out if I have anemia?

Your doctor can tell if you have anemia by a blood test called a complete blood count (CBC). Your doctor also will do a physical exam and talk to you about the food you eat, the medicines you are taking, and your family health history. If you have anemia, your doctor may want to do other tests to find out what's causing it.

What is the treatment for anemia?

With any type of anemia, there are two treatment goals:

- To get red blood cell counts or hemoglobin levels back to normal so that your organs and tissues can get enough oxygen

- To treat the underlying cause of the anemia

The treatment your doctor prescribes for you will depend on the cause of the anemia. For example, treatment for sickle cell anemia is different than treatment for anemia caused by low iron or folic acid intake. Treatment may include changes in foods you eat, taking dietary supplements (like vitamins or iron pills), changing the medicines you are taking, or in more severe forms of anemia, medical procedures such as blood transfusion or surgery.

What will happen if my anemia goes untreated?

Some types of anemia may be life threatening if not diagnosed and treated. Too little oxygen in the body can damage organs. With anemia, the heart must work harder to make up for the lack of red blood cells or hemoglobin. This extra work can harm the heart and even lead to heart failure.

How do I prevent anemia?

There are steps you can take to help prevent some types of anemia:

- Eat foods high in iron:

  - Cereal/breads with iron in it (100 percent iron-fortified is best. Check food label.)

  - Liver

  - Lentils and beans

  - Oysters

  - Tofu

  - Green, leafy vegetables such as spinach

  - Red meat (lean only)

  - Fish

  - Dried fruits such as apricots, prunes, and raisins

- Eat and drink foods that help your body absorb iron, like orange juice, strawberries, broccoli, or other fruits and vegetables with vitamin C.

- Don't drink coffee or tea with meals. These drinks make it harder for your body to absorb iron.

- Calcium can hurt your absorption of iron. If you have a hard time getting enough iron, talk to your doctor about the best way to also get enough calcium.

- Make sure you consume enough folic acid and vitamin B_{12}.

- Make balanced food choices. Most people who make healthy, balanced food choices get the iron and vitamins their bodies need from the foods they eat. Food fads and dieting can lead to anemia.

- Talk to your doctor about taking iron pills (supplements). Do *not* take these pills without talking to your doctor first. These pills come in two forms: ferrous and ferric. The ferrous form is better absorbed by your body. But taking iron pills can cause side effects, like nausea, vomiting, constipation, and diarrhea. Reduce these side effects by taking these steps:

  - Start with half of the recommended dose. Gradually increase to the full dose.

  - Take the pill in divided doses. For example, if you are prescribed two pills daily, take one in morning with breakfast and the other after dinner.

  - Take the pill with food.

  - If one type of iron pill is causing problems, ask your doctor for another brand.

- If you are a nonpregnant woman of childbearing age, get tested for anemia every five to ten years. This can be done during a regular health exam. Testing should start in adolescence.

- If you are a nonpregnant woman of childbearing age with these risk factors for iron deficiency, get tested every year:

  - heavy periods

  - low iron intake

  - have been diagnosed with anemia in the past

- Follow your doctor's orders for treating the underlying cause of your anemia. This will prevent the anemia from coming back or becoming serious.

It is important to keep iron pills tightly capped and away from children's reach. In children, death has occurred from ingesting 200 mg of iron.

How much iron do I need every day?

Most people get enough iron by making healthy, balanced food choices and eating iron-rich foods. But some groups of people are at greater risk for low iron levels:

- Teenage girls/women of childbearing age (who have heavy bleeding during their period, who have had more than one child, or use an intrauterine device [IUD])

- Older infants and toddlers (mainly those who drink a lot of milk or are having a growth spurt)

- Pregnant women (about half of pregnant women have iron-deficiency anemia)

- Female athletes who engage in regular, intense exercise

These groups of people should be screened at times for iron deficiency. If the tests show that the body isn't getting enough iron, iron pills (supplements) may be prescribed. In extreme cases of iron deficiency, your doctor might prescribe iron shots. Many doctors prescribe iron pills during pregnancy because many pregnant women don't get enough iron. Iron pills can help when diet alone can't restore the iron level back to normal. Talk with your doctor to find out if you are getting enough iron through the foods you eat or if you or your child needs to be taking iron pills.

How much iron do I need if I am pregnant?

Pregnant women need to consume twice as much iron as women who are not pregnant. But about half of all pregnant women do not get enough iron. During pregnancy, your body needs more iron because of the growing fetus, the higher volume of blood, and blood loss during delivery. If a pregnant woman does not get enough iron for herself or her growing baby, she has an increased chance of having preterm birth and a low-birth-weight baby. If you're pregnant, follow these tips:

- Make sure you get 27 mg of iron every day. Take an iron supplement (pill). It may be part of your prenatal vitamin. Start taking it at your first prenatal visit.

- Get tested for anemia at your first prenatal visit.

- Ask if you need to be tested for anemia four to six weeks after delivery.

Section 15.2

Anemia of Chronic Disease

Excerpted from "Anemia of Inflammation and Chronic Disease," National Institute of Diabetes and Digestive and Kidney Diseases, National Institutes of Health, NIH Publication No. 09-6181, December 2008.

What is anemia?

Anemia is a condition in which the blood has a lower-than-normal number of red blood cells (RBCs). RBCs contain hemoglobin, an iron-rich protein that gives blood its red color and allows RBCs to transport oxygen from the lungs to the tissues of the body. Because RBC numbers are low in anemia, blood hemoglobin levels are also low.

What is anemia of inflammation and chronic disease (AI/ACD)?

AI/ACD is a type of anemia that commonly occurs with chronic, or long-term, illnesses or infections. Cancer and inflammatory disorders, in which abnormal activation of the immune system occurs, can also cause AI/ACD. Some people develop AI/ACD without having any signs of these health problems.

AI/ACD is easily confused with iron-deficiency anemia because in both forms of anemia, levels of iron circulating in the blood are low. Circulating iron is necessary for RBC production. Low blood iron levels occur in iron-deficiency anemia because levels of iron stored in the body's tissues are depleted. In AI/ACD, however, iron stores are normal or high. Low blood levels occur in AI/ACD, despite normal iron stores, because inflammatory and chronic diseases interfere with the body's ability to use stored iron and absorb iron from the diet. Certain treatments for chronic diseases may also impair RBC production and contribute to AI/ACD. AI/ACD is the second most common form of anemia, after iron-deficiency anemia, but it is rarely severe.

While AI/ACD can affect people at any age, older adults are especially susceptible because they have the highest rates of chronic disease. AI/ACD is also common among hospitalized patients, particularly those with chronic illnesses.

135

What causes AI/ACD?

A number of chronic diseases can cause anemia for different reasons.

Infectious and inflammatory diseases. As part of the immune response that occurs with infection and noninfectious inflammatory diseases, cells of the immune system release proteins called cytokines. These proteins help heal and defend the body against infection. But they can also affect normal body functions. In AI/ACD, immune cytokines interfere with the body's ability to absorb and use iron. Cytokines may also interfere with the production and normal activity of erythropoietin (EPO), a hormone made by the kidneys that stimulates bone marrow to produce RBCs.

Infectious diseases that cause AI/ACD include tuberculosis, human immunodeficiency virus (HIV), endocarditis—infection in the heart—and osteomyelitis, a bone infection. Sometimes acute infections—those that develop quickly and may not last long—can also cause AI/ACD.

Inflammatory diseases that can lead to AI/ACD include rheumatoid arthritis, lupus, diabetes, heart failure, degenerative joint disease, and inflammatory bowel disease (IBD). IBD, including Crohn disease, can also cause iron deficiency due to poor absorption of iron by the diseased intestine and bleeding from the gastrointestinal tract.

Kidney disease. People with kidney disease can develop anemia for several different reasons. For one, diseased kidneys often fail to make enough EPO. In addition, kidney disease results in abnormal absorption and use of iron, which is typical of AI/ACD. Because anemia worsens as kidney disease advances, nearly everyone with end-stage kidney disease has anemia.

People with kidney failure can also develop iron deficiency due to blood loss during hemodialysis, a procedure that removes blood from an artery, purifies it, and returns it to a vein, thereby doing the job that the kidneys no longer can. Low levels of iron and of folic acid—another nutrient required for normal RBC production—may also contribute to anemia in people with kidney disease.

Cancer. AI/ACD can occur with certain types of cancer, including Hodgkin disease, non-Hodgkin lymphoma, and breast cancer. Like chronic inflammatory disorders and infections, these types of cancer cause inflammatory cytokines to be released in the body. The anemia of AI/ACD can also be made worse by cancer chemotherapy and radiation treatments that damage the bone marrow—where RBCs are produced—and by the cancer's invasion of bone marrow.

What are the symptoms of AI/ACD?

AI/ACD typically develops slowly and, because it is usually mild, may cause few or no symptoms. Or its symptoms may be masked by the symptoms of the underlying disease. Sometimes AI/ACD can cause or contribute to the following problems:

- Tiredness

- Low energy and listlessness

- Weakness

- Pale skin

- Fast heartbeat

- Shortness of breath

- Exercise intolerance

How is AI/ACD diagnosed?

Healthcare providers can test people with chronic illnesses for AI/ACD during their regular appointments. A complete blood count (CBC)—a laboratory test performed on a sample of a patient's blood—can reveal anemia by determining the hematocrit level, which reflects the number of RBCs in the blood. A CBC also measures the level of blood hemoglobin. Low hematocrit and hemoglobin levels indicate anemia. Blood tests can also show low iron levels in the blood but normal measures of iron stores in the body—a hallmark of AI/ACD.

How is AI/ACD treated?

AI/ACD often is not treated separately from the condition with which it occurs. In general, doctors focus on treating the underlying illness. If this treatment is successful, the anemia usually resolves. For example, antibiotics prescribed for infection and anti-inflammatory drugs prescribed for rheumatoid arthritis or IBD can cause the anemia of AI/ACD to disappear. However, AI/ACD is increasingly being viewed as a medical condition that merits direct treatment.

For people with cancer or kidney disease who have low levels of EPO, a synthetic form of this normal hormone may be prescribed. People with kidney disease and AI/ACD may also be advised to take vitamin B_{12} and folic acid supplements. If iron deficiency has a role in causing the anemia, iron supplements may be given.

Section 15.3

Aplastic Anemia

Excerpted from "Aplastic Anemia," National Heart Lung and Blood Institute, National Institutes of Health, February 2009.

What Is Aplastic Anemia?

Aplastic anemia is a blood disorder in which the body's bone marrow doesn't make enough new blood cells. Bone marrow is a sponge-like tissue inside the bones. It makes stem cells that develop into red blood cells, white blood cells, and platelets.

Red blood cells carry oxygen to all parts of your body. They also remove carbon dioxide (a waste product) from your body's cells and carry it to the lungs to be exhaled. White blood cells help your body fight infections. Platelets are blood cell fragments that stick together to seal small cuts or breaks on blood vessel walls and stop bleeding.

It's normal for blood cells to die. The lifespan of red blood cells is about 120 days. White blood cells live less than 1 day. Platelets live about 6 days. As a result, your bone marrow must constantly make new blood cells.

If your bone marrow is unable to make enough new blood cells, a number of health problems can occur. These include arrhythmias, an enlarged heart, heart failure, infections, and bleeding. Severe aplastic anemia can even cause death.

What Causes Aplastic Anemia?

Damage to the bone marrow's stem cells causes aplastic anemia. When stem cells are damaged, they don't grow into healthy blood cells.

The cause of the damage can be acquired or inherited. Acquired aplastic anemia is more common, and sometimes it's only temporary. Aplastic anemia that's inherited is rare.

In more than half of the people who have aplastic anemia, the cause of the disorder is unknown. Some research suggests that stem cell damage may occur because the body's immune system attacks its own cells by mistake.

Acquired Causes

A number of diseases, conditions, and factors can cause aplastic anemia, including the following:

- Toxins, such as pesticides, arsenic, and benzene
- Radiation and chemotherapy (treatments for cancer)
- Medicines, such as chloramphenicol (an antibiotic rarely used in the United States)
- Infectious diseases, such as hepatitis, Epstein-Barr virus, cytomegalovirus, parvovirus B19, and human immunodeficiency virus (HIV)
- Autoimmune disorders, such as lupus and rheumatoid arthritis

In some cases, cancer from another part of the body can spread to the bone and cause aplastic anemia.

Inherited Causes

Certain inherited conditions can damage the stem cells and lead to aplastic anemia. Examples include Fanconi anemia, Shwachman-Diamond syndrome, dyskeratosis congenita, and Diamond-Blackfan anemia.

What Are the Signs and Symptoms of Aplastic Anemia?

Low numbers of red blood cells, white blood cells, and platelets cause most of the signs and symptoms of aplastic anemia.

Signs and Symptoms of Low Blood Cell Counts

Red blood cells. The most common symptom of a low red blood cell count is fatigue (feeling tired or weak). Not having enough hemoglobin in the blood causes fatigue. Hemoglobin is an iron-rich protein in red blood cells that carries oxygen to the body.

A low red blood cell count also can cause shortness of breath; dizziness, especially when standing up; headache; coldness in your hands or feet; pale skin, gums, and nail beds; and chest pain.

If you don't have enough hemoglobin-carrying red blood cells, your heart has to work harder to circulate the reduced amount of oxygen in your blood. This can lead to arrhythmias, heart murmur, an enlarged heart, or even heart failure.

White blood cells. White blood cells help fight infections. Signs and symptoms of a low white blood cell count include fevers, frequent infections that can be severe, and flu-like illnesses that linger.

Platelets. Platelets stick together to seal small cuts on blood vessel walls and stop bleeding. People who have low platelet counts tend to bruise and bleed easily, and the bleeding may be hard to stop.

Common types of bleeding linked to a low platelet count include nosebleeds, bleeding gums, pinpoint red bleeding spots on the skin, and blood in the stool. Women also may have heavy menstrual bleeding.

Other Signs and Symptoms

Aplastic anemia can cause signs and symptoms that aren't directly related to low blood cell counts. Examples include nausea (feeling sick to your stomach) and skin rashes.

Paroxysmal Nocturnal Hemoglobinuria

About one-third of people who have aplastic anemia have a condition called paroxysmal nocturnal hemoglobinuria (PNH). This is a red blood cell disorder. Most people who have PNH don't have any signs or symptoms.

If symptoms do occur, they may include the following:

- Shortness of breath

- Swelling or pain in the abdomen or swelling in the legs caused by blood clots

- Blood in the urine

- Headache

- Jaundice (a yellowish color of the eyes or skin)

In people who have aplastic anemia with PNH, either condition can develop first.

How Is Aplastic Anemia Diagnosed?

Your doctor will diagnose aplastic anemia based on your medical and family histories, a physical exam, and test results.

Once your doctor knows the cause and severity of the condition, he or she can create a treatment plan for you.

Diagnostic Tests

A number of tests are used to diagnose aplastic anemia. These tests help do the following:

- Confirm a diagnosis of aplastic anemia, look for its cause, and find out how severe it is
- Rule out other conditions that may cause similar symptoms
- Check for paroxysmal nocturnal hemoglobinuria (PNH)

Complete blood count. Often, the first test used to diagnose aplastic anemia is a complete blood count (CBC). The CBC measures many different parts of your blood.

This test checks your hemoglobin and hematocrit levels. Hemoglobin is an iron-rich protein in red blood cells that carries oxygen to the body. Hematocrit is a measure of how much space red blood cells take up in your blood. A low level of hemoglobin or hematocrit is a sign of anemia.

The CBC also checks the number of red blood cells, white blood cells, and platelets in your blood. Abnormal results may be a sign of aplastic anemia, an infection, or another condition.

Finally, the CBC looks at mean corpuscular volume (MCV). MCV is a measure of the average size of your red blood cells. The results may be a clue as to the cause of your anemia.

Reticulocyte count. A reticulocyte count measures the number of young red blood cells in your blood. The test shows whether your bone marrow is making red blood cells at the correct rate. People who have aplastic anemia have low reticulocyte levels.

Bone marrow tests. Bone marrow tests show whether your bone marrow is healthy and making enough blood cells. The two bone marrow tests are aspiration and biopsy.

Bone marrow aspiration may be done to find out if and why your bone marrow isn't making enough blood cells. For this test, your doctor removes a small amount of bone marrow fluid through a needle. The sample is examined under a microscope to check for faulty cells.

A bone marrow biopsy may be done at the same time as an aspiration or afterward. For this test, your doctor removes a small amount of bone marrow tissue through a needle.

The tissue is examined to check the number and types of cells in the bone marrow. In aplastic anemia, the bone marrow has a lower than normal number of all three types of blood cells.

Other tests. Other conditions can cause symptoms similar to those of aplastic anemia. Thus, other tests may be needed to rule out those conditions. These tests may include the following:

- *X-ray, computed tomography (CT) scan, or ultrasound imaging tests:* Your doctor may use these tests to look for enlarged lymph nodes in your abdomen. Enlarged lymph nodes may be a sign of blood cancer. These tests also may be used to examine the kidneys and the bones in the arms and hands, which are sometimes abnormal in young people who have Fanconi anemia. This type of anemia can lead to aplastic anemia.

- *Chest x-ray:* This test creates pictures of the structures inside your chest, such as your heart and lungs. A chest x-ray may be used to rule out infections.

- *Liver tests and viral studies:* These tests are used to check for liver diseases and viruses.

- *Tests that check vitamin B$_{12}$ and folate levels in the blood:* These tests can help rule out anemia due to vitamin deficiency.

Your doctor also may recommend blood tests for PNH and to check your immune system for antibodies. (Antibodies in the immune system that attack your own bone marrow cells may cause aplastic anemia.)

How Is Aplastic Anemia Treated?

Treatments for aplastic anemia include blood transfusions, blood and marrow stem cell transplants, and medicines. These treatments can prevent or limit complications, relieve symptoms, and improve quality of life.

In some cases, a cure may be possible. Blood and marrow stem cell transplants may cure the disorder in people who are eligible for a transplant. Removing a known cause of aplastic anemia, such as exposure to a toxin, also may cure the condition.

Who Needs Treatment

People who have mild or moderate aplastic anemia may not need treatment as long as the condition doesn't get worse. People who have severe aplastic anemia need medical treatment right away to prevent complications.

People who have very severe aplastic anemia need emergency medical care in a hospital. Very severe aplastic anemia can be fatal if it's not treated right away.

Blood Transfusions

People who have aplastic anemia may need blood transfusions to keep their blood cell counts at acceptable levels.

A blood transfusion is a common procedure in which blood is given to you through an intravenous (IV) line in one of your blood vessels. Transfusions require careful matching of donated blood with the recipient's blood.

Blood transfusions help relieve the symptoms of aplastic anemia, but they're not a permanent treatment.

Blood and Marrow Stem Cell Transplants

A blood and marrow stem cell transplant replaces damaged stem cells with healthy ones from another person (a donor).

During the transplant, which is like a blood transfusion, you get donated stem cells through a tube placed in a vein in your chest. Once the stem cells are in your body, they travel to your bone marrow and begin making new blood cells.

Blood and marrow stem cell transplants often cure aplastic anemia in people who are eligible for this type of transplant. The transplant works best in children and young adults with severe aplastic anemia who are in good health and who have matched donors.

Older people may be less able to handle the treatments needed to prepare the body for the transplant. They're also more likely to have complications after the transplant.

Medicines

If you have aplastic anemia, your doctor may prescribe medicines to do the following:

- Stimulate your bone marrow

- Suppress your immune system

- Prevent and treat infections

Medicines to stimulate bone marrow. Man-made versions of substances that occur naturally in the body can stimulate the bone marrow to make more blood cells. Examples of these types of medicines include erythropoietin and colony-stimulating factors.

These medicines have some risks. You and your doctor will work together to decide whether the benefits of these medicines outweigh the risks. If this treatment works well, it can help you avoid the need for blood transfusions.

Medicines to suppress the immune system. Research suggests that some cases of aplastic anemia may occur because the body's immune system attacks its own cells by mistake. For this reason, your doctor may prescribe medicines to suppress your immune system.

These medicines can allow your bone marrow to start making blood cells again. These medicines also may help you avoid the need for blood transfusions.

Medicines that suppress the immune system don't cure aplastic anemia. However, they can relieve its symptoms and reduce its complications.

These medicines often are used for people who aren't eligible for a bone and marrow stem cell transplant or who are waiting for a transplant.

Three medicines—often given together—can suppress the body's immune system. They are antithymocyte globulin (ATG), cyclosporine, and methylprednisolone.

It may take a few months to notice the effects of these medicines. Most often, as blood cell counts rise, symptoms lessen. Blood cell counts in people who respond well to these medicines usually don't reach normal levels. However, the blood cell counts often are high enough to allow people to do their normal activities.

People who have aplastic anemia may need long-term treatment with these medicines.

Medicines that suppress the immune system can have side effects. They also may increase the risk of developing leukemia or myelodysplasia (MDS). Leukemia is a cancer of the blood cells. MDS is a condition in which the bone marrow makes too many faulty blood cells.

Medicines to prevent and treat infections. People who have aplastic anemia may be at risk for infections due to a low number of white blood cells. Your doctor may prescribe antibiotic and antiviral medicines to prevent and treat infections.

Section 15.4

Fanconi Anemia

Excerpted from "Fanconi Anemia," National Heart Lung and Blood Institute, National Institutes of Health, December 2007.

What Is Fanconi Anemia?

Fanconi anemia, or FA, is a rare, inherited blood disorder that leads to bone marrow failure. FA causes your bone marrow to stop making enough new blood cells for your body to work normally. FA also can cause your bone marrow to make many abnormal blood cells. This can lead to serious health problems such as cancer.

FA is a blood disorder, but it also can affect many of your body's organs, tissues, and systems. Children who inherit FA are at higher risk of being born with birth defects. People with FA are at higher risk for some cancers and other serious health problems.

FA is different from Fanconi syndrome. Fanconi syndrome affects a person's kidneys. It's a rare and serious condition found mostly in children. Children with Fanconi syndrome pass high amounts of key nutrients and chemicals through their urine, which leads to serious health and developmental problems.

Bone Marrow and Your Blood

Bone marrow is the spongy red tissue inside the large bones of your body. Healthy bone marrow makes three types of blood cells:

- Red blood cells (also called RBCs), which carry oxygen to all parts of your body. They also remove carbon dioxide (a waste product) from your body's cells and carry it to the lungs to be exhaled.

- White blood cells (also called WBCs), which help your body fight infections.

- Platelets, which help your blood clot.

Blood cells live for a limited time. Then, they are replaced with new blood cells from your bone marrow. If your bone marrow can't make enough new blood cells to replace the ones that die, you can suffer from serious health problems.

Fanconi Anemia and Your Body

FA is one of many different types of anemia. The term "anemia" is used to describe conditions in which the number of red blood cells in a person's blood is lower than normal.

FA is a type of aplastic anemia. In aplastic anemia, the bone marrow slows down or stops making all three types of blood cells. Low levels of the three blood cell types can harm many of the body's organs, tissues, and systems.

With too few red blood cells, your body's tissues won't receive enough oxygen to work well.

With too few white blood cells, your body may have problems fighting infections. This can make you sick more often and make infections worse.

With too few platelets, you may suffer from excessive bleeding.

Outlook

If you or your child has FA, you face a greater risk than other people for some cancers. About 10 percent of people with FA develop leukemia, a type of blood cancer.

People with FA who survive to be adults are much more likely than others to develop cancerous solid tumors. The risk for solid tumors increases with age in those who have FA. These tumors can develop in your mouth, tongue, throat, or esophagus (the tube leading from your mouth to your stomach). Women who have FA are at much greater risk than women who don't have the disease for developing tumors in the reproductive organs.

FA is an unpredictable disease. The average life span for people who have FA is between twenty and thirty years. The most common causes of death related to FA are bone marrow failure, leukemia, and solid tumors.

New medical advances have improved the chances of surviving FA. Bone marrow transplant is the major advance in treatment. However, even with a bone marrow transplant, the risk for some cancers is greater in people who have FA.

What Causes Fanconi Anemia?

Fanconi anemia (FA) is an inherited disease. "Inherited" means that the disease is passed from parents to children through abnormal genes. At least eleven genes can cause FA if they're not normal. FA develops when both parents pass the same abnormal gene for FA to their child.

People who have only one abnormal FA gene are "carriers" of FA. Carriers don't have FA, but they can pass the abnormal gene to their children.

If both of your parents have an abnormal FA gene, you have:

- a 25 percent chance of having FA;

- a 25 percent chance of not having FA;

- a 50 percent chance of being a carrier of FA and passing the gene to any children you have.

If only one of your parents has a defective FA gene, you won't develop the disorder. However, there is a 50 percent chance that you will be a carrier and pass the gene to any children you have.

What Are the Signs and Symptoms of Fanconi Anemia?

Major Signs and Symptoms

Your doctor may suspect you or your child has Fanconi anemia (FA) if there are signs and symptoms of the following:

- Anemia

- Bone marrow failure

- Birth defects

- Developmental or eating problems

Because FA is an inherited disease, children may be tested if one of their brothers or sisters has the disease.

Anemia

If you have anemia, you have a lower than normal number of healthy red blood cells. This means that your blood isn't able to get enough oxygen to your body's cells, so they can't work normally. Symptoms of anemia include the following:

- Fatigue (tiredness)

- Weakness

- Dizziness

- Coldness in your hands and feet
- Chest pains
- Headaches
- Pale skin

Bone Marrow Failure

When your bone marrow fails, it can't make enough of the three types of blood cells—red and white blood cells and platelets—that your body needs to work normally. This can cause many problems, with various signs and symptoms.

With too few red blood cells, you can develop anemia. In FA, the size of your red blood cells also can be much larger than normal. This makes it more difficult for these cells to work well.

With too few white blood cells, you may have infections more often and they may last longer and be more serious than in people who don't have FA.

With too few platelets, you may bleed and bruise easily, suffer from internal bleeding, or have petechiae. Petechiae are tiny red spots caused by bleeding in small blood vessels just below your skin.

Sometimes when you have FA, your bone marrow makes a lot of harmful, immature white blood cells called blasts. These blasts don't work like normal blood cells. As they build up in your bone marrow, they block the production of normal blood cells. A large number of blasts in your bone marrow can lead to a type of blood cancer called acute myeloid leukemia (AML).

Birth Defects

Many different birth defects can be signs of FA. These include the following:

- **Bone or skeleton defects:** FA can cause missing, oddly shaped, or three or more thumbs. Arm bones, hips, legs, hands, and toes may not form fully or normally. The spine may be curved—a condition called scoliosis.

- **Eye and ear defects:** The eyes, eyelids, and ears may not be normally shaped. A child also may be born deaf.

- **Skin discoloration:** This includes coffee-colored areas or odd-looking patches of lighter skin.

- **Kidney problems:** A child might be born with a missing kidney or kidneys that aren't shaped normally.

- **Congenital heart defects:** The most common congenital heart defect linked to FA is a ventricular septal defect (VSD). VSD is when the wall that s separates the left and right chambers of the heart (the ventricles) is deformed or has a hole in it.

Developmental Problems

Other signs and symptoms of FA are related to physical and mental development. These include the following:

- Low birth weight

- Poor appetite

- Slower growth than other children

- Lower than normal height

- Small head size

- Mental retardation or learning disabilities

Signs and Symptoms of Fanconi Anemia in Adults

Some signs and symptoms of FA may develop as you or your child gets older.
Women with FA may experience some or all of the following:

- Sex organs that are less developed than normal

- Starting menstruation later than women who don't have FA

- Starting menopause earlier than women who don't have FA

- Difficulty becoming pregnant and carrying a pregnancy to full term

Men who have FA may have male sex organs that are less developed and may be less fertile than men who don't have the disease.

How Is Fanconi Anemia Diagnosed?

People who have Fanconi anemia (FA) are born with the disease. They may or may not show signs or symptoms of it at birth. For this reason, FA isn't always diagnosed when a person is born. In fact, most people with the disease are diagnosed between the ages of two and fifteen years.

The tests used to diagnose FA depend on a person's age and symptoms. In all cases, medical history and family history are an important part of diagnosing FA. However, because FA has many of the same signs and symptoms as other diseases, only genetic testing can confirm its diagnosis.

Diagnostic Tests and Procedures

The signs and symptoms for FA aren't unique to the disease. They're also linked to many other diseases and conditions, such as aplastic anemia. For this reason, genetic testing is needed to confirm a diagnosis of FA. Genetic tests for FA include the following.

Chromosome breakage test. This is the most common test for FA. It's available only in special laboratories. It shows whether your chromosomes (long chains of genes) break more easily than normal.

Sometimes, skin cells are used for the test, but usually a small amount of blood is taken from a vein in your arm with a needle. A technician combines some of the blood cells that were taken out with certain chemicals. If you have FA, the chromosomes in your blood sample break and rearrange when mixed with the test chemicals. This doesn't happen in the cells of people who don't have FA.

Cytometric flow analysis. Cytometric flow analysis, or CFA, is done in a laboratory to see how chemicals affect your chromosomes as your cells grow and divide. Skin cells are used for this test. A technician mixes the skin cells with chemicals that can cause the chromosomes in those cells to act abnormally. If you have FA, your cells are much more sensitive to these chemicals. The chromosomes in your skin cells will break at a high rate as they go through the cycle in this test. This doesn't happen in the cells of people who don't have FA.

Mutation screening. A mutation is an abnormality in a gene or genes. Geneticists and other specialists can examine genes in your cells, usually from a sample of your skin cells. With special equipment and laboratory processes, they can look for mutations in your genes that are linked to FA.

How Is Fanconi Anemia Treated?

Doctors decide how to treat Fanconi anemia (FA) based on a patient's age and how well (or how poorly) the patient's bone marrow is producing new blood cells.

Goals of Treatment

Long-term treatments for FA can do either of the following:

- Cure the anemia. Damaged bone marrow cells are replaced with healthy ones that can make enough of all three types of blood cells on their own.

- Treat the symptoms without curing the cause. This is done using medicines and other substances that can help your body make more blood cells for a limited time.

Observation and Short-Term Treatment

If you or your child has FA, but your bone marrow is still able to make many of the new blood cells your body needs, your doctor may perform frequent blood count checks. During this period of observation, your doctor will probably want you to have bone marrow exams once a year. Your doctor also will screen you closely for any signs of cancer or tumors.

If your blood counts begin to drop sharply and stay low, your doctor may assume your bone marrow is failing. He or she may give you antibiotics to help your body fight infections.

In the short term, your doctor also may want to give you blood transfusions to increase your blood cell counts to normal levels. However, long-term use of blood transfusions can reduce the chances that other treatments, which can help your body make enough blood cells on its own, will work.

Long-Term Treatment

There are four main types of long-term treatment for FA:

- Bone marrow transplant

- Androgen therapy

- Synthetic growth factors

- Gene therapy

Bone marrow transplant: Bone marrow transplant, also called stem cell transplant, is the current standard treatment for patients with FA that's causing major bone marrow failure. Healthy bone marrow cells from another person, called a donor, are used to replace the abnormal cells in your bone marrow.

Bone marrow transplant is most successful in younger people who have few or no serious health problems, a brother or sister donor, and few or no previous blood transfusions.

Successful bone marrow transplants will allow your body to make enough of all three types of blood cells to work normally. However, if you've had a transplant to treat FA, you will still be at risk for some types of blood cancer and for developing cancerous solid tumors. Your doctor will check your health regularly and often after the procedure.

Androgen therapy. Before improvements made bone marrow transplants more effective, androgen therapy was the standard treatment for people with FA. Androgens are artificial male hormones that can help your body make more blood cells for long periods.

Androgens are effective in increasing your red blood cell count. They also help to increase your platelet count. They're less effective in making more white blood cells in your body.

Unlike bone marrow transplant, androgens don't enable your bone marrow to produce enough of all three types of blood cells on its own. You may need ongoing treatment with androgens to control the effects of FA. Also, androgens eventually lose their ability to help your body make more blood cells, which means you will need other treatments.

Androgen treatment can have serious side effects, such as liver disease, and it can't prevent you from developing leukemia.

Synthetic growth factors. Your doctor may choose to treat your FA with substances known as growth factors. These are substances found in your body, but they also can be man-made. They help your body make more red and white blood cells. Growth factors that can help your body make more platelets are still being researched. One of the more common growth factors used to treat FA is called EPO, or erythropoietin. EPO has some risks. Based on your situation, your doctor will decide whether EPO's benefits outweigh its risks.

More research is needed on growth factor treatment for FA. Early results suggest that growth factors may have fewer and less serious side effects than androgens.

Gene therapy. Researchers are looking for ways to replace abnormal FA genes with normal, healthy genes. They believe that the replacement genes will be able to make the proteins needed to repair and protect your bone marrow cells.

Gene therapy uses viruses that have been altered so that they can deliver normal genes to replace abnormal ones in FA patients' bone marrow stem cells.

Early results hold promise, but this form of treatment for FA is still in the experimental stage.

Surgery

Surgery may be needed to improve the use of arms, thumbs, hips, legs, and other parts of the body that are malformed or underdeveloped due to birth defects caused by FA.

If your child is born with a heart defect linked to FA called ventricular septal defect, he or she may need surgery to close the hole in the heart's wall so the heart can function normally.

Children with FA also may need surgery to correct problems in the digestive system that can harm their nutrition, growth, and survival. One of the most common problems is an FA-related birth defect where the windpipe (trachea), which carries air to the lungs, is connected to the esophagus, which carries food to the stomach. This can cause serious breathing, swallowing, and eating problems and can lead to lung infections. Surgery is needed to separate the two organs to allow normal eating and breathing.

Living with Fanconi Anemia

If you or your child has Fanconi anemia (FA), your chances for survival have increased due to improvements in bone marrow transplantation. In addition, other new treatments are being developed that hold promise. But FA still presents serious challenges to patients and their families.

Special Concerns and Needs

Many people with FA live into adulthood. If you have FA, you will require regular and ongoing medical attention. Your blood counts will need to be monitored regularly. Although your body can use healthy bone marrow cells from a donor to make the blood cells you need, you remain at risk for many cancers. You will need to be screened for FA-related cancers more often than people who don't have FA.

If FA has left you with very low levels of platelets in your blood, your doctor may advise you to avoid contact sports and other activities that carry the risk of physical injury.

If your child has FA, he or she may have problems eating or keeping food down. Your doctor may recommend additional special feedings to keep your child's weight at a level needed for ongoing development and good health.

Section 15.5

Glucose-6-Phosphate Dehydrogenase (G6PD) Deficiency

"G6PD Deficiency," August 2006, reprinted with permission from www
.kidshealth.org. Copyright © 2006 The Nemours Foundation. This information was provided by KidsHealth, one of the largest resources
online for medically reviewed health information written for parents,
kids, and teens. For more articles like this one, visit www.KidsHealth
.org or www.TeensHealth.org.

G6PD deficiency is an inherited condition in which the body doesn't
have enough of the enzyme glucose-6-phosphate dehydrogenase, or
G6PD, which helps red blood cells (RBCs) function normally. This deficiency can cause hemolytic anemia, usually after exposure to certain
medications, foods, or even infections.

Most people with G6PD deficiency don't have any symptoms, while
others develop symptoms of anemia only after RBCs have been destroyed, a condition called hemolysis. In these cases, the symptoms
disappear once the cause, or trigger, is removed. In rare cases, G6PD
deficiency leads to chronic anemia.

With the right precautions, a child with G6PD deficiency can lead
a healthy and active life.

About G6PD Deficiency

G6PD is one of many enzymes that help the body process carbohydrates and turn them into energy. G6PD also protects red blood
cells from potentially harmful by-products that can accumulate when
a person takes certain medications or when the body is fighting an
infection.

In people with G6PD deficiency, either the RBCs do not make
enough G6PD or what is produced cannot properly function. Without
enough G6PD to protect them, RBCs can be damaged or destroyed.
Hemolytic anemia occurs when the bone marrow (the soft, spongy part
of the bone that produces new blood cells) cannot compensate for this
destruction by increasing its production of RBCs.

Causes of G6PD Deficiency

G6PD deficiency is passed along in genes from one or both parents to a child. The gene responsible for this deficiency is on the X chromosome.

G6PD deficiency is most common in African American males. Many African American females are carriers of G6PD deficiency, meaning they can pass the gene for the deficiency to their children but do not have symptoms; only a few are actually affected by G6PD deficiency.

People of Mediterranean heritage, including Italians, Greeks, Arabs, and Sephardic Jews, also are commonly affected. The severity of G6PD deficiency varies among these groups—it tends to be milder in African Americans and more severe in people of Mediterranean descent.

Why does G6PD deficiency occur more often in certain groups of people? It is known that Africa and the Mediterranean basin are high-risk areas for the infectious disease malaria. Researchers have found evidence that the parasite that causes this disease does not survive well in G6PD-deficient cells. So they believe that the deficiency may have developed as a protection against malaria.

G6PD Deficiency Symptom Triggers

Kids with G6PD deficiency typically do not show any symptoms of the disorder until their red blood cells are exposed to certain triggers, which can be:

- illness, such as bacterial and viral infections;

- certain painkillers and fever-reducing drugs;

- certain antibiotics (especially those that have "sulf" in their names);

- certain antimalarial drugs (especially those that have "quine" in their names).

Some kids with G6PD deficiency can tolerate the medications in small amounts; others cannot take them at all. Check with your doctor for more specific instructions, as well as a complete list of medications that could pose a problem for a child with G6PD deficiency.

Other substances can be harmful to kids with this condition when consumed—or even touched—such as fava beans and naphthalene (a chemical found in mothballs and moth crystals). Mothballs can be particularly harmful if a child accidentally swallows one, so *any* contact should be avoided.

Symptoms of G6PD Deficiency

A child with G6PD deficiency who is exposed to a medication or infection that triggers the destruction of RBCs may have no symptoms at all. In more serious cases, a child may exhibit symptoms of anemia (also known as a hemolytic crisis), including:

- paleness (in darker-skinned children paleness is sometimes best seen in the mouth, especially on the lips or tongue);

- extreme tiredness;

- rapid heartbeat;

- rapid breathing or shortness of breath;

- jaundice, or yellowing of the skin and eyes, particularly in newborns;

- an enlarged spleen;

- dark, tea-colored urine.

Once the trigger is removed or resolved, the symptoms of G6PD deficiency usually disappear fairly quickly, typically within a few weeks.

If symptoms are mild, no medical treatment is usually needed. As the body naturally makes new red blood cells, the anemia will improve. If symptoms are more severe, a child may need to be hospitalized for supportive medical care.

Diagnosing and Treating G6PD Deficiency

In most cases, cases of G6PD deficiency go undiagnosed until a child develops symptoms. If doctors suspect G6PD deficiency, blood tests usually are done to confirm the diagnosis and to rule out other possible causes of the anemia.

If you feel that your child may be at risk because of either a family history or your ethnic background, talk to your doctor about performing a screening with blood tests to check for G6PD deficiency.

Treating the symptoms associated with G6PD deficiency is usually as simple as removing the trigger—that is, treating the illness or infection or stopping the use of a certain drug. However, a child with severe anemia may require treatment in the hospital to receive oxygen, fluids, and, if needed, a transfusion of healthy blood cells. In rare cases, the deficiency can lead to other more serious health problems.

Caring for Your Child

The best way to care for a child with G6PD deficiency is to limit exposure to the triggers of its symptoms. With the proper precautions, G6PD deficiency should not keep your child from living a healthy, active life.

Section 15.6

Hemoglobin C Disease

"Hemoglobin C Disease," © 2009 A.D.A.M., Inc. Reprinted with permission.

Alternative Names

Clinical hemoglobin C

Definition

Hemoglobin C disease is a blood disorder passed down through families. It leads to a type of anemia, which causes red blood cells to break down earlier than normal.

Causes

Hemoglobin C is a problem with hemoglobin, the part of red blood cells that carry oxygen. It is a type of hemoglobinopathy. The disease is caused by problems with a gene called beta globin.

The disease most often occurs in African Americans. You are more likely to develop hemoglobin C disease if someone in your family has had it.

Symptoms

Most people do not have symptoms. Occasionally, jaundice may occur. Some persons with this disease may develop gallstones that require treatment.

Exams and Tests

Physical examination reveals an enlarged spleen.
Tests that may be done include:

- complete blood count;
- hemoglobin electrophoresis;
- peripheral smear;
- serum hemoglobin.

Treatment

Usually no treatment is needed. Folic acid supplementation may help your body produce normal red blood cells and improve the symptoms of the anemia.

Outlook (Prognosis)

People with hemoglobin C disease can expect to lead a normal life.

Possible Complications

Complications include episodes of pain, hip problems, vision problems, and gallbladder disease.

When to Contact a Medical Professional

Call your health care provider if you have symptoms of hemoglobin C disease.

Prevention

Genetic counseling may be appropriate for high-risk couples who wish to have a baby.

References

Goldman L, Ausiello D. *Cecil Textbook of Medicine*. 23rd. Philadelphia, Pa: WB Saunders; 2007:1225–26.

Section 15.7

Hemoglobin E Disease

You have just learned that your infant has hemoglobin E disease. Naturally you are concerned and have many questions. This section will help answer some of your questions. However, it should not take the place of an informed discussion with your baby's doctor (primary care provider).

What is hemoglobin?

Hemoglobin is a protein in the red blood cells. It carries oxygen to all parts of the body and gives blood its red color. There are many hemoglobin types (this is not the same as a blood type). Hemoglobin is inherited through genes, one from each parent. Most people have hemoglobin A, also called adult or normal hemoglobin. The presence of hemoglobin A makes the red blood cells smooth and round. These cells move easily through the blood vessels and deliver oxygen normally to the body.

What is hemoglobin E disease?

Hemoglobin E in the red blood cells is responsible for causing hemoglobin E disease. Children inherit this disease from their parents as a recessive genetic disorder. This means a hemoglobin E gene is passed from both mom and dad to the baby causing hemoglobin E disease (hemoglobin EE). When both parents have one hemoglobin E gene, there is a one in four or 25 percent chance with each pregnancy that an infant will inherit two hemoglobin E genes. Persons with hemoglobin EE have red blood cells that are smaller than usual. There are no associated health problems with hemoglobin EE, but the gene for hemoglobin E is passed on to each of one of your future grandchildren. Hemoglobin E disease is not contagious.

What is hemoglobin E/beta-thalassemia disease?

Children with hemoglobin E/beta-thalassemia inherit one gene for hemoglobin E from one parent and one beta-thalassemia gene from the other parent. The beta-thalassemia gene causes the body to make less than the usual amount of hemoglobin. The combination of hemoglobin E/ beta-thalassemia is a disease that can be life threatening. Persons with this disease will need special medical care throughout their life.

How common are hemoglobin E and beta-thalassemia?

The highest frequency of hemoglobin E is among people of Southeast Asian descent, especially those living in or having ancestors from Cambodia, Laos, and Thailand. Hemoglobin E is also found in people who live in Vietnam, Malaysia, northeastern India, Bangladesh, Pakistan, Nepal, and Sri Lanka and their descendants. Beta-thalassemia is highest among people living in Mediterranean countries and their descendants, such as Greece and Italy. Other areas for beta-thalassemia include the Arabian Peninsula, Turkey, Iran, Africa, India, Southeast Asia, and southern China.

What are the signs and symptoms of hemoglobin E/beta-thalassemia?

Hemoglobin E/beta-thalassemia disease causes severe destruction of red blood cells. If this condition is left untreated, severe anemia occurs. Other problems are heart failure, an enlarged liver and spleen, poor growth, and changes in the bones.

What can be done to treat hemoglobin E/beta-thalassemia disease?

There is no known cure for hemoglobin E/beta-thalassemia. Treatment for this disease includes repeated blood transfusions.

What are the chances of having a child with hemoglobin E/beta-thalassemia?

When one parent has hemoglobin E trait (one hemoglobin E gene and one hemoglobin A gene) and the other parent has beta-thalassemia trait (one hemoglobin beta-thalassemia gene and one hemoglobin A gene), there is a one in four or 25 percent chance with each pregnancy that your child will inherit:

- two hemoglobin A (normal) genes; or

- one hemoglobin A gene and one hemoglobin E gene; or

- one hemoglobin A gene and one beta-thalassemia gene; or

- one hemoglobin E gene and one beta-thalassemia gene.

What are the most important things to remember with hemoglobin E/beta-thalassemia?

- Work closely with your child's doctor and hematologist (a doctor who is a blood specialist). Make sure your child has regular checkups with him or her.

- Call your child's doctor when you have questions and have your child seen if you have any medical concerns.

How do I get more information?

Talk with your baby's doctor. You may also want to have a genetic consultation for you and your family to see how these diseases might affect future children or grandchildren.

Section 15.8

Iron-Deficiency Anemia

What is iron-deficiency anemia?

Iron-deficiency anemia is when lack of iron means that the blood does not contain enough hemoglobin—the iron-based pigment in red blood cells that gives them their color and carries oxygen. Severe and prolonged iron deficiency is needed to cause anemia.

Iron-deficiency anemia is one of several types of anemia. This type of anemia is common, particularly in women near menopause, teenage girls, premature or very small babies, and the elderly, and is usually easy to treat.

Why did I get iron-deficiency anemia?

The reasons for getting iron-deficiency anemia include:

- losing a lot of blood from heavy periods or stomach and bowel problems, including ulcers or cancer;

- lack of iron in the diet over a long period of time;

- fast growth in children;

- being born early (premature);

- being pregnant—the mother's iron stores go to her baby;

- excessive exercise—the body needs more iron than usual and iron is lost in sweat;

- being unable to absorb iron in the bowel, for example in Crohn disease or celiac disease;

- regular use of medicines that can cause stomach bleeding (for example, aspirin and anti-inflammatories); and

- damaged veins or bleeding piles (hemorrhoids).

What happens in iron-deficiency anemia?

Iron is one of twenty minerals found in food. It is stored in your liver, spleen, and bone marrow and is vital for mental and physical wellbeing. While most of the body's iron is recycled from dead red blood cells, a small but essential amount comes from food. If your body does not have enough iron, it can't make enough hemoglobin.

What does iron-deficiency anemia feel like?

The symptoms of iron-deficiency anemia are caused by the lack of oxygen being supplied to the tissues. You may feel tired, short of breath when exercising, or unable to concentrate, have headaches, or get irritable. Your skin and the inside of your mouth may be pale. You may also be likely to pick up infections. Eventually, your nails can become spoon-shaped and brittle, the corners of your mouth may crack, and you may have difficulty swallowing. Some people also get cravings for unusual substances, such as ice or earth.

Older people with iron-deficiency anemia may get angina (pain in the chest) because the heart has to work harder to supply enough oxygen to the body.

Children with low iron levels may be slow to learn or develop.

While symptoms can be severe, in the early stages of iron deficiency you may have no symptoms or just mild fatigue.

How is iron-deficiency anemia diagnosed?

Anemia may be diagnosed if you have some of the symptoms listed above, but if the anemia is not severe you may not feel anything and will be diagnosed only if you have a routine blood test. Blood tests will show how much iron is in your blood and what type of anemia you have. Other tests may be needed to see if there is any bleeding in your stomach or bowel.

What makes iron-deficiency anemia better?

What will help the condition depends on the cause of your anemia. However, iron-deficiency anemia is usually easily treated with iron supplements and a good diet. Your blood count will be checked regularly to make sure anemia has not returned.

Iron supplements. Iron supplements are usually given as tablets, but if you need a high dose of iron, you may have an injection. Iron tablets can turn your bowel motions black—this is harmless. They may also cause indigestion, nausea, diarrhea, or constipation. If so, your doctor may change the tablets or suggest other ways of reducing the indigestion. Take your tablets as prescribed.

Take iron tablets on an empty stomach unless you get bad indigestion, in which case you should take them with food.

Don't take iron supplements with milk, tea, or coffee—these can reduce the amount of iron your body absorbs.

Wait two hours after taking iron tablets before taking other medicines.

Keep taking the tablets for at least three months or until your doctor tells you to stop. You must take them until well after your hemoglobin is normal.

If you are pregnant you may be given iron tablets. A healthy diet is also recommended.

Children should be given their iron medicine (usually in liquid form) before meals with orange juice (not milk), as vitamin C increases iron absorption. They should use a straw because liquid iron can discolor the mouth.

Diet. Your body absorbs only a small amount of iron, so it is important to eat a lot of iron-rich foods (meat, fish, or poultry, whole or enriched grains) every day.

Eating a lot of foods rich in vitamin C (e.g., citrus fruits, kiwi fruit, red capsicum, leafy green vegetables) will help iron absorption.

Limit your milk intake to 500 mL daily. Talk with your doctor, dietitian, or community health nurse about other ways to get enough calcium.

Don't drink tea with meals—it prevents iron absorption.

Your doctor or community health nurse can tell you how much iron you need daily. A dietitian can plan a diet for you.

What happens if anemia is not treated?

The anemia can get worse and you can feel more and more unwell, particularly if the underlying cause, such as stomach bleeding, is not treated.

For severe iron-deficiency anemia, you may need a blood transfusion.

Iron deficiency due to pregnancy may improve on its own if your diet is good; however, iron supplements may be needed. Researchers are still looking into when and how to treat iron-deficiency anemia in pregnancy.

If you have heavy periods your doctor may be able to suggest medicines to reduce blood loss.

The material provided by CMPMedica Australia Pty Ltd is intended for Australian residents only, is of a general nature, and is provided for information purposes only. The material is not a substitute for independent professional medical advice from a qualified healthcare professional. It is not intended to be used by anyone to diagnose, treat, cure, or prevent any disease or medical condition. No person should act in reliance solely on any statement contained in the material provided, and at all times should obtain specific advice from a qualified healthcare professional.

Section 15.9

Pernicious (Megaloblastic) Anemia

Excerpted from "Pernicious Anemia," National Heart Lung and Blood Institute, National Institutes of Health, February 2009.

Pernicious anemia is a condition in which the body can't make enough healthy red blood cells because it doesn't have enough vitamin B_{12}.

People who have pernicious anemia can't absorb enough vitamin B_{12} due to a lack of intrinsic factor, a protein made in the stomach. This leads to vitamin B_{12} deficiency. In people who have pernicious anemia, the cells that make intrinsic factor are destroyed.

Other conditions and factors also can cause vitamin B^{12} deficiency. Examples include infections, surgery, medicines, and diet. Technically, the term "pernicious anemia" refers to vitamin B_{12} deficiency due to a lack of intrinsic factor. Often, vitamin B_{12} deficiency due to other causes also is called pernicious anemia.

Without enough red blood cells to carry oxygen to your body, you may feel tired and weak. Severe or long-lasting pernicious anemia can damage the heart, brain, and other organs in the body. The condition also can cause other complications, such as nerve damage, neurological problems (such as memory loss), and digestive tract problems.

Pernicious anemia is more common in people of Northern European and African descent. In the United States, older people are at higher risk for the condition. Pernicious anemia also can occur in younger people and other population groups.

The signs and symptoms of pernicious anemia are due to a lack of vitamin B_{12} (vitamin B_{12} deficiency). Without enough vitamin B_{12}, your body can't make enough healthy red blood cells. This causes anemia.

Some of the signs and symptoms of pernicious anemia, such as fatigue (tiredness), shortness of breath, and dizziness, apply to all types of anemia. Other signs and symptoms, such as muscle weakness, memory loss, and nausea (feeling sick to your stomach), are specific to a lack of vitamin B_{12}.

Your doctor will diagnose pernicious anemia based on your medical and family histories, a physical exam, and the results from tests. Your doctor will want to find out whether the condition is due to a lack of intrinsic factor or another cause.

Doctors treat pernicious anemia by replacing the missing vitamin B_{12} in your body. This is done using vitamin B_{12} pills or shots. People who have pernicious anemia may need lifelong treatment. If your doctor can find the cause of your pernicious anemia, you may get treatment for that problem.

You can't prevent pernicious anemia that's due to a lack of intrinsic factor. However, if you have pernicious anemia because of dietary factors, you can take steps to prevent it. Eating foods high in vitamin B_{12} can help prevent low vitamin B_{12} levels. Your doctor also may advise taking vitamin B_{12} supplements.

With proper treatment, people who have pernicious anemia can recover, feel well, and live normal lives. See your doctor regularly for checkups and ongoing treatment. Take vitamin B_{12} supplements as your doctor advises. This may help prevent anemia symptoms and complications.

If you have pernicious anemia, tell your family members. Pernicious anemia can run in families, so they may be more likely to develop the condition.

Section 15.10

Sickle Cell Disease

Reprinted from "Facts about Sickle Cell Disease," Centers for Disease Control and Prevention. The text of this document is available online at http://www.cdc.gov/ncbddd/sicklecell/faq_sicklecell.htm; accessed April 23, 2009.

Sickle cell disease (SCD) is a group of inherited red blood cell disorders. Healthy red blood cells are round, and they move through small blood vessels to carry oxygen to all parts of the body. In sickle cell disease, the red blood cells become hard and sticky and look like a C-shaped farm tool called a "sickle." The sickle cells die early, which causes a constant shortage of red blood cells. Also, when they travel through small blood vessels, they get stuck and clog the blood flow. This can cause pain and other serious problems.

What Causes Sickle Cell Disease?

Sickle cell disease is a genetic condition that is present at birth. It is inherited when a child receives two sickle cell genes—one from each parent.

How Is It Diagnosed?

Sickle cell disease is diagnosed with a simple blood test. It is most often found at birth during routine newborn screening tests at the hospital. In addition, sickle cell disease can be diagnosed before birth.

Because children with sickle cell disease are at an increased risk of infection and other health problems, early diagnosis and treatment are important.

What Are the Symptoms and Complications and How Are They Treated?

People with sickle cell disease start to have symptoms during the first year of life, usually around five months of age. Symptoms and complications of sickle cell disease are different for each person and can range from mild to severe:

- Hand-foot syndrome
- Pain "episode" or "crisis"
- Anemia
- Infection
- Acute chest syndrome
- Splenic sequestration
- Vision loss
- Leg ulcers
- Stroke
- Other

Hand-Foot Syndrome

This is usually the first symptom of sickle cell disease. Swelling in the hands and feet, often along with a fever, is caused by the sickle cells getting stuck in the blood vessels and blocking the flow of blood in and out of the hands and feet.

Treatment. Pain medicine and fluids, such as water.

Pain "Episode" or "Crisis"

This is the most common complication, and the top reason that people with sickle cell disease go to the emergency room or hospital. When sickle cells travel through small blood vessels, they can get stuck and clog the blood flow. This causes pain that can start suddenly, be mild to severe, and can last for any length of time.

Prevention. There are simple steps that people with sickle cell disease can take to help prevent and reduce the number of pain crises:

- Drink plenty of water.
- Try not to get too hot or too cold.
- Try to avoid places with high altitudes (flying, mountain climbing, or cities with a high altitude).
- Try to avoid places or situations with low oxygen (mountain climbing or exercising extremely hard, such as in military boot camp or when training for an athletic competition).

- Adults with severe sickle cell disease can take a medicine called hydroxyurea to help reduce the number of pain crises.

- People taking hydroxyurea must be checked often by a doctor because the medicine can cause serious side effects, including an increased risk of dangerous infections.

Treatment. Pain medicine.

Anemia

This is a very common complication. With sickle cell disease, the red blood cells die early. This means there are not enough healthy red blood cells to carry oxygen throughout the body. When this happens, a person might have the following symptoms:

- Tiredness

- Irritability

- Dizziness and lightheadedness

- Fast heart rate

- Difficulty breathing

- Pale skin color

- Jaundice (yellow color to the skin and whites of the eyes)

- Slow growth

- Delayed puberty

Treatment. Blood transfusions are used to treat severe anemia. A sudden worsening of anemia resulting from infection or enlargement of the spleen is a common reason for a transfusion.

Infection

People with sickle cell disease, especially infants and children, are more at risk for harmful infections. Pneumonia is a leading cause of death in infants and young children with sickle cell disease.

Prevention. Vaccinations can protect against harmful infections. Babies and children with sickle cell disease should have all of the regular childhood vaccinations, plus a few extra. The extra ones are as follows:

- Flu vaccine (influenza vaccine) every year after six months of age

- A special pneumococcal vaccine (called 23-valent pneumococcal vaccine) at two and five years of age

- Meningococcal vaccine, if recommended by a doctor

Adults with sickle cell disease should have the flu vaccine every year, as well as the pneumococcal vaccine and any others recommended by a doctor.

In addition, children with sickle cell disease should receive a daily dose of penicillin, an antibiotic medicine, to help prevent infections. This can begin at two months of age and continue until the child is at least five years of age.

Treatment. Infections are treated with antibiotic medicines and sometimes blood transfusions. At the first sign of an infection, such as a fever, it is important for people with sickle cell disease to see a doctor. Early treatment of infection can help prevent problems.

Acute Chest Syndrome

This can be life-threatening and should be treated in a hospital. It is similar to pneumonia and symptoms include chest pain, coughing, difficulty breathing, and fever.

Prevention. Adults with severe sickle cell disease can take a medicine called hydroxyurea to help prevent acute chest syndrome. People taking hydroxyurea must be watched closely because the medicine can cause serious side effects, including an increased risk of dangerous infections.

A person who is on bed rest or has recently had surgery can use an incentive spirometer, also called "blow bottle," to help prevent acute chest syndrome.

Treatment. Depending on the cause, treatment might include oxygen, medicine to treat an infection, medicine to open up blood vessels to improve blood flow, and blood transfusions.

Splenic Sequestration

This can be life-threatening and should be treated in a hospital. It happens when a large number of sickle cells get trapped in the spleen and cause it to suddenly get large. Symptoms include sudden weakness, pale lips, fast breathing, extreme thirst, abdominal (belly) pain on the left side of body, and fast heart beat.

Parents of a child with sickle cell disease should learn how to feel and measure the size of their child's spleen.

Prevention. For those who have had a very severe, life-threatening episode of splenic sequestration or who have had many episodes in the past, it might be necessary to have regular blood transfusions or the spleen can be removed (called splenectomy) to stop it from happening again.

Treatment. Treatment typically is a blood transfusion.

Vision Loss

Vision loss, including blindness, can occur when blood vessels in the eye become blocked with sickle cells and the retina (the thin layer of tissue inside the back of the eye) gets damaged.

Prevention. People with sickle cell disease should have their eyes checked every year to look for damage to the retina. If possible, this should be done by an eye doctor who specializes in diseases of the retina.

Treatment. If the retina is damaged, laser treatment often can prevent further vision loss.

Leg Ulcers

This usually occurs on the lower part of the leg. They happen more often in males than in females and usually appear from ten through fifty years of age. The cause of leg ulcers is unclear.

Treatment. Leg ulcers can be treated with medicated creams and ointments. Leg ulcers can be painful, and patients can be given strong pain medicine. Bed rest and keeping the leg (or legs) raised to reduce swelling is helpful, although not always possible.

Stroke

A stroke can happen if sickle cells get stuck in a blood vessel and clog blood flow to the brain. About 10 percent of children with sickle cell disease will have a stroke. Stroke can cause lifelong disabilities and learning problems.

Prevention. Doctors can sometimes identify children who are at risk for stroke using a special type of exam called "transcranial Doppler ultrasound." In some cases, a doctor might recommend frequent blood transfusions to help prevent a stroke. People who have frequent blood transfusions must be watched closely because there are serious side effects. For example, too much iron can build up in the body, causing life-threatening damage to the organs.

Other Possible Complications

- Damage to body organs, tissues, or bones because not enough blood is flowing to the affected area(s).

- Gallstones.

- Painful erection of the penis, called priapism, that can last less than two hours or more than four hours. If it lasts more than four hours, the person should get urgent medical help. It can lead to impotence.

Is There a Cure?

The only cure for SCD is bone marrow/stem cell transplant.

Bone marrow is a soft, fatty tissue inside the center of the bones where blood cells are made. A bone marrow/stem cell transplant is a procedure that takes healthy cells that form blood from one person—the donor—and puts them into someone whose bone marrow is not working properly.

Bone marrow/stem cell transplants are very risky, and can have serious side effects, including death. For the transplant to work, the bone marrow must be a close match. Usually, the best donor is a brother or sister. Bone marrow/stem cell transplants are used only in cases of severe sickle cell disease for children who have minimal organ damage from the disease.

Can a Person "Catch" Sickle Cell Disease from Someone Who Has It?

No, a person cannot "catch" sickle cell disease from another person. Sickle cell disease is a genetic condition that is inherited when a child receives two sickle cell genes—one from each parent.

Can a Woman with Sickle Cell Disease Have a Healthy Pregnancy?

Yes; however, women with sickle cell disease are more likely to have problems during pregnancy that can affect their health and the health of their unborn baby. During pregnancy, the disease can become more severe and pain episodes can occur more frequently. A pregnant woman with sickle cell disease is at a higher risk of preterm labor and of having a low birth weight baby. However, with early prenatal care and careful monitoring throughout pregnancy, women with sickle cell disease can have a healthy pregnancy.

During pregnancy, there is a test to find out if the baby will have sickle cell disease, sickle cell trait, or neither one. The test is usually done after the second month of pregnancy.

Women with sickle cell disease might want to see a genetic counselor to find information about the disease and the chances that sickle cell disease will be passed to the baby.

Section 15.11

Spherocytosis

What Is Hereditary Spherocytosis?

Spherocytosis, in most cases, is an inherited disease that destroys red blood cells. This destruction of the red blood cells causes anemia.

The shape of a normal red blood cell resembles a disk. Normal red blood cells easily change shape to move effectively through the small blood vessels between organs of the body. A person with spherocytosis has red blood cells that are very round and have difficulty changing this shape. The lack of ability to change shapes makes moving through the small blood vessels difficult. Therefore, the red blood cells stay in the spleen longer than normal. This lengthy stay in the spleen damages the cell membranes. Eventually, the spleen will destroy these abnormal red blood cells.

What Causes Spherocytosis?

Spherocytosis can be caused by a number of different genetic defects all of which have in common the production of a faulty protein component of the cell membrane. The faulty component leads to the weakness of the red blood cell wall. In addition to being fragile, these red blood cells are less resistant to stress and rupture easily. In some rare cases, spherocytosis is not inherited; the cause of this blood disease is considered to be a spontaneous mutation of the gene. Infection, fever, and stress can stimulate the spleen to destroy more red blood cells than usual. If this occurs, the skin and whites of the eyes will turn yellow because the hemoglobin level will drop and the bilirubin level will rise.

Signs and Symptoms

Spherocytosis is frequently a mild disorder with very few symptoms. The symptoms associated with anemia and spherocytosis are the following:

- Paleness or yellow color of the skin or eyes
- Stomach pain
- Shortness of breath
- Lack of energy
- Lack of appetite
- Irritability in children
- Fever
- Vomiting

In more severe cases, patients may:

- develop gallstones;
- experience aplastic crises (severe decrease in red blood cell production) caused by a viral infection.

How Is Spherocytosis Diagnosed?

Doctors have several ways to test for spherocytosis including blood tests and examination of the spleen. Due to the hereditary nature of spherocytosis, parents with a family history of spherocytosis should have their children tested.

Treatment for Spherocytosis

- Young children (up to five years of age) should take folic acid supplements.

- Blood transfusions may help with severe anemia.

- Surgical removal of the spleen (splenectomy) in children five years of age or older. This does not cure that patient of spherocytosis; rather it allows red blood cells to live longer. Without a spleen, a person has an increased risk for some serious infections. Therefore, patients who have their spleen removed need to take penicillin (or another antibiotic) for the rest of their lives. Several special immunizations (pneumococcal and meningococcal) are also required to help prevent some infections.
Call the doctor if the patient:

- has a fever of greater than 101.5° F;

- has had their spleen removed and skin is pale and/or yellow or if eyes are yellow;

- still has their spleen and skin is more pale and/or yellow than usual or if eyes are more yellow than normal;

- is having difficulty taking prescribed medication.

Section 15.12

Thalassemia

"Thalassemias," November 2008, reprinted with permission from www.kids health.org. Copyright © 2008 The Nemours Foundation. This information was provided by KidsHealth, one of the largest resources online for medically reviewed health information written for parents, kids, and teens. For more articles like this one, visit www.KidsHealth.org, or www.TeensHealth.org.

What Are Thalassemias?

Thalassemias are genetic disorders that involve the decreased and defective production of hemoglobin, a molecule found inside all red blood cells (RBCs) that transports oxygen throughout the body.

As frightening as thalassemias can be, the outlook is encouraging. In the past twenty years, new therapies have greatly improved the quality of life and life expectancy in kids who have these diseases.

The two types of thalassemia are alpha-thalassemia and beta-thalassemia. Their names describe which part of the hemoglobin molecule that is affected, the alpha or the beta chain. Hemoglobin contains two different kinds of protein chains named alpha and beta chains. Any deficiency in these chains causes abnormalities in the formation, size, and shape of RBCs.

Thalassemia can cause ineffective production of RBCs and their destruction. As a result, people with thalassemia often have a reduced number of RBCs in the bloodstream (anemia), which can affect the transportation of oxygen to body tissues. In addition, thalassemia can cause RBCs to be smaller than normal or drop hemoglobin in the RBCs to below-normal levels.

Kids who have different forms of thalassemia have different kinds of health problems. Some only have mild anemia with little or no effects, while others require frequent serious medical treatment.

Causes

Thalassemia is always inherited, passed on from parents to children through their genes. A child usually does not develop symptoms unless both parents carry a thalassemia gene.

If only one parent passes a gene for thalassemia on to the child, then the child is said to have thalassemia trait. Thalassemia trait will not develop into the full-blown disease, and no medical treatment is necessary.

Many families have thalassemia carriers, but the trait often goes undiagnosed because it produces no or few symptoms. Frequently, thalassemia is not diagnosed in a family until a baby is born with it. So if someone in your family carries a thalassemia gene, it's wise to have genetic counseling if you're thinking of having children.

At one time it was believed that the disease affected only people of Italian or Greek descent, but it's now known that many people with thalassemia also come from or are descended from Africa, Malaysia, China, and many parts of Southeast Asia.

Because of a recent pattern of migration from Southeast Asia, there has been an increase in the past decade of thalassemia in North America. Testing for thalassemia is generally recommended for anyone from Southeast Asia with unexplained anemia.

If your doctor determines that your child is at risk for thalassemia, prenatal tests can find out if your unborn child is affected.

Types of Thalassemias

Alpha-Thalassemia

Children with alpha-thalassemia trait do not have thalassemia disease. People normally have four genes for alpha globin, two inherited from each parent. If one or two of these four genes are affected, the child is said to have alpha-thalassemia trait.

A specific blood test called a hemoglobin electrophoresis is used to screen for alpha-thalassemia trait and can be done in infancy. Sometimes, alpha-thalassemia trait can be detected through routine newborn blood screening, which is required in most states in the U.S.

Often, results of the hemoglobin electrophoresis test are normal in people who have alpha-thalassemia trait and a diagnosis of alpha-thalassemia is done only after other conditions are ruled out and after the parents are screened. The disease can be harder to detect in older kids and adults.

Kids who have the alpha-thalassemia trait usually have no significant health problems except mild anemia, which can cause slight fatigue.

Alpha-thalassemia trait is often mistaken for an iron-deficiency anemia because RBCs will appear small when viewed under a microscope.

Other cases can cause more severe anemia where three genes are affected. People with this form of alpha-thalassemia may require occasional blood transfusions during times of physical stress, like fevers or other illnesses, or when the anemia is severe enough to cause symptoms such as fatigue.

The most severe form of the disorder is called alpha-thalassemia major. This type is extremely rare, and women carrying fetuses with this form of thalassemia have a high incidence of miscarriage because the fetuses cannot survive.

Beta-Thalassemia

Beta-thalassemia, the most common form of the disorder seen in the United States, is grouped into three categories: beta-thalassemia minor (trait), intermedia, and major (Cooley anemia). A person who carries a beta-thalassemia gene has a 25 percent (one in four) chance of having a child with the disease if his or her partner also carries the trait.

Beta-Thalassemia Minor (Trait)

Beta-thalassemia minor often goes undiagnosed because kids with the condition have no real symptoms other than mild anemia and small red blood cells. It is often suspected based on routine blood tests such as a complete blood count (CBC) and can be confirmed with a hemoglobin electrophoresis. No treatment is usually needed.

As with alpha-thalassemia trait, the anemia associated with this condition may be misdiagnosed as an iron deficiency.

Beta-Thalassemia Intermedia

Children with beta-thalassemia intermedia have varying effects from the disease—mild anemia might be their only symptom or they might require regular blood transfusions.

The most common complaint is fatigue or shortness of breath. Some kids also experience heart palpitations, also due to the anemia, and mild jaundice, which is caused by the destruction of abnormal red blood cells that result from the disease. The liver and spleen may be enlarged, which can feel uncomfortable for a child. Severe anemia can also affect growth.

Another symptom of beta-thalassemia intermedia can be bone abnormalities. Because the bone marrow is working overtime to make more RBCs to counteract the anemia, kids can experience enlargement of their cheekbones, foreheads, and other bones. Gallstones are a frequent complication because of abnormalities in bile production that involve the liver and the gallbladder.

Some kids with beta-thalassemia intermedia may require a blood transfusion only occasionally. They will always have anemia, but may not need transfusions except during illness, medical complications, or later on during pregnancy.

Other children with this form of the disease require regular blood transfusions. In these kids, low or falling hemoglobin levels greatly reduce the blood's ability to carry oxygen to the body, resulting in extreme fatigue, poor growth, and facial abnormalities. Regular transfusions can help alleviate these problems. Sometimes, kids who have this form of the disease have their spleens removed.

Beta-thalassemia intermedia is often diagnosed in the first year of life. Doctors may be prompted to test for it when a child has chronic anemia or a family history of the condition. As long as it is diagnosed while the child is still doing well and has not experienced any serious complications, it can be successfully treated and managed.

Beta-Thalassemia Major

Beta-thalassemia major, also called Cooley anemia, is a severe condition in which regular blood transfusions are necessary for the child to survive.

Although multiple lifelong transfusions save lives, they also cause a serious side effect: an overload of iron in the bodies of thalassemia patients. Over time, people with thalassemia accumulate deposits of iron, especially in the liver, heart, and endocrine (hormone-producing) glands. The deposits eventually can affect the normal functioning of the heart and liver, in addition to delaying growth and sexual maturation.

To minimize iron deposits, kids must undergo chelation (iron-removing) therapy. This can be done by taking daily medication by mouth or by subcutaneous or intravenous administration.

Daily chelation therapy is given five to seven days a week and has been proven to prevent liver and heart damage from iron overload, allow for normal growth and sexual development, and increase life span. Iron concentrations are monitored every few months. Sometimes liver biopsies are needed to get a more accurate picture of the body's iron load.

Children on regular transfusions are monitored closely for iron levels and complications of iron overload on the chelation medications.

Other risks associated with chronic blood transfusions for thalassemia major include blood-borne diseases like hepatitis B and C. Blood banks screen for such infections, in addition to rarer infections such as human immunodeficiency virus (HIV). In addition, kids who have many transfusions can develop allergic reactions that can prevent further transfusions and cause serious illnesses.

179

For kids and teens with thalassemia, adolescence can be a difficult time, particularly because of the amount of time required for transfusions and chelation therapy.

Recently, some kids have successfully undergone bone marrow transplants to treat thalassemia major; however, this is considered only in cases of severely disabling thalassemia disease. There is considerable risk to bone marrow transplants: the procedure involves the destruction of all of the blood-forming cells in the bone marrow and repopulating the marrow space with donor cells that must match perfectly (the closest match is usually from a sibling).

The procedure is usually done in children younger than sixteen years of age who have no existing evidence of liver scarring or serious liver disease. Results have been encouraging so far, with disease-free survival in many patients.

Blood-forming stem cells taken from umbilical cord blood have also been successfully transplanted, and research using this technique is expected to increase. Currently bone marrow treatment is the only known cure for the disease.

Talking to the Doctor

If you know the thalassemia trait exists in your family, it's important to meet with your doctor, particularly if you notice any of the symptoms of thalassemia major—anemia, listlessness, or bone abnormalities—in your child.

If you're thinking of having children, speak with a genetic counselor to determine your risk of passing on the disease.

Chapter 16

Hemochromatosis

What is hemochromatosis?

Hemochromatosis is the most common form of iron overload disease. Primary hemochromatosis, also called hereditary hemochromatosis, is an inherited disease. Secondary hemochromatosis is caused by anemia, alcoholism, and other disorders.

Juvenile hemochromatosis and neonatal hemochromatosis are two additional forms of the disease. Juvenile hemochromatosis leads to severe iron overload and liver and heart disease in adolescents and young adults between the ages of fifteen and thirty. The neonatal form causes rapid iron buildup in a baby's liver that can lead to death.

Hemochromatosis causes the body to absorb and store too much iron. The extra iron builds up in the body's organs and damages them. Without treatment, the disease can cause the liver, heart, and pancreas to fail.

Iron is an essential nutrient found in many foods. The greatest amount is found in red meat and iron-fortified breads and cereals. In the body, iron becomes part of hemoglobin, a molecule in the blood that transports oxygen from the lungs to all body tissues.

Healthy people usually absorb about 10 percent of the iron contained in the food they eat, which meets normal dietary requirements. People with hemochromatosis absorb up to 30 percent of iron. Over time, they absorb and retain between five and twenty times more iron than the body needs.

Reprinted from "Hemochromatosis," National Institute of Diabetes and Digestive and Kidney Diseases, National Institutes of Health, NIH Publication No. 07-4621, April 2007.

Because the body has no natural way to rid itself of the excess iron, it is stored in body tissues, specifically the liver, heart, and pancreas.

What causes hemochromatosis?

Hereditary hemochromatosis is mainly caused by a defect in a gene called HFE, which helps regulate the amount of iron absorbed from food. The two known mutations of HFE are C282Y and H63D. C282Y is the most important. In people who inherit C282Y from both parents, the body absorbs too much iron and hemochromatosis can result. Those who inherit the defective gene from only one parent are carriers for the disease but usually do not develop it; however, they still may have higher than average iron absorption. Neither juvenile hemochromatosis nor neonatal hemochromatosis are caused by an HFE defect. Juvenile and neonatal hemochromatosis are caused by a mutation in a gene called hemojuvelin.

What are the risk factors for hemochromatosis?

Hereditary hemochromatosis is one of the most common genetic disorders in the United States. It most often affects Caucasians of Northern European descent, although other ethnic groups are also affected. About five people out of one thousand—0.5 percent—of the U.S. Caucasian population carry two copies of the hemochromatosis gene and are susceptible to developing the disease. One out of every eight to twelve people is a carrier of one abnormal gene. Hemochromatosis is less common in African Americans, Asian Americans, Hispanics/Latinos, and American Indians.

Although both men and women can inherit the gene defect, men are more likely than women to be diagnosed with hereditary hemochromatosis at a younger age. On average, men develop symptoms and are diagnosed between thirty and fifty years of age. For women, the average age of diagnosis is about fifty.

What are the symptoms of hemochromatosis?

Joint pain is the most common complaint of people with hemochromatosis. Other common symptoms include fatigue, lack of energy, abdominal pain, loss of sex drive, and heart problems. However, many people have no symptoms when they are diagnosed.

If the disease is not detected and treated early, iron may accumulate in body tissues and eventually lead to serious problems such as the following:

- Arthritis
- Liver disease, including an enlarged liver, cirrhosis, cancer, and liver failure
- Damage to the pancreas, possibly causing diabetes
- Heart abnormalities, such as irregular heart rhythms or congestive heart failure
- Impotence
- Early menopause
- Abnormal pigmentation of the skin, making it look gray or bronze
- Thyroid deficiency
- Damage to the adrenal glands

How is hemochromatosis diagnosed?

A thorough medical history, physical examination, and routine blood tests help rule out other conditions that could be causing the symptoms. This information often provides helpful clues, such as a family history of arthritis or unexplained liver disease.

Blood tests can determine whether the amount of iron stored in the body is too high. The transferrin saturation test reveals how much iron is bound to the protein that carries iron in the blood. Transferrin saturation values higher than 45 percent are considered too high.

The total iron binding capacity test measures how well your blood can transport iron, and the serum ferritin test shows the level of iron in the liver. If either of these tests shows higher than normal levels of iron in the body, doctors can order a special blood test to detect the HFE mutation, which will confirm the diagnosis. If the mutation is not present, hereditary hemochromatosis is not the reason for the iron buildup and the doctor will look for other causes.

A liver biopsy may be needed, in which case a tiny piece of liver tissue is removed and examined with a microscope. The biopsy will show how much iron has accumulated in the liver and whether the liver is damaged.

Hemochromatosis is considered rare and doctors may not think to test for it. Thus, the disease is often not diagnosed or treated. The initial symptoms can be diverse, vague, and mimic the symptoms of many other diseases. The doctors also may focus on the conditions caused by hemochromatosis—arthritis, liver disease, heart disease, or diabetes—

rather than on the underlying iron overload. However, if the iron over-load caused by hemochromatosis is diagnosed and treated before organ damage has occurred, a person can live a normal, healthy life.

Hemochromatosis is usually treated by a specialist in liver disorders called a hepatologist, a specialist in digestive disorders called a gas-troenterologist, or a specialist in blood disorders called a hematologist. Because of the other problems associated with hemochromatosis, other specialists may be involved in treatment, such as an endocrinologist, cardiologist, or rheumatologist. Internists or family practitioners can also treat the disease.

How is hemochromatosis treated?

Treatment is simple, inexpensive, and safe. The first step is to rid the body of excess iron. This process is called phlebotomy, which means removing blood the same way it is drawn from donors at blood banks. Based on the severity of the iron overload, a pint of blood will be taken once or twice a week for several months to a year, and occasionally longer. Blood ferritin levels will be tested periodically to monitor iron levels. The goal is to bring blood ferritin levels to the low end of nor-mal and keep them there. Depending on the lab, that means 25 to 50 micrograms of ferritin per liter of serum.

Once iron levels return to normal, maintenance therapy begins, which involves giving a pint of blood every two to four months for life. Some people may need phlebotomies more often. An annual blood ferritin test will help determine how often blood should be removed. Regular follow-up with a specialist is also necessary.

If treatment begins before organs are damaged, associated condi-tions—such as liver disease, heart disease, arthritis, and diabetes—can be prevented. The outlook for people who already have these conditions at diagnosis depends on the degree of organ damage. For example, treat-ing hemochromatosis can stop the progression of liver disease in its early stages, which leads to a normal life expectancy. However, if cirrhosis, or scarring of the liver, has developed, the person's risk of developing liver cancer increases, even if iron stores are reduced to normal levels.

People with complications of hemochromatosis may want to receive treatment from a specialized hemochromatosis center. These centers are located throughout the country.

People with hemochromatosis should not take iron or vitamin C supplements. And those who have liver damage should not consume alcoholic beverages or raw seafood because they may further dam-age the liver.

Treatment cannot cure the conditions associated with established hemochromatosis, but it will help most of them improve. The main exception is arthritis, which does not improve even after excess iron is removed.

How is hemochromatosis tested?

Screening for hemochromatosis—testing people who have no symptoms—is not a routine part of medical care or checkups. However, researchers and public health officials do have some suggestions:

- Siblings of people who have hemochromatosis should have their blood tested to see if they have the disease or are carriers.

- Parents, children, and other close relatives of people who have the disease should consider being tested.

- Doctors should consider testing people who have joint disease, severe and continuing fatigue, heart disease, elevated liver enzymes, impotence, and diabetes because these conditions may result from hemochromatosis.

Since the genetic defect is common and early detection and treatment are so effective, some researchers and education and advocacy groups have suggested that widespread screening for hemochromatosis would be cost-effective and should be conducted. However, a simple, inexpensive, and accurate test for routine screening does not yet exist and the available options have limitations. For example, the genetic test provides a definitive diagnosis, but it is expensive. The blood test for transferrin saturation is widely available and relatively inexpensive, but it may have to be done twice with careful handling to confirm a diagnosis and show that the result is the consequence of iron overload.

Hope through Research

Scientists hope further study of the HFE gene will reveal how the body normally metabolizes iron. They also want to learn how iron injures cells and contributes to organ damage in other diseases, such as alcoholic liver disease, hepatitis C, porphyria cutanea tarda, heart disease, reproductive disorders, cancer, autoimmune hepatitis, diabetes, and joint disease.

Scientists are working to find out why only some patients with HFE mutations develop the disease. In addition, hemochromatosis research includes the following areas:

- **Genetics:** Researchers are examining how the HFE gene normally regulates iron levels and why not everyone with an abnormal pair of genes develops the disease.

- **Pathogenesis:** Scientists are studying how iron injures body cells. Iron is an essential nutrient, but above a certain level it can damage or even kill cells.

- **Epidemiology:** Research is underway to explain why the amounts of iron people normally store in their bodies differ. Research is also being conducted to determine how many people with the defective HFE gene go on to develop symptoms and why some people develop symptoms and others do not.

- **Screening and testing:** Scientists are working to determine at what age testing is most effective, which groups should be tested, and which are the best tests for widespread screening.

Chapter 17

Leukemia

Chapter Contents

Section 17.1

Acute Lymphocytic Leukemia

"Acute Lymphocytic Leukemia," Leukemia and Lymphoma Society, 2008. Reprinted with permission. For additional help and the most current information, contact the Leukemia and Lymphoma Society, 1311 Mamaroneck Avenue, Suite 310 White Plains, NY 10605, www.leukemialymphoma.org, 800-955-4572, infocenter@LLS.org. The prevalence and incidence statistics in this document were updated by Leukemia and Lymphoma Society from the National Cancer Institute's Surveillance, Epidemiology and End Results (SEER) Program, Cancer Statistics Review 1975–2006, published online by SEER, www.seer.cancer.gov, in April 2009.

Understanding Acute Lymphocytic Leukemia

Acute lymphocytic leukemia (ALL) is a type of blood cancer. Other names for ALL are acute lymphoblastic leukemia and acute lymphoid leukemia.

About 5,760 people in the United States are expected to be diagnosed with ALL in 2009. It is the most common type of leukemia in children under age fifteen. The risk of getting ALL increases in people ages forty-five and older. However, people can get ALL at any age.

Most children with ALL are cured of their disease after treatment.

Causes and Risk Factors

ALL starts with a change to a single cell in the bone marrow. Scientists are studying the exact genetic changes that cause a normal cell to become an ALL cell.

Few factors have been associated with an increased risk of developing ALL. Exposure to high doses of radiation therapy used to treat other types of cancer is one known risk factor. Other possible risk factors are continually under study. ALL is not contagious (catching).

ALL occurs at different rates in different geographic locations. There are higher rates in more developed countries and in higher socioeconomic groups. Scientists continue to explore possible relationships with lifestyle or environmental factors but no firm conclusions have yet been reached. This suggests that many factors may be involved. At the present time there is no known way to prevent most cases of the disease.

Information about Phosphocol P32: Phosphocol P32 is a prescription drug approved to treat adults with fluid in the abdominal or chest cavity caused by cancer or infection. Safety and effectiveness in children has not been established. The United States Food & Drug Administration (FDA) updated the safety information of this drug in August 2008 following reports linking Phosphocol P32 to leukemia, when used in an unapproved way to treat children with bleeding between the joints caused by hemophilia. The labeling of Phosphocol P 32 was modified by the manufacturer, Covidien Ltd., in August 2008 to reflect this risk. Information about the leukemia cases (two children, ages nine and fourteen, with hemophilia developed acute lymphocytic leukemia approximately ten months after intra-articular injections of Phosphocol P 32 [0.6 and 1.5 mCi total dose]) was added to the "Warnings" section of the Phosphocol P 32 label. Also, "leukemia in children" is now noted as a risk in the label's "Adverse Events" section. Safety information is posted on the FDA Medwatch Web site (August 2008). The manufacturer strongly encourages medical professionals and their patients to follow the guidelines outlined in the prescribing information included with Phosphocol P 32.

Signs and Symptoms

Some signs or symptoms of ALL are similar to other more common and less severe illnesses. Specific blood tests and bone marrow tests are needed to make a diagnosis. A person with ALL may have:

- aches in arms, legs, back;
- black-and-blue marks for no apparent reason;
- enlarged lymph nodes;
- fever without obvious cause;
- headaches;
- pale-looking skin;
- pinhead-size red spots under the skin;
- prolonged bleeding from minor cuts;
- shortness of breath during physical activity;

- tiredness;

- vomiting.

The best advice for any person troubled by symptoms such as a lasting, low-grade fever, unexplained weight loss, tiredness, or shortness of breath is to see a healthcare provider.

Diagnosis

Blood and bone marrow tests are done to look for leukemia cells. A CBC (complete blood count) is used to help diagnose ALL. A bone marrow aspirate and a bone marrow biopsy are two of the tests that are done. An aspirate is done to take a close look at the cells in the marrow in order to look for abnormal cells such as leukemic blast cells. It can also be used for cytogenetic analysis, immunophenotyping, and other tests. The biopsy gives information about how much disease is in the marrow. Immunophenotyping is used to find out if the patient's leukemia cells are B cells or T cells. Most people with ALL have the B-cell type. Most cases of the B-cell type are called precursor B-cell type.

The doctor uses information from these tests to decide the type of drug therapy a patient needs and how long treatment will last. Bone marrow tests are also done to see if treatment is destroying leukemic blast cells.

To decide the best treatment for the patient, the doctor may also consider:

- the patient's age;

- the number of ALL cells in the blood;

- if the ALL has spread to the covering of the brain or spinal cord;

- if there are certain chromosomal changes.

Treatment

Patients with ALL need to start chemotherapy right away. It is important to get medical care in a center where doctors are experienced in treating patients with ALL.

The goal of treatment for ALL is to cure the disease. Children with ALL are likely to be cured of their disease. The number of adult patients who have remissions has increased. The length of remissions in adults has improved.

There are two parts of treatment for ALL, called induction therapy and post-induction therapy. The aim of induction therapy is to:

- kill as many ALL cells as possible;

- get blood counts back to normal;

- and to get rid of all signs of the disease for an extended period of time.

This is called a remission.

Some drugs used to treat ALL are given by mouth. Other drugs are given by placing a catheter in a vein—usually in the patient's upper chest. During induction therapy most patients are treated with more than one drug and they may be given several drugs in combination. Each drug type works in a different way to kill the cells. Combining drug types can strengthen the effects of the drugs. Some of the drugs used to treat ALL are clofarabine, cytarabine, daunorubicin, methotrexate, mitoxantrone, cyclophosphamide, vincristine, pegaspargase, imatinib mesylate, prednisone, and dexamethasone.

Patients with ALL often have leukemic cells in the lining of the spinal cord and brain. The procedure used to check the spinal fluid for leukemic cells is called a spinal tap. The cells cannot always be found in an exam of the spinal fluid.

To prevent leukemia in the central nervous system (CNS) leukemia, all patients who are in remission have the lining of the spinal cord and brain treated. In some cases, treatment is needed for ALL that has already affected the lining of the spinal cord and brain (CNS leukemia) and is causing problems such as headache, nausea and vomiting, and blurred vision. Parts of the body that aren't easily reached with chemotherapy given by mouth or intravenous (IV) line—such as the lining of the spinal cord and brain—are treated by injection into the spinal fluid. Drugs such as methotrexate or cytarabine are injected into the spinal fluid either to prevent or treat CNS leukemia.

When the treatment is for CNS leukemia, a spinal tap is done. Then spinal fluid is removed and chemotherapy is injected into the spinal canal.

Radiation therapy may be given to the spine or brain. Spinal taps are done from time to time to check if leukemic cells are being killed and to give more doses of chemotherapy. Sometimes both chemotherapy and radiation therapy are used.

Many ALL patients build up uric acid in their blood from their disease. Uric acid is a chemical made in the body. The use of chemotherapy also increases the uric acid. A high level of uric acid can cause kidney stones. Patients with high uric acid levels may be given a drug called allopurinol (Aloprim®, Zyloprim®) by mouth or IV. Another drug used to treat high uric acid levels is called rasburicase (Elitek®).

Post-induction therapy: More treatment is needed even after a patient with ALL is in remission. This is called post-induction therapy. It is given in cycles for two to three years. Post-induction therapy is given because some ALL cells remain that are not found by common blood or marrow tests. For most people, the post-remission therapy drugs used are not the same drugs used during induction therapy. The doctor considers many things to decide the kind of post-induction therapy a patient needs, such as:

- the patient's response to induction therapy;

- whether the patient has certain chromosomal abnormalities.

High-risk types of ALL—such as T-cell ALL, infant ALL, and adult ALL—are usually treated with higher doses of drugs during induction and post-induction therapy. One treatment plan is to use higher doses of drugs and give them for a longer time. Allogeneic stem cell transplant may be a good treatment for some high-risk ALL patients.

Ph-positive ALL-induction/post-induction: About one out of five adults with ALL and a small number of children with ALL have a type called Ph-positive (or Philadelphia-positive) ALL.

Ph-positive ALL may be treated with imatinib mesylate, also called Gleevec® or with other related drugs, such as dasatinib (Sprycel®) or nilotinib (Tasigna®). These drugs are given with chemotherapy. Gleevec® (or Sprycel® or Tasigna®) is given by mouth. Doctors are studying how well this treatment works in patients with Ph-positive ALL.

During post-induction therapy, Gleevec® (or another related drug) is given with other drugs. Usually people with Ph-positive ALL stay on Gleevec® (or another related drug) after post-induction therapy is completed.

Allogeneic stem cell transplant: Allogeneic stem cell transplant is a treatment used for some patients with ALL.

The main purpose of doing the transplant is to give strong doses of chemotherapy or radiation therapy to kill the ALL cells. This will also kill the healthy stem cells in the marrow. The transplanted donor stem cells help start a new supply of red cells, white cells, and platelets.

Allogeneic stem cell transplant is a high-risk procedure. For this reason, it may not be a good treatment for some ALL patients. Allogeneic stem cell transplant may be a choice for adult ALL patients if:

- they are not doing well with other treatments;
- the expected benefits of stem cell transplant exceed the risks;
- there is a donor.

Stem cell transplant is usually not considered for a child unless:

- Doctors have determined that the child's type of ALL is not likely to respond well to chemotherapy;
- chemotherapy has not worked well;
- the child has relapsed ALL.

Side Effects of Treatment

Not all patients have treatment side effects. Patients who experience side effects should speak to their treatment teams about how to manage their side effects.

Possible side effects of treatment for ALL include:

- The number of red cells may decrease (called anemia). Transfusions of red cells (blood cells that are donated and given to the patient) may be needed to increase red cells.

- Patients also may have a drop in the number of platelets. If a patient's platelet count is very low he or she may need a platelet transfusion to prevent bleeding.

- A big drop in white cells may lead to an infection. Such infections are usually treated with antibiotics, until the white cell count goes up and the infection clears up. For adults, growth factors are sometimes given to increase white cells. G-CSF (Neulasta® or Neupogen®) and GM-CSF (Leukine®) are drugs that increase the number of white cells. The doctor may talk about the absolute neutrophil count or ANC, which is the number of neutrophils, a type of white cell, a person has to fight an infection. Fever or chills may be the only signs of infection. Patients with an infection may also have coughing, sore throat, pain when urinating, or frequent loose bowel movements.

To lower the risk of infection:

- The patient, the patient's visitors, and medical staff need to wash their hands well.
- The patient's central line must be kept clean. Patients on chemotherapy should take good care of their teeth and gums.

Chemotherapy affects the parts of the body where new cells form quickly. This includes the inside of the mouth and bowel, and the skin and hair. Some other chemotherapy side effects are:

- mouth sores;
- diarrhea;
- hair loss;
- rashes;
- nausea;
- vomiting.

Drugs and other therapies can be given to prevent or treat nausea or vomiting.

Follow-Up Visits

Patients who have finished all of their therapy still need to go to their doctors regularly for exams and tests. The doctor may recommend longer periods of time between follow-up visits if a patient continues to be disease free.

Treatment for ALL can cause long-term or late effects. Children should be checked for treatment effects on growth or learning that may not take place right away. It is important to identify problems early. Talk to the doctor about when your child's learning skills should be assessed. Some children will need special help with schoolwork during and after treatment.

Relapsed or Refractory ALL

Some patients have a remission after treatment but then ALL cells return later—this is called a relapse. Other patients with ALL may still have ALL cells in the marrow even after treatment (refractory leukemia).

For patients who relapse, the same or different drugs may be given, or be used. A drug called clofarabine (Clolar®) is being used to treat some children (ages one to twenty-one) with relapsed and refractory ALL.

In refractory leukemia, drugs that were not used to treat the patient's ALL in the first round of treatment may be given. Allogeneic stem cell transplantation also may be used.

Clinical Trials

Clinical trials are used to study new drugs, new treatments, or new uses for approved drugs or treatments. These are some of the types of trials under way:

- Leukemia-specific therapy, based on a patient's specific type of leukemia—such as the type of chromosome changes—is being studied.

- The ALL cells of some patients are not as easily killed by drugs as those of other patients. This is called drug resistance. Scientists are trying to understand why some ALL cells are resistant to the effects of chemotherapy. This will help them develop better treatments.

- Scientists are studying ways to boost the body's natural defenses, called immunotherapy. The goal is to kill or prevent the growth of ALL cells.

- Blood cell growth factors can be used to help restore normal blood cells during treatment.

- Scientists are studying the exact genetic changes that cause a normal cell to become an ALL cell. This research is leading to the development of new treatments. These treatments could block the effects of cancer-causing genes called oncogenes.

- Gene profiling will be used more in the future to design more specific treatments for the different types of leukemia. New targeted treatments are being developed for ALL.

- Many therapies, such as nilotinib, are being studied in clinical trials for Ph-positive ALL and other high-risk types of ALL. T-cell ALL, infant ALL, and adult ALL are other high-risk types of ALL.

- Doctors are studying a type of stem cell transplant, called a nonmyeloablative stem cell transplant (also called a reduced-intensity transplant).

Talk to the Doctor

It may be helpful to write down questions to ask your doctor. You can also write down or record your doctor's answers and review them later. You may want to bring a family member or friend with you to the doctor. This person can listen, take notes, and offer support. Some patients record information and listen to it at home.

Section 17.2

Chronic Lymphocytic Leukemia

Excerpted from "Chronic Lymphocytic Leukemia Treatment (PDQ®), Patient Version," PDQ® Cancer Information Summary. National Cancer Institute, Bethesda, MD. Updated October 2008. Available at http://cancer.gov. Accessed April 22, 2009.

Chronic lymphocytic leukemia is a type of cancer in which the bone marrow makes too many lymphocytes (a type of white blood cell).

Chronic lymphocytic leukemia (also called CLL) is a blood and bone marrow disease that usually gets worse slowly. CLL is the second most common type of leukemia in adults. It often occurs during or after middle age; it rarely occurs in children.

Normally, the body makes blood stem cells (immature cells) that develop into mature blood cells over time. A blood stem cell may become a myeloid stem cell or a lymphoid stem cell.

The myeloid stem cell develops into one of three types of mature blood cells:

- Red blood cells that carry oxygen and other materials to all tissues of the body

- White blood cells that fight infection and disease

- Platelets that help prevent bleeding by causing blood clots to form

The lymphoid stem cell develops into a lymphoblast cell and then into one of three types of lymphocytes (white blood cells):

- B lymphocytes that make antibodies to help fight infection

- T lymphocytes that help B lymphocytes make antibodies to fight infection

- Natural killer cells that attack cancer cells and viruses

In CLL, too many blood stem cells develop into abnormal lymphocytes and do not become healthy white blood cells. The abnormal lymphocytes may also be called leukemic cells. The lymphocytes are not able to fight infection very well. Also, as the number of lymphocytes increases in the blood and bone marrow, there is less room for healthy white blood cells, red blood cells, and platelets. This may result in infection, anemia, and easy bleeding.

Older age can affect the risk of developing chronic lymphocytic leukemia.

Anything that increases your risk of getting a disease is called a risk factor. Having a risk factor does not mean that you will get cancer; not having risk factors doesn't mean that you will not get cancer. People who think they may be at risk should discuss this with their doctor. Risk factors for CLL include the following:

- Being middle-aged or older, male, or white

- A family history of CLL or cancer of the lymph system

- Having relatives who are Russian Jews or Eastern European Jews

Possible signs of chronic lymphocytic leukemia include swollen lymph nodes and tiredness.

Usually CLL does not cause any symptoms and is found during a routine blood test. Sometimes symptoms occur that may be caused by CLL or by other conditions. A doctor should be consulted if any of the following problems occur:

- Painless swelling of the lymph nodes in the neck, underarm, stomach, or groin

- Feeling very tired

- Pain or fullness below the ribs

- Fever and infection

- Weight loss for no known reason

Tests that examine the blood, bone marrow, and lymph nodes are used to detect (find) and diagnose chronic lymphocytic leukemia.

The following tests and procedures may be used:

- **Physical exam and history:** An exam of the body to check general signs of health, including checking for signs of disease, such as lumps or anything else that seems unusual. A history of the patient's health habits and past illnesses and treatments will also be taken.

- **Complete blood count (CBC):** A procedure in which a sample of blood is drawn and checked for the following:

  - The number of red blood cells, white blood cells, and platelets

  - The amount of hemoglobin (the protein that carries oxygen) in the red blood cells

  - The portion of the blood sample made up of red blood cells

- **Cytogenetic analysis:** A test in which cells in a sample of blood or bone marrow are viewed under a microscope to look for changes in the structure or number of chromosomes in the lymphocytes.

- **Immunophenotyping:** A test in which the cells in a sample of blood or bone marrow are looked at under a microscope to find out if malignant lymphocytes (cancer) began from the B lymphocytes or the T lymphocytes.

- **Bone marrow aspiration and biopsy:** The removal of bone marrow, blood, and a small piece of bone by inserting a hollow needle into the hipbone or breastbone. A pathologist views the bone marrow, blood, and bone under a microscope to look for abnormal cells.

Stages of Chronic Lymphocytic Leukemia

After chronic lymphocytic leukemia has been diagnosed, tests are done to find out how far the cancer has spread in the blood and bone marrow. Staging is the process used to find out how far the cancer has spread. It is important to know the stage of the disease in order to plan the best treatment. The following tests may be used in the staging process:

- **Bone marrow aspiration and biopsy:** The removal of bone marrow, blood, and a small piece of bone by inserting a hollow needle into the hipbone or breastbone. A pathologist views the bone marrow, blood, and bone under a microscope to look for abnormal cells.

- **Chest x-ray:** An x-ray of the organs and bones inside the chest. An x-ray is a type of energy beam that can go through the body and onto film, making a picture of areas inside the body, such as the lymph nodes.

- **MRI (magnetic resonance imaging):** A procedure that uses a magnet, radio waves, and a computer to make a series of detailed pictures of areas inside the body, such as the brain and spinal cord. This procedure is also called nuclear magnetic resonance imaging (NMRI).

- **Computed Tomography (CT) scan (also called a CAT scan):** A procedure that makes a series of detailed pictures of areas inside the body, taken from different angles. The pictures are made by a computer linked to an x-ray machine. A dye may be injected into a vein or swallowed to help the organs or tissues show up more clearly. This procedure is also called computed tomography, computerized tomography, or computerized axial tomography.

- **Blood chemistry studies:** A procedure in which a blood sample is checked to measure the amounts of certain substances released into the blood by organs and tissues in the body. An unusual (higher or lower than normal) amount of a substance can be a sign of disease in the organ or tissue that makes it.

- **Antiglobulin test:** A test in which a sample of blood is looked at under a microscope to find out if there are any antibodies on the surface of red blood cells or platelets. These antibodies may react with and destroy the red blood cells and platelets. This test is also called a Coombs test.

The following stages are used for chronic lymphocytic leukemia.

Stage 0. In stage 0 chronic lymphocytic leukemia, there are too many lymphocytes in the blood, but there are no other symptoms of leukemia. Stage 0 chronic lymphocytic leukemia is indolent (slow-growing).

Stage I. In stage I chronic lymphocytic leukemia, there are too many lymphocytes in the blood and the lymph nodes are larger than normal.

Stage II. In stage II chronic lymphocytic leukemia, there are too many lymphocytes in the blood, the liver or spleen is larger than normal, and the lymph nodes may be larger than normal.

Stage III. In stage III chronic lymphocytic leukemia, there are too many lymphocytes in the blood and there are too few red blood cells. The lymph nodes, liver, or spleen may be larger than normal.

Stage IV. In stage IV chronic lymphocytic leukemia, there are too many lymphocytes in the blood and too few platelets. The lymph nodes, liver, or spleen may be larger than normal and there may be too few red blood cells.

Refractory Chronic Lymphocytic Leukemia

Refractory chronic lymphocytic leukemia is cancer that does not get better with treatment.

Treatment Option Overview

There are different types of treatment for patients with chronic lymphocytic leukemia.

Different types of treatment are available for patients with chronic lymphocytic leukemia. Some treatments are standard (the currently used treatment), and some are being tested in clinical trials. A treatment clinical trial is a research study meant to help improve current treatments or obtain information on new treatments for patients with cancer. When clinical trials show that a new treatment is better than the standard treatment, the new treatment may become the standard treatment. Patients may want to think about taking part in a clinical trial. Some clinical trials are open only to patients who have not started treatment.

Standard Treatments

Five types of standard treatment are used.

Watchful waiting. Watchful waiting is closely monitoring a patient's condition without giving any treatment until symptoms appear or change. This is also called observation. During this time, problems caused by the disease, such as infection, are treated.

Radiation therapy. Radiation therapy is a cancer treatment that uses high-energy x-rays or other types of radiation to kill cancer cells or keep them from growing. There are two types of radiation therapy. External radiation therapy uses a machine outside the body to send radiation toward the cancer. Internal radiation therapy uses a radioactive substance sealed in needles, seeds, wires, or catheters that are placed directly into or near the cancer. The way the radiation therapy is given depends on the type and stage of the cancer being treated.

Chemotherapy. Chemotherapy is a cancer treatment that uses drugs to stop the growth of cancer cells, either by killing the cells or by stopping them from dividing. When chemotherapy is taken by mouth or injected into a vein or muscle, the drugs enter the bloodstream and can reach cancer cells throughout the body (systemic chemotherapy). When chemotherapy is placed directly into the spinal column, an organ, or a body cavity such as the abdomen, the drugs mainly affect cancer cells in those areas (regional chemotherapy). The way the chemotherapy is given depends on the type and stage of the cancer being treated.

Surgery. Splenectomy is surgery to remove the spleen.

Monoclonal antibody therapy. Monoclonal antibody therapy is a cancer treatment that uses antibodies made in the laboratory from a single type of immune system cell. These antibodies can identify substances on cancer cells or normal substances in the body that may help cancer cells grow. The antibodies attach to the substances and kill the cancer cells, block their growth, or keep them from spreading. Monoclonal antibodies are given by infusion. They may be used alone or to carry drugs, toxins, or radioactive material directly to cancer cells.

New Treatments

New types of treatment are being tested in clinical trials. One example of this is chemotherapy with stem cell transplant.

Chemotherapy with stem cell transplant. Chemotherapy with stem cell transplant is a method of giving chemotherapy and replacing blood-forming cells destroyed by the cancer treatment. Stem cells (immature blood cells) are removed from the blood or bone marrow of the patient or a donor and are frozen and stored. After the chemotherapy is completed, the stored stem cells are thawed and given back to the patient through an infusion. These reinfused stem cells grow into (and restore) the body's blood cells.

Clinical Trials

For some patients, taking part in a clinical trial may be the best treatment choice. Clinical trials are part of the cancer research process. Clinical trials are done to find out if new cancer treatments are safe and effective or better than the standard treatment.

Many of today's standard treatments for cancer are based on earlier clinical trials. Patients who take part in a clinical trial may receive the standard treatment or be among the first to receive a new treatment.

Patients who take part in clinical trials also help improve the way cancer will be treated in the future. Even when clinical trials do not lead to effective new treatments, they often answer important questions and help move research forward.

Follow-Up

Some of the tests that were done to diagnose the cancer or to find out the stage of the cancer may be repeated. Some tests will be repeated in order to see how well the treatment is working. Decisions about whether to continue, change, or stop treatment may be based on the results of these tests. This is sometimes called re-staging.

Some of the tests will continue to be done from time to time after treatment has ended. The results of these tests can show if your condition has changed or if the cancer has recurred (come back). These tests are sometimes called follow-up tests or check-ups.

Treatment Options by Stage

Stage 0 Chronic Lymphocytic Leukemia

Treatment of stage 0 chronic lymphocytic leukemia is usually watchful waiting.

Stage I, Stage II, Stage III, and Stage IV Chronic Lymphocytic Leukemia

Treatment of stage I, stage II, stage III, and stage IV chronic lymphocytic leukemia may include the following:

- Watchful waiting when there are few or no symptoms
- Monoclonal antibody therapy
- Chemotherapy with 1 or more drugs, with or without steroids or monoclonal antibody therapy
- Low- dose external radiation therapy to areas of the body where cancer is found, such as the spleen or lymph nodes
- A clinical trial of chemotherapy and biologic therapy with stem cell transplant

Treatment Options for Refractory Chronic Lymphocytic Leukemia

Treatment of refractory chronic lymphocytic leukemia may include the following:

- A clinical trial of chemotherapy with stem cell transplant
- A clinical trial of a new treatment

Section 17.3

Acute Myelogenous Leukemia

"Acute Myelogenous Leukemia," The Leukemia & Lymphoma Society; 2008. Reprinted with permission. For additional help and the most current information, contact the Leukemia and Lymphoma Society, 1311 Mamaroneck Avenue, Suite 310 White Plains, NY 10605, www.leukemia-lymphoma.org, 800-955-4572, infocenter@LLS.org. The prevalence and incidence statistics in this document were updated by Leukemia and Lymphoma Society from the National Cancer Institute's Surveillance, Epidemiology and End Results (SEER) Program, Cancer Statistics Review 1975–2006, published online by SEER, www.seer.cancer.gov, in April 2009.

Understanding Acute Myelogenous Leukemia

About 12,810 people living in the Unites States are expected to be diagnosed with acute myelogenous leukemia (AML) in 2009. The chance of getting AML increases with age. However, children and adults of any age can develop AML. About one in five children with leukemia has AML. The goal of treatment for AML is to bring about a remission or to cure the disease.

The number of patients with AML who enter remission, stay in remission for years, or are cured has increased significantly over the past thirty years.

Causes and Risk Factors

AML starts with a change to a single cell in the bone marrow. With AML, the leukemic cells are often referred to as blast cells.

Medical researchers are working to understand the cell changes that lead to AML.

Down syndrome and other uncommon genetic disorders such as Fanconi anemia and Shwachman-Diamond syndrome and others are associated with an increased risk of AML.

Some other risk factors associated with AML are:

• some types of chemotherapy;

• radiation therapy used to treat other cancers;

- tobacco smoke;

- exposure to large amounts of benzene.

Most people who have these risk factors do not get AML—and most people with AML do not have these risk factors.

You cannot catch AML from someone else. Very rarely, more cases of AML than would be expected are diagnosed within the same family. It is thought that children in these families inherit a gene that makes them more susceptible to developing AML. Research to improve the understanding of familial cancers and effective medical management of them is underway.

Signs and Symptoms

Some of the signs and symptoms for AML are common to many illnesses. Some changes that a person with AML may have are:

- tiredness or no energy;

- shortness of breath during physical activity;

- pale skin;

- swollen gums;

- slow healing of cuts;

- pinhead-size red spots under the skin;

- prolonged bleeding from minor cuts;

- mild fever;

- black-and-blue marks (bruises) with no clear cause;

- aches in bones or knees, hips, or shoulder.

The best advice for any person troubled by any of these symptoms is to see a healthcare provider.

Diagnosis

Blood and bone marrow tests are done to diagnose AML. A bone marrow aspiration and a bone marrow biopsy are two of the tests that are done. A bone marrow aspiration shows the cell type and certain abnormalities by looking at proteins on the cell's surface. It can be used for cytogenetic analysis and other tests.

Cytogenetic analysis is a lab test to examine the chromosomes of the leukemic blast cells. Some changes to chromosomes give doctors information about how to treat their AML patients.

A bone marrow biopsy shows chromosome and gene abnormalities and how much disease is in the marrow. Both tests are also done to see if treatment is destroying leukemic blast cells. The doctor uses information from these tests to decide if leukemia is present, the type of treatment the patient needs, and the best treatment for the patient.

The doctor will also consider the patient's age, the general health of the patient, and the presence of certain changes to chromosomes to determine the best treatment for the patient.

Subtypes of AML

There are different types of AML. These are called subtypes. Most patients diagnosed with AML have one of eight different subtypes, as shown in table 17.1.

Table 17.1. Subtypes of AML

Designation	Cell Subtype
M0	Myeloblastic, on special analysis
M1	Myeloblastic, without maturation
M2	Myeloblastic, with maturation
M3	Promyelocytic
M4	Myelomonocytic
M5	Monocytic
M6	Erythroleukemia
M7	Megakaryocytic

Doctors look at the AML cells in a patient's marrow or blood to identify the patient's subtype of AML. Treatment for AML may vary by subtype. For example, acute promyelocytic leukemia (APL) and acute monocytic leukemia are subtypes of AML that need different treatment than other subtypes of AML.

Treatment

Patients with AML need to start chemotherapy right away. It is important to get medical care in a center where doctors are experienced in treating AML patients.

There are two parts of AML treatment, called induction therapy and consolidation therapy. The aim of induction therapy is to kill as many AML cells as possible and get blood cell counts back to normal over time. When the aim of induction therapy is achieved it is called a remission. A patient in remission feels better over time and leukemia cells can't be seen in his or her blood or marrow.

Induction therapy is done in the hospital. Patients are often in the hospital for three to four weeks. Some patients may need to be in the hospital longer.

Many different drugs are used to kill leukemic cells. Each drug type works in a different way to kill the cells. Combining drug types can strengthen the effects of the drugs. New drug combinations are being studied. Two or more chemotherapies are usually used together to treat AML. Some drugs are given by mouth. Most chemotherapies are given through a catheter placed into a vein, usually in the patient's upper chest.

The first round of chemotherapy usually does not get rid of all the AML cells. Most patients will need more treatment. Usually the same drugs are used for more rounds of treatment to complete induction therapy.

More treatment is usually needed even after a patient with AML is in remission. This second part of treatment is called consolidation therapy. It is needed because some AML cells remain that are not found by common blood or marrow tests. Consolidation therapy is also done in the hospital. As with induction therapy, patients may be in the hospital for three to four weeks, or sometimes longer. Consolidation therapy may include chemotherapy with or without an allogeneic stem cell transplant or autologous stem cell transplant.

Follow-up visits: Patients who are in remission still need to see the doctor regularly for exams and blood tests. Bone marrow tests may be needed too. The doctor may recommend longer waits between follow-up visits if a patient continues to be disease-free.

Refractory leukemia and relapsed leukemia: Some patients still have AML cells in their marrow after treatment. This is called refractory AML. With refractory AML, drugs that were not used to treat the patient's AML in the first part of treatment may be given. Allogeneic stem cell transplantation also may be used for certain patients.

For patients who relapse, the same or different drugs may be given, or stem cell transplantation may be used. A drug called gemtuzumab ozogamicin (Mylotarg®) is being used to treat some older patients who have relapsed AML.

Treatment in Children

About 3,509 new cases of childhood leukemia were expected to be diagnosed in 2009 in the United States (for children zero to fourteen years of age). Induction therapy for children with AML starts with two or three drugs. Stronger treatment is needed after a child with AML is in remission. This is called intensive consolidation therapy. It is given because usually some AML cells remain after induction therapy. These AML cells do not show up in standard blood or marrow tests. Consolidation therapy in children includes a number of chemotherapies.

About four out of five children with AML go into remission. About half of children with AML have no signs of disease after five years. Most of these children are considered cured.

AML treatment is less likely to bring about a remission or cure when children:

- have acute myelogenous leukemia with very high white cell counts;

- are younger than one year of age;

- have certain chromosomes in their AML cells that are not normal.

Allogeneic stem cell transplants may be used in children who are not doing well or who relapse after high-dose chemotherapy. Doctors will discuss the benefits and risks with parents and older children.

Long-term and late effects of treatment for children: Transplant and other treatment can cause long-term or late effects involving a child's growth, hormones, heart, and other parts of the body. Treatment for leukemia can also cause problems with learning skills. But special education methods can help these children learn. It is important to identify problems early. Talk to the doctor about when your child's learning skills should be assessed.

Treatment in Older Adults

At least half of patients are over sixty-five years old when their disease is diagnosed. Some healthy older patients can be treated with the same doses of chemotherapy as younger adults. Sometimes older patients have other medical problems, such as heart disease, kidney or lung disease, or diabetes. The doctor takes these other medical conditions into account to decide which drugs and dosages to use. The doctor will also consider the patient's type of AML, his or her physical ability to handle the treatment, and his or her feelings about the treatment approach.

Treating Special AML Subtypes

Acute promyelocytic leukemia treatment: Acute promyelocytic leukemia is the most curable form of AML. People with acute promyelocytic leukemia are treated with a substance that comes from vitamin A called all-trans retinoic acid (ATRA). This treatment is given along with chemotherapy. It is often successful in bringing this type of leukemia into remission. Another treatment for acute promyelocytic leukemia is arsenic trioxide (ATO). It may be given to patients whose leukemia has returned or cannot be brought under control with chemotherapy and ATRA.

Acute monocytic leukemia treatment: In one type of AML, called acute monocytic leukemia, the leukemia cells are more likely to invade the lining of the spinal canal or brain. The patient gets chemotherapy directly into the spinal canal to treat these hard-to-reach cells. A needle is placed into the spinal canal during a procedure called a spinal tap. Spinal fluid is removed and chemotherapy is injected into the spinal canal. Sometimes radiation therapy may be used to treat a large mass of leukemia cells in the spine or brain.

Allogeneic Stem Cell Transplantation

Chemotherapy used to treat AML also kills the healthy stem cells in the marrow. Allogeneic stem cell transplant is used to treat some AML patients.

There are two reasons for doing an allogeneic stem cell transplant:

- To give strong doses of chemotherapy to kill more AML cells

- To give the patient the donor immune cells to attack any AML cells that remain

When the donor cells attack the AML cells it is called graft versus leukemia or GVL. GVL is also called graft versus cancer.

Allogeneic stem cell transplant can be a high-risk procedure. For this reason, it may not be a good treatment for some AML patients. The decision to do a transplant depends on the patient's age and overall health, the chances that chemotherapy alone will cure his or her

AML, and the patient's understanding of the benefits and risks of the transplant. Doctors will discuss these with patients and parents of young children with AML.

AML patients who have an allogeneic stem cell transplant are usually between the ages of one and fifty and are in remission. In addition, the patient needs to have a matched donor.

Doctors are studying a type of stem cell transplant called a nonmyeloablative stem cell transplant. This treatment may be helpful for older patients.

Autologous Stem Cell Transplantation

Patients who do not have a matched donor for a stem cell transplant may be given very high doses of chemotherapy and an autologous stem cell transplant instead. The goal of an autologous stem cell transplant is to restore the body's ability to make normal blood cells after high-dose chemotherapy.

Disease and Treatment Side Effects

Not all patients have side effects.

However, chemotherapy and radiation therapy often affect a person's blood counts. The number of red cells may decrease (called anemia). Transfusions of red cells (blood cells that are donated and given to the patient) are usually needed to increase the red cell count. Patients usually have a drop in the number of platelets. If a patient's platelet count is very low he or she usually needs a platelet transfusion to prevent or treat bleeding. A long-lasting and big drop in white cells may lead to an infection. Such infections are usually treated with antibiotics, until the normal white cell count goes up and the infection clears up. Patients with an infection may also have coughing, sore throat, pain when urinating, or frequent loose bowel movements. Or, fever or chills may be the only signs of infection.

To lower the risk of bacterial, viral, and fungal infections, patients, visitors, and medical staff need to wash their hands well. Also, the patient's central line must be kept clean and patients should follow all medical advice for taking care of their teeth and gums.

Complete blood counts are usually done throughout treatment. If the red cell counts or platelet counts are too low transfusions may be necessary. Growth factors are sometimes given to increase the number of white cells if they are too low. G-CSF (Neupogen® or Neulasta®) and GM-CSF (Leukine®) are drugs that increase white cell counts. Your doctor may talk about neutropenia (a lower than normal neutrophil

209

count) and absolute neutrophil count or ANC, which is the number of white cells that are neutrophils.

Other side effects of treatment include: mouth sores, rashes, dry mouth, diarrhea, nausea, constipation, hair loss, vomiting, or changes in the way certain foods taste. Drugs or other therapies may be helpful to prevent or treat nausea, vomiting, and other side effects.

Chemotherapy may cause the amount of uric acid to increase in the blood of some AML patients. (Some patients also have a buildup of uric acid from the disease itself.) Uric acid is a chemical made in the body. A high level of uric acid can cause kidney stones. Patients with high uric acid levels may be given a drug called allopurinol (Aloprim®, Zyloprim®) by mouth. Another drug used to treat high uric acid levels is called rasburicase (Elitek®), which is given by vein.

Clinical Trials

Clinical trials are used to study new drugs, new treatments, or new uses for approved drugs or treatments. Research has contributed to the growing number of patients with AML who enter remission, stay in remission for years, or are cured. One of the challenges for future research is to develop treatments that help more patients.

Scientists are trying to create new drugs or find them from natural sources. They are also studying new combinations of drugs already being used. Scientists are studying ways to boost the body's natural defenses, called immunotherapy. The goal is to kill or prevent the growth of AML cells.

Scientists are studying a type of stem cell transplant, called a non-myeloablative stem cell transplant.

Scientists are studying cytokines, natural substances made by cells. Cytokines can also be made in the lab. They can be used to help restore normal blood cell counts during treatment or boost the immune system to better attack the leukemia cells.

Leukemia-specific therapy, based on a patient's specific subtype of leukemia, such as the type of chromosome changes, is being studied.

The AML cells of some patients are not as easily killed by drugs as those of other patients. This is called drug resistance. Scientists are trying to understand why some AML cells are resistant to the effects of chemotherapy. This will help them develop better treatments.

Scientists are studying the exact genetic changes that cause a normal cell to become an AML cell. This research is leading to the development of new treatments. These treatments could block the effects of cancer-causing genes (called oncogenes).

Gemtuzumab ozogamicin (Mylotarg®) is approved by the U.S. Food and Drug Administration (FDA) to treat CD33-positive AML patients in first relapse who are sixty years of age or older and who are not considered candidates for cytotoxic chemotherapy. This drug is being studied in combination with other drugs to treat relapsed AML and is also being studied in combination with all-trans retinoic acid (ATRA) and arsenic trioxide (ATO) to treat acute promyelocytic leukemia.

Some other drugs under study for future use in AML treatment include:

- Farnesyl transferase inhibitors, for example tipifarnib (Zarnestra®) or lonafarnib;

- FLT-3 inhibitors;

- Proteosome inhibitors, such as bortezomib (Velcade®);

- Multi-drug resistance modulators, such as cyclosporine A or PSC-833;

- Antisense molecules (Genasense®, GTI-2040);

- Hypomethylating agents, such as decitabine (Dacogen®);

- Histone deacetylase inhibitors, such as depsipeptide.

Talk to the Doctor

It may be helpful to write down questions to ask your doctor. Then you can write down your doctor's answers and review them later. You may want to bring a family member or friend with you to the doctor. This person can listen, take notes, and offer support. Some patients record information and listen to it at home.

Section 17.4

Chronic Myelogenous Leukemia

Excerpted from "Chronic Myelogenous Leukemia Treatment (PDQ®), Patient Version," PDQ® Cancer Information Summary, National Cancer Institute, Bethesda, MD. Updated August 2008. Available at: http://cancer.gov. Accessed April 22, 2009.

Chronic myelogenous leukemia is a disease in which the bone marrow makes too many white blood cells.

Chronic myelogenous leukemia (also called CML or chronic granulocytic leukemia) is a slowly progressing blood and bone marrow disease that usually occurs during or after middle age, and rarely occurs in children.

Normally, the bone marrow makes blood stem cells (immature cells) that develop into mature blood cells over time. A blood stem cell may become a myeloid stem cell or a lymphoid stem cell. The lymphoid stem cell develops into a white blood cell. The myeloid stem cell develops into one of three types of mature blood cells:

- Red blood cells that carry oxygen and other materials to all tissues of the body

- Platelets that help prevent bleeding by causing blood clots to form

- Granulocytes (white blood cells) that fight infection and disease

In CML, too many blood stem cells develop into a type of white blood cell called granulocytes. These granulocytes are abnormal and do not become healthy white blood cells. They may also be called leukemic cells. The leukemic cells can build up in the blood and bone marrow so there is less room for healthy white blood cells, red blood cells, and platelets. When this happens, infection, anemia, or easy bleeding may occur.

These and other symptoms may be caused by CML. Other conditions may cause the same symptoms. A doctor should be consulted if any of the following problems occur:

- Feeling very tired

- Weight loss for no known reason

- Night sweats

- Fever
- Pain or a feeling of fullness below the ribs on the left side

Sometimes CML does not cause any symptoms at all.

Most people with CML have a gene mutation (change) called the Philadelphia chromosome. Every cell in the body contains deoxyribonucleic acid (DNA), genetic material that determines how the cell looks and acts. DNA is contained inside chromosomes. In CML, part of the DNA from one chromosome moves to another chromosome. This change is called the " Philadelphia chromosome." It results in the bone marrow making an enzyme, called tyrosine kinase, that causes too many stem cells to develop into white blood cells (granulocytes or blasts).

The Philadelphia chromosome is not passed from parent to child.

Tests that examine the blood and bone marrow are used to detect (find) and diagnose chronic myelogenous leukemia.

The following tests and procedures may be used:

- **Physical exam and history:** An exam of the body to check general signs of health, including checking for signs of disease such as an enlarged spleen. A history of the patient's health habits and past illnesses and treatments will also be taken.

- **Complete blood count (CBC):** A procedure in which a sample of blood is drawn and checked for the following:

  - The number of red blood cells, white blood cells, and platelets

  - The amount of hemoglobin (the protein that carries oxygen) in the red blood cells

  - The portion of the sample made up of red blood cells

- **Blood chemistry studies:** A procedure in which a blood sample is checked to measure the amounts of certain substances released into the blood by organs and tissues in the body. An unusual (higher or lower than normal) amount of a substance can be a sign of disease in the organ or tissue that makes it.

- **Cytogenetic analysis:** A test in which cells in a sample of blood or bone marrow are viewed under a microscope to look for certain changes in the chromosomes, such as the Philadelphia chromosome.

- **Bone marrow aspiration and biopsy:** The removal of bone marrow, blood, and a small piece of bone by inserting a needle into the hipbone or breastbone. A pathologist views the bone marrow, blood, and bone under a microscope to look for abnormal cells.

Stages of Chronic Myelogenous Leukemia

After chronic myelogenous leukemia has been diagnosed, tests are done to find out if the cancer has spread.

Staging is the process used to find out how far the cancer has spread. There is no standard staging system for chronic myelogenous leukemia (CML). Instead, the disease is classified by phase: chronic phase, accelerated phase, or blastic phase. It is important to know the phase in order to plan treatment. The following tests and procedures may be used to find out the phase:

- Cytogenetic analysis

- Bone marrow aspiration and biopsy

Chronic myelogenous leukemia has three phases.

As the amount of blast cells increases in the blood and bone marrow, there is less room for healthy white blood cells, red blood cells, and platelets. This may result in infections, anemia, and easy bleeding, as well as bone pain and pain or a feeling of fullness below the ribs on the left side. The number of blast cells in the blood and bone marrow and the severity of symptoms determine the phase of the disease.

Chronic Phase

In chronic phase CML, fewer than 10 percent of the cells in the blood and bone marrow are blast cells.

Accelerated Phase

In accelerated phase CML, 10 to 19 percent of the cells in the blood and bone marrow are blast cells.

Blastic Phase

In blastic phase CML, 20 percent or more of the cells in the blood or bone marrow are blast cells. When tiredness, fever, and an enlarged spleen occur during the blastic phase, it is called blast crisis.

Relapsed Chronic Myelogenous Leukemia

In relapsed CML, the number of blast cells increases after a remission.

Treatment Option Overview

Different types of treatment are available for patients with chronic my-elogenous leukemia (CML). Some treatments are standard (the currently used treatment), and some are being tested in clinical trials. A treatment clinical trial is a research study meant to help improve current treatments or obtain information on new treatments for patients with cancer. When clinical trials show that a new treatment is better than the standard treatment, the new treatment may become the standard treatment. Patients may want to think about taking part in a clinical trial. Some clinical trials are open only to patients who have not started treatment.

Six types of standard treatment are used.

Tyrosine kinase inhibitor therapy. A drug called imatinib mesy-late is used as initial treatment for certain types of chronic myelogenous leukemia in newly diagnosed patients. It blocks an enzyme called tyrosine kinase that causes stem cells to develop into more white blood cells (granulocytes or blasts) than the body needs. Another tyrosine kinase inhibitor called dasatinib is used to treat patients with certain types of CML that have progressed, and is being studied as an initial treatment.

Chemotherapy. Chemotherapy is a cancer treatment that uses drugs to stop the growth of cancer cells, either by killing the cells or by stopping them from dividing. When chemotherapy is taken by mouth or injected into a vein or muscle, the drugs enter the bloodstream and can reach cancer cells throughout the body (systemic chemotherapy). When chemotherapy is placed directly into the spinal column, an organ, or a body cavity such as the abdomen, the drugs mainly affect cancer cells in those areas (regional chemotherapy). The way the chemotherapy is given depends on the type and stage of the cancer being treated.

Biologic therapy. Biologic therapy is a treatment that uses the patient's immune system to fight cancer. Substances made by the body or made in a laboratory are used to boost, direct, or restore the body's natural defenses against cancer. This type of cancer treatment is also called biotherapy or immunotherapy.

High-dose chemotherapy with stem cell transplant. High-dose chemotherapy with stem cell transplant is a method of giving high doses of chemotherapy and replacing blood-forming cells destroyed by the cancer treatment. Stem cells (immature blood cells) are removed from the blood or bone marrow of the patient or a donor and are frozen and stored. After the chemotherapy is completed, the stored stem cells are thawed and given back to the patient through an infusion. These reinfused stem cells grow into (and restore) the body's blood cells.

Donor lymphocyte infusion (DLI). Donor lymphocyte infusion (DLI) is a cancer treatment that may be used after stem cell transplant. Lymphocytes (a type of white blood cell) from the stem cell transplant donor are removed from the donor's blood and may be frozen for storage. The donor's lymphocytes are thawed if they were frozen and then given to the patient through one or more infusions. The lymphocytes see the patient's cancer cells as not belonging to the body and attack them.

Surgery. Splenectomy is surgery to remove the spleen.

For some patients, taking part in a clinical trial may be the best treatment choice. Clinical trials are part of the cancer research process. Clinical trials are done to find out if new cancer treatments are safe and effective or better than the standard treatment.

Many of today's standard treatments for cancer are based on earlier clinical trials. Patients who take part in a clinical trial may receive the standard treatment or be among the first to receive a new treatment.

Patients who take part in clinical trials also help improve the way cancer will be treated in the future. Even when clinical trials do not lead to effective new treatments, they often answer important questions and help move research forward.

Follow-Up

Some of the tests that were done to diagnose the cancer or to find out the stage of the cancer may be repeated. Some tests will be repeated in order to see how well the treatment is working. Decisions about whether to continue, change, or stop treatment may be based on the results of these tests. This is sometimes called re-staging.

Some of the tests will continue to be done from time to time after treatment has ended. The results of these tests can show if your condition has changed or if the cancer has recurred (come back). These tests are sometimes called follow-up tests or check-ups.

Treatment Options for Chronic Myelogenous Leukemia
Chronic Phase Chronic Myelogenous Leukemia

Treatment of chronic phase chronic myelogenous leukemia may include the following:

- Drug therapy with a tyrosine kinase inhibitor
- High-dose chemotherapy with donor stem cell transplant
- Biologic therapy (interferon) with or without chemotherapy
- Chemotherapy
- Splenectomy
- A clinical trial of lower-dose chemotherapy with donor stem cell transplant
- A clinical trial of a new treatment

Accelerated Phase Chronic Myelogenous Leukemia

Treatment of accelerated phase chronic myelogenous leukemia may include the following:

- Stem cell transplant
- Drug therapy with a tyrosine kinase inhibitor
- Biologic therapy (interferon) with or without chemotherapy
- High-dose chemotherapy
- Chemotherapy
- Transfusion therapy to replace red blood cells, platelets, and sometimes white blood cells, to relieve symptoms and improve quality of life
- A clinical trial of a new treatment

Blastic Phase Chronic Myelogenous Leukemia

Treatment of blastic phase chronic myelogenous leukemia may include the following:

- Drug therapy with a tyrosine kinase inhibitor
- Chemotherapy using one or more drugs
- High-dose chemotherapy
- Donor stem cell transplant
- Chemotherapy as palliative therapy to relieve symptoms and improve quality of life
- A clinical trial of a new treatment

Relapsed Chronic Myelogenous Leukemia

Treatment of relapsed chronic myelogenous leukemia may include the following:

- Drug therapy with a tyrosine kinase inhibitor
- Donor stem cell transplant
- Donor lymphocyte infusion
- Biologic therapy (interferon)
- A clinical trial of biologic therapy, combination chemotherapy, or other drug therapy

Section 17.5

Hairy Cell Leukemia

Excerpted from "Hairy Cell Leukemia Treatment (PDQ®), Patient Version," PDQ® Cancer Information Summery, National Cancer Institute, Bethesda, MD. Updated August 2008. Available at http://cancer.gov. Accessed April 22, 2009.

Hairy cell leukemia is a type of cancer in which the bone marrow makes too many lymphocytes (a type of white blood cell).

Hairy cell leukemia is a cancer of the blood and bone marrow. This rare type of leukemia gets worse slowly or does not get worse at all. The disease is called hairy cell leukemia because the leukemia cells look "hairy" when viewed under a microscope.

Normally, the bone marrow makes blood stem cells (immature cells) that develop into mature blood cells over time. A blood stem cell may become a myeloid stem cell or a lymphoid stem cell.

The myeloid stem cell develops into one of three types of mature blood cells:

- Red blood cells that carry oxygen and other materials to all tissues of the body
- White blood cells that fight infection and disease
- Platelets that help prevent bleeding by causing blood clots to form

The lymphoid stem cell develops into a lymphoblast cell and then into one of three types of lymphocytes (white blood cells):

- B lymphocytes that make antibodies to help fight infection

- T lymphocytes that help B lymphocytes make antibodies to help fight infection

- Natural killer cells that attack cancer cells and viruses

In hairy cell leukemia, too many blood stem cells develop into lymphocytes. These lymphocytes are abnormal and do not become healthy white blood cells. They may also be called leukemic cells. The leukemic cells can build up in the blood and bone marrow so there is less room for healthy white blood cells, red blood cells, and platelets. This may cause infection, anemia, and easy bleeding. Some of the leukemia cells may collect in the spleen and cause it to swell.

Risk Factors

Gender and age may affect the risk of developing hairy cell leukemia. Anything that increases your chance of getting a disease is called a risk factor. Having a risk factor does not mean that you will get cancer; not having risk factors doesn't mean that you will not get cancer. People who think they may be at risk should discuss this with their doctor. The cause of hairy cell leukemia is unknown. It occurs more often in older men.

Symptoms

Possible signs of hairy cell leukemia include tiredness, infections, and pain below the ribs. These and other symptoms may be caused by hairy cell leukemia. Other conditions may cause the same symptoms. A doctor should be consulted if any of the following problems occur:

- Weakness or feeling tired

- Fever or frequent infections

- Easy bruising or bleeding

- Shortness of breath

- Weight loss for no known reason

- Pain or a feeling of fullness below the ribs

- Painless lumps in the neck, underarm, stomach, or groin

219

Diagnosis

Tests that examine the blood and bone marrow are used to detect (find) and diagnose hairy cell leukemia.

The following tests and procedures may be used:

- **Physical exam and history:** An exam of the body to check general signs of health, including checking for signs of disease, such as a swollen spleen, lumps, or anything else that seems unusual. A history of the patient's health habits and past illnesses and treatments will also be taken.

- **Complete blood count (CBC):** A procedure in which a sample of blood is drawn and checked for the following:

  - The number of red blood cells, white blood cells, and platelets

  - The amount of hemoglobin (the protein that carries oxygen) in the red blood cells

  - The portion of the sample made up of red blood cells

- **Peripheral blood smear:** A procedure in which a sample of blood is checked for cells that look "hairy," the number and kinds of white blood cells, the number of platelets, and changes in the shape of blood cells.

- **Bone marrow aspiration and biopsy:** The removal of bone marrow, blood, and a small piece of bone by inserting a hollow needle into the hipbone or breastbone. A pathologist views the bone marrow, blood, and bone under a microscope to look for signs of cancer.

- **Immunophenotyping:** A test in which the cells in a sample of blood or bone marrow are looked at under a microscope to check the pattern of proteins that are on the surface of the cells. Hairy cells have a certain pattern.

- **Computed tomography (CT) scan (also called a CAT scan):** A procedure that makes a series of detailed pictures of areas inside the body, taken from different angles. The pictures are made by a computer linked to an x-ray machine. A dye may be injected into a vein or swallowed to help the organs or tissues show up more clearly. This procedure is also called computed tomography, computerized tomography, or computerized axial tomography. A CT scan of the abdomen may be done to check for swollen lymph nodes or a swollen spleen.

Stages of Hairy Cell Leukemia

There is no standard staging system for hairy cell leukemia. Staging is the process used to find out how far the cancer has spread. Groups are used in place of stages for hairy cell leukemia. The disease is grouped as untreated, progressive, or refractory.

Untreated Hairy Cell Leukemia

The hairy cell leukemia is newly diagnosed and has not been treated except to relieve symptoms such as weight loss and infections. In untreated hairy cell leukemia, some or all of the following conditions occur:

- Hairy (leukemia) cells are found in the blood and bone marrow.
- The number of red blood cells, white blood cells, or platelets may be lower than normal.
- The spleen may be larger than normal.

Progressive Hairy Cell Leukemia

In progressive hairy cell leukemia, the leukemia has been treated with either chemotherapy or splenectomy (removal of the spleen) and one or both of the following conditions occur:

- There is an increase in the number of hairy cells in the blood or bone marrow.
- The number of red blood cells, white blood cells, or platelets in the blood is lower than normal.

Relapsed or Refractory Hairy Cell Leukemia

Relapsed hairy cell leukemia has come back after treatment. Refractory hairy cell leukemia has not responded to treatment.

Treatment Option Overview

Different types of treatment are available for patients with hairy cell leukemia. Some treatments are standard (the currently used treatment), and some are being tested in clinical trials. A treatment clinical trial is a research study meant to help improve current treatments or obtain information on new treatments for patients with cancer. When clinical trials show that a new treatment is better than the standard treatment, the new treatment may become the standard treatment. Patients may want to think about taking part in a clinical trial. Some clinical trials are open only to patients who have not started treatment.

Four types of standard treatment are used.

Watchful waiting. Watchful waiting is closely monitoring a patient's condition, without giving any treatment until symptoms appear or change.

Chemotherapy. Chemotherapy is a cancer treatment that uses drugs to stop the growth of cancer cells, either by killing the cells or by stopping them from dividing. When chemotherapy is taken by mouth or injected into a vein or muscle, the drugs enter the bloodstream and can reach cancer cells throughout the body (systemic chemotherapy). When chemotherapy is placed directly into the spinal column, an organ, or a body cavity such as the abdomen, the drugs mainly affect cancer cells in those areas (regional chemotherapy). The way the chemotherapy is given depends on the type and stage of the cancer being treated. Cladribine and pentostatin are anticancer drugs commonly used to treat hairy cell leukemia. These drugs may increase the risk of developing other types of cancer, especially Hodgkin lymphoma and non-Hodgkin lymphoma. Long-term follow up for second cancers is very important.

Biologic therapy. Biologic therapy is a cancer treatment that uses the patient's immune system to fight cancer. Substances made by the body or made in a laboratory are used to boost, direct, or restore the body's natural defenses against cancer. This type of cancer treatment is also called biotherapy or immunotherapy. Interferon-alpha is a biologic agent commonly used to treat hairy cell leukemia. For relapsed or refractory patients, a biologic agent called rituximab may be used.

Surgery. Splenectomy is a surgical procedure to remove the spleen.

New Treatments

Stem cell transplant. Stem cell transplant is a method of giving chemotherapy and replacing blood-forming cells destroyed by the cancer or cancer treatment. Stem cells (immature blood cells) are removed from the blood or bone marrow of a brother or sister and are frozen and stored. After the chemotherapy is completed, the stored stem cells are thawed and given back to the patient through an infusion. These reinfused stem cells grow into (and restore) the body's blood cells.

Clinical Trials

For some patients, taking part in a clinical trial may be the best treatment choice. Clinical trials are part of the cancer research process. Clinical trials are done to find out if new cancer treatments are safe and effective or better than the standard treatment.

Many of today's standard treatments for cancer are based on earlier clinical trials. Patients who take part in a clinical trial may receive the standard treatment or be among the first to receive a new treatment.

Patients who take part in clinical trials also help improve the way cancer will be treated in the future. Even when clinical trials do not lead to effective new treatments, they often answer important questions and help move research forward.

Follow-Up

Some of the tests that were done to diagnose the cancer or to find out the stage of the cancer may be repeated. Some tests will be repeated in order to see how well the treatment is working. Decisions about whether to continue, change, or stop treatment may be based on the results of these tests. This is sometimes called re-staging.

Some of the tests will continue to be done from time to time after treatment has ended. The results of these tests can show if your condition has changed or if the cancer has recurred (come back). These tests are sometimes called follow-up tests or check-ups.

Treatment Options for Hairy Cell Leukemia

Untreated Hairy Cell Leukemia

If the patient's blood cell counts are not too low and there are no symptoms, treatment may not be needed and the patient is carefully watched for changes in his or her condition. If blood cell counts become too low or symptoms appear, initial treatment may include the following:

- Chemotherapy
- Splenectomy

Progressive Hairy Cell Leukemia

Treatment for progressive hairy cell leukemia may include the following:

- Chemotherapy
- Biologic therapy
- Splenectomy

Relapsed or Refractory Hairy Cell Leukemia

Treatment of relapsed or refractory hairy cell leukemia may include the following:

- Chemotherapy
- Biologic therapy
- A clinical trial of stem cell transplant
- A clinical trial of high-dose chemotherapy
- A clinical trial of biologic therapy

Chapter 18

Lymphoma

Chapter Contents

Section 18.1

Hodgkin Lymphoma

"Hodgkin Lymphoma," The Leukemia & Lymphoma Society, 2008. Reprinted with permission. For additional help and the most current information, contact The Leukemia & Lymphoma Society, 1311 Mamaroneck Avenue, Suite 310 White Plains, NY 10605, www.leukemia-lymphoma.org, 800-955-4572, infocenter@LLS.org.Understanding Lymphoma

Lymphoma is the name for a group of blood cancers. Hodgkin lymphoma and non-Hodgkin lymphoma (NHL) are the two main types of lymphoma. About 11.1 percent of people with lymphoma have Hodgkin lymphoma. The rest have one of many different kinds of NHL.

Lymphoma starts in the lymphatic system. The lymphatic system is part of the body's immune system. The marrow and lymphocytes are part of the immune system. Some other parts of the immune system are the lymph nodes, the lymphatic vessels, and the spleen.

Hodgkin Lymphoma

Hodgkin lymphoma is one of the most curable forms of cancer. It is most likely to be diagnosed in people in their twenties or thirties. It is less common in middle age and becomes more common again after age sixty.

Hodgkin lymphoma is distinguished from other types of lymphoma by the presence of the Reed-Sternberg cell (named for the scientists who first identified it). Although they are found within the lymph nodes, Reed-Sternberg cells may not be lymphocytes. Other related cells associated with the disease are called "Hodgkin cells."

Causes and Risk Factors

Lymphoma starts with a change to a lymphocyte. The change to the lymphocyte causes it to become a lymphoma cell. The lymphoma cells pile up and form masses that gather in the lymph nodes or other parts of the lymphatic system. Researchers are working to better understand the causes of the different types of lymphoma.

Most cases of Hodgkin lymphoma occur in people who do not have identifiable risk factors, and most people with these risk factors do not get the disease. Many environmental and occupational studies have been conducted, without showing clear links between exposures and the disease. Some possible risk factors are:

- Epstein-Barr virus has been associated with nearly half of cases of Hodgkin lymphoma. This virus has not been conclusively established as a cause.

- People infected with human T-cell lymphocytotropic virus (HTLV) or human immunodeficiency virus (HIV) have an increased probability of developing Hodgkin lymphoma.

- There are occasional cases of familial clustering, as with some other cancers. There is an increase in incidence of Hodgkin lymphoma in siblings of patients with the disease.

Signs and Symptoms

The most common sign of Hodgkin lymphoma is one or more enlarged lymph nodes. The enlarged lymph node is painless and may be in the neck, upper chest, armpit, abdomen, or groin.

Signs and symptoms of Hodgkin lymphoma may also include:

- fever;

- night sweats;

- tiredness;

- weight loss;

- itchy skin.

Diagnosis and Staging

Doctors do a test called a lymph node biopsy to diagnose Hodgkin lymphoma. To do the biopsy, a surgeon removes an enlarged lymph node. The lymph node is examined under a microscope by a pathologist.

The diagnosis of Hodgkin lymphoma can be difficult and often requires an experienced pathologist to analyze the biopsy slides. In some cases, the use of immunophenotyping can help distinguish Hodgkin lymphoma from the other types of lymphoma or other lymph node reactions that are not cancerous. The pathologist also looks for the presence of Reed-Sternberg cells and other related cells called Hodgkin cells.

The patient's doctor will do other tests to see how widespread the disease is. This is called "staging." The tests are:

- **Blood tests:** To look for low red cells, white cells, or platelets.

- **Bone marrow aspiration and bone marrow biopsy:** To look for Hodgkin lymphoma cells in the marrow.

- **Imaging tests:** To create pictures of the chest and abdomen and see if there are lymphoma masses in the deep lymph nodes, liver, spleen, or lungs.
  Examples of imaging tests are:

- CT scans (computed tomography);

- MRI (magnetic resonance imaging);

- PET scans (positron emission tomography).

Stage 1: Hodgkin lymphoma is in just one lymph node region.

Stage 2: Hodgkin lymphoma is in two or three lymph node regions that are near each other. For example, the lymphoma is in the upper body regions (neck, chest, and armpit) or the lymphoma is in the lower body regions (abdomen and groin).

Stage 3: Hodgkin lymphoma is in several lymph node regions such as the neck, chest, and abdomen.

Stage 4: Hodgkin lymphoma is widespread in the lymph nodes and other parts of the body, such as the lungs, liver, or bone.

Patients are also divided into either "A" or "B" categories. "A" patients don't have fever, a lot of sweating or weight loss. "B" patients have fever, a lot of sweating, or weight loss.

Treatment

Hodgkin lymphoma can be cured in about 86 percent of all patients. The cure rate in younger patients is about 90 percent.

A patient with Hodgkin lymphoma is usually treated by a doctor called a hematologist or oncologist. It is important to get treatment in a center where doctors are experienced in the care of patients with Hodgkin lymphoma. Each patient should talk to the doctor about his or her disease and treatment plan. Some patients may want to get a second medical opinion.

Some factors that may affect the type of treatment for a patient are:

- enlarged chest nodes or abdominal lymph nodes;

- enlarged spleen;

- many affected groups of lymph nodes;

- affected lungs, liver, bone, or other parts of the body;

- very low red cell count (anemia);

- other problems such as diabetes mellitus or heart or kidney disease.

Treatment includes chemotherapy or chemotherapy and involved field radiation therapy, which targets the Hodgkin lymphoma masses. Other parts of the body are protected to prevent harm. Chemotherapy is used with radiation to kill nearby lymphoma cells.

Four or more drugs may be used together. Drugs may be injected, given through a catheter, or taken by mouth.

Examples of drugs used to treat Hodgkin lymphoma:

- Bleomycin (Blenoxane®)

- Cyclophosphamide (Cytoxan®)

- Dacarbazine (DTIC-Dome®)

- Doxorubicin (Adriamycin®)

- Lomustine (CeeNU®)

- Prednisone

- Procarbazine (Matulane®)

- Vinblastine (Velban®)

- Vincristine (Oncovin®)

Treatment may include at least four drugs, for example, ABVD— Adriamycin® (doxorubicin), bleomycin, vinblastine, and dacarbazine.

Chemotherapy may be the only treatment used for a patient if the Hodgkin lymphoma is widespread and the patient has fever, night sweats, or weight loss. Chemotherapy is given in "cycles," usually several weeks apart. A number of cycles are needed. The treatment is outpatient for most patients and may last from six to ten months. Some patients may have to be in the hospital for a short time (if the patient develops a fever or other signs of infection). Some patients who need antibiotics may stay in the hospital until the infection is gone.

High doses of chemotherapy may also kill normal blood-forming cells in the marrow. Chemotherapy may cause red cells, white cells, or platelets to drop to very low counts in the blood. A red blood cell transfusion or drugs called "blood cell growth factors" may be needed until the effect of chemotherapy wears off.

Examples of growth factors are:

- **Darbepoetin alfa (Aranesp®) and epoetin alfa (Procrit®, EPO):** These can increase the red cell count.

- **G-CSF (Neupogen® or Neulasta®) and GM-CSF (Leukine®):** These can increase the number of neutrophils.

Hodgkin lymphoma makes it harder for the body's immune system to fight off infection. Chemotherapy and radiation can add to the problem since they also lower the immune system's ability to fight infection. Following the doctor's advice about how to prevent infection will help lower the risk of developing an infection. Also, when patients are cured, their immune responses may improve.

A patient who has high-dose chemotherapy may need an autologous stem cell transplant. High-dose chemotherapy plus autologous stem cell transplant is not a cure. However, it may give a patient a longer disease-free period than standard-dose chemotherapy without a stem cell transplant.

Relapsed Hodgkin Lymphoma

In some patients, Hodgkin lymphoma may come back (called a recurrence or relapse). The doctor will treat these patients again with chemotherapy. The treatment often gives patients very long disease-free periods.

Treatment Side Effects

There are many possible side effects of treatment for Hodgkin lymphoma. Patients react to treatment in different ways. Most side effects are mild and last only a short time. Other side effects may be serious or last a long time. When side effects occur, most:

- can be helped with treatment;

- do not last long;

- clear up when treatment ends.

The number of red cells may decrease in patients (this is called anemia) treated with chemotherapy. Blood transfusions or growth factors to increase red cells may be needed. Darbepoetin alfa (Aranesp®) and epoetin alfa (Procrit®, EPO) are drugs that might be given to increase red cell count.

A severe drop in white cells may lead to an infection. Infections caused by bacteria or fungi are treated with antibiotics. To help a patient's white cell count to improve:

- The amount of chemotherapy drugs may be reduced.

- The time between treatments may be increased.

- Growth factors to increase neutrophils may be given. A neutrophil is a type of white cell that fights infection in the body. G-CSF (Neupogen® or Neulasta®) and GM-CSF (Leukine®) are drugs that increase the number of neutrophils.

Some common side effects from treatment for Hodgkin lymphoma are:

- mouth sores;

- nausea;

- vomiting;

- diarrhea;

- constipation;

- bladder irritation;

- blood in the urine.

Other side effects from treatment may include:

- extreme tiredness;

- fever;

- cough;

- rash;

- hair loss;

- weakness;

- tingling sensation;

- lung, heart, or nerve problems.

Long-Term and Late Effects

Patients should talk with their health care providers about any possible long-term effects or late effects of treatment.

Fertility (the ability to conceive a baby) may be affected by treatment in both men and women. Patients may want to talk to their doctors about this before treatment begins. For example, men who plan to have children in the future may want to consider banking sperm before starting treatment. If a couple's ability to have children is not affected by treatment, their chance of having a healthy baby is the same as for a healthy couple.

Cancer-related fatigue is another example of a possible long-term effect.

Follow-up Care

Regular medical follow-up for Hodgkin lymphoma survivors enables doctors to assess the effects of therapy, identify recurrence of the disease, and detect long-term or late effects. Cancer survivors should see their primary care physicians for general health examinations and an oncologist for follow-up care related to cancer. Some treatment centers have follow-up clinics, which provide a comprehensive, multidisciplinary approach to monitoring and supporting cancer survivors.

Clinical Trials

Clinical trials are used to study new drugs, new treatments, or new uses for approved drugs or treatments.

There are clinical trials for:

• newly diagnosed Hodgkin lymphoma patients;

• patients who do not get a good response to treatment;

• patients who relapse after treatment;

• patients who continue treatment after remission (maintenance).

Talking to the Doctor

It may be helpful to write down questions to ask your doctor. Then you can write down your doctor's answers and review them later. You may want to bring a family member or friend with you to the doctor. This person can listen, take notes, and offer support. Some patients record information and listen to it at home.

Section 18.2

Non-Hodgkin Lymphoma

"Non-Hodgkin Lymphoma," The Leukemia & Lymphoma Society, 2008. Reprinted with permission. For additional help and the most current information, contact The Leukemia & Lymphoma Society, 1311 Mamaroneck Avenue, Suite 310 White Plains, NY 10605, www.leukemia-lymphoma.org, 800-955-4572, infocenter@LLS.org. The prevalence and incidence statistics in this document were updated by The Leukemia & Lymphoma Society from the National Cancer Institute's Surveillance, Epidemiology and End Results (SEER) Program, Cancer Statistics Review 1975–2006, published online by SEER, www.seer.cancer.gov, in April 2009.

Understanding Lymphoma

About 65,980 new cases of non-Hodgkin lymphoma (NHL) are expected to occur United States in 2009. About 74,490 people in the United States will be diagnosed with lymphoma this year. As of 2009, an estimated 601,184 people are living with lymphoma (active disease or in remission).

Hodgkin lymphoma and non-Hodgkin lymphoma (NHL) are the two main types. Most people with lymphoma have one of many different kinds of NHL. About 11.1 percent of people with lymphoma have Hodgkin lymphoma.

Lymphoma is the name for a group of blood cancers that start in the lymphatic system. The lymphatic system is part of the body's immune system—the body's defense against infection. The marrow and lymphocytes are part of the immune system. Some other parts of the immune system are the lymph nodes, the lymphatic vessels, which connect the lymph nodes and contain lymph (a liquid that carries lymphocytes), and the spleen.

Lymphoma generally starts in lymph nodes or lymphatic tissue in sites of the body such as the stomach or intestines. Lymphoma may involve the marrow and the blood in some cases.

Causes and Risk Factors

The reasons for the development of lymphoma are not certain. Lymphoma starts with a change to a type of white blood cell called

233

a lymphocyte. The change to the lymphocyte causes it to become a lymphoma cell. The lymphoma cells pile up and form lymphoma cell masses. These masses gather in the lymph nodes or other parts of the lymphatic system. For NHL, immune response plays a role in some patients.

Types of Non-Hodgkin Lymphoma

There are many types of non-Hodgkin lymphoma. Most NHLs are B-cell lymphomas (about 90 percent). The other types are T-cell and NK-cell lymphomas and immunodeficiency-associated lymphoproliferative disorders.

NHL that is:

• slow-growing is also called low-grade or indolent;

• fast-growing is also called high-grade or aggressive.

A patient should talk to his or her doctor about the type of NHL he or she has and its treatment. A patient with NHL is usually treated by a doctor called a hematologist or oncologist.

It is important to get treatment in a center where doctors are experienced in the care of the patient's type of NHL. Some patients may want to get a second medical opinion.

B-cell non-Hodgkin lymphoma: There are fourteen different types of B-cell non-Hodgkin lymphoma. Diffuse large B-cell lymphoma (a fast-growing lymphoma) and follicular lymphoma (a slow-growing lymphoma) are the two most common B-cell lymphomas. Together these two types make up more than half of all NHL.

Some patients with fast-growing lymphoma can be cured. For patients with slow-growing lymphoma, treatment may keep the disease in check for many years. This can be true even when tests show disease remains in some parts of the body.

Examples of NHL are:

• Slow-growing B-cell or T-Cell NHL:

  • small cell lymphocytic lymphoma;

  • follicular lymphoma;

  • cutaneous T-cell lymphoma.

• Fast-growing B-cell or T-cell NHL:

- diffuse large B-cell lymphoma;

- mantle cell lymphoma;

- Burkitt lymphoma;

- acute adult T-cell lymphoma;

- human immunodeficiency virus/acquired immunodeficiency syndrome (HIV/AIDS)–associated lymphoma.

Sometimes NHL is described by its location in the body. Primary central nervous system lymphoma forms in the brain and/or the spinal cord. Secondary central nervous system lymphoma starts with lymphoma in other parts of the body, which spreads to the brain and/or the spinal cord.

Signs and Symptoms

The most common sign of NHL is one or more enlarged lymph nodes in the neck, armpit, or groin. Enlarged lymph nodes also can be near the ears or elbow.

Some signs and symptoms of NHL are:

- swollen lymph nodes;

- fever;

- night sweats;

- feeling tired;

- loss of appetite;

- weight loss;

- rash.

Diagnosis and Staging

Doctors do a test called a biopsy to find out if a patient has NHL. To do the biopsy, a surgeon removes an enlarged lymph node and a pathologist studies the lymph node under a microscope to see if the patient has NHL. Sometimes the biopsy is done to examine cells from a tumor or the skin.

The doctor may do a cytogenetic analysis of the cells from the biopsy. This is a lab test that looks to see if there are changes in the chromosomes of the NHL cells.

Blood tests are done to look for low counts of red cells, white cells, or platelets. Bone marrow tests are done to look for NHL cells in the marrow.

A lab test called immunophenotyping can also be used to find out if the patient's NHL cells are B cells or T cells.

These lab tests help the doctor to diagnose the patient's type of NHL and the best way to treat the patient's disease.

Imaging tests are done to create pictures of the chest and abdomen and see if there are lymphoma masses in the deep lymph nodes, liver, spleen, or lungs.

Examples of imaging tests are:

- CT scans (computed tomography);

- MRI (magnetic resonance imaging);

- PET scans (positron emission tomography).

The next step after the doctor makes a diagnosis of NHL is to find out how widespread the disease is. This is called "staging." Blood, marrow, and imaging tests also help the doctor to see how advanced the disease is. The doctor looks for the signs below to identify the stage:

- The number of lymph nodes that are affected

- Where the affected lymph nodes are (for example, in the abdomen or the chest or both parts of the body)

- Whether any cancer cells are in other parts of the body besides the lymph nodes or lymphatic system, such as the lungs or liver

Non-Hodgkin lymphoma stages:

- **Stage 1:** The lymphoma is in just one lymph node region.

- **Stage 2:** The lymphoma is in two or three lymph node regions that are near each other. For example, the lymphoma is in the upper body regions (neck, chest, or armpit) or the lymphoma is in the lower body regions (abdomen and groin).

- **Stage 3:** The lymphoma is in several lymph node regions in the neck and chest and abdomen.

- **Stage 4:** The lymphoma is widespread in the lymph nodes and other parts of the body, such as the lungs, liver, or bone.

Treatment

The doctor has to take into account many factors to make a treatment plan for NHL:

- The type of NHL

- How fast the lymphoma is growing

- The stage of the disease

- The type of lymphocyte affected (such as T cells or B cells)

- Whether parts of the body besides the lymph nodes are involved—such as the lungs, liver, or bones

- The patient's age and overall health

- The patient's symptoms—such as fever, sweating, and weight loss

Examples of Drugs Used to Treat Non-Hodgkin Lymphoma

- Bendamustine (Treanda®)

- Bleomycin (Blenoxane®)

- Carboplatin (Paraplatin®)

- Chlorambucil (Leukeran®)

- Cyclophosphamide (Cytoxan®)

- Cytarabine (Cytosar-U®)

- Dacarbazine (DTIC-Dome®)

- Dexamethasone (Decadron®)

- Doxorubicin (Adriamycin®)

- Etoposide (Etopophos®)

- Fludarabine (Fludara®)

- Ifosfamide (Ifex®)

- Methotrexate

- Prednisone

- Rituximab (Rituxan®)

- Vincristine (Oncovin®)

Chemotherapy is given in "cycles," usually several weeks apart. Patients need a number of cycles. The treatment may last from six to ten months—it is outpatient treatment for most patients. Some patients may have to be in the hospital for a short time if the patient develops a fever or other signs of infection. Some patients who need antibiotics may stay in the hospital until the infection is gone.

Drug treatments may include up to five drugs. For example, R-CHOP is Rituxan®, cyclophosphamide, doxorubicin, Oncovin® (vincristine), prednisone, and is a common drug combination for some types of NHL.

Rituxan® is a monoclonal antibody therapy. It is used alone or with chemotherapy to treat some types and treatment stages of NHL. Rituxan® does not attack stem cells in bone marrow. This lets healthy B cells grow back after treatment. Antibody-producing B cells (plasma cells) that help fight infection are not harmed by Rituxan.

High doses of chemotherapy may also kill normal blood-forming cells in the marrow. Chemotherapy may cause red cells, white cells, or platelets to drop to very low counts in the blood. A red blood cell transfusion or drugs called "blood cell growth factors" may be needed until the effect of chemotherapy wears off.

Examples of growth factors are:

- **Darbepoetin alfa (Aranesp®) and epoetin alfa (Procrit®, EPO):** These can increase red cell count;

- **G-CSF (Neupogen® or Neulasta®) and GM-CSF (Leukine®):** These can increase the number of neutrophils.

Radiation Therapy

Radiation therapy can be used along with chemotherapy when there are very large masses of lymphoma cells in a small area of the body. Radiation also can be used when large lymph nodes are pressing on an organ (such as the bowel) and chemotherapy can't control the problem. Radiation usually isn't the only treatment for NHL because the lymphoma cells are likely to be in many areas of the body.

Stem Cell Transplantation

A stem cell transplant (sometimes called a bone marrow transplant) is used for some patients with NHL. Donated stem cells (allogeneic transplant) or the patient's own stem cells (autologous infusion) are injected into the patient's blood after chemotherapy ends.

Allogeneic stem cell transplantation: The decision to include treatment with allogeneic stem cell transplantation depends on:

- patient age;

- overall health;

- how well the donor cells and patient cells "match";

- the patient's response to drug therapy.

The decision also depends on the patient's understanding of the benefits and risks of the transplant. If the doctor thinks a patient might benefit from a transplant, he or she will talk about these factors with the patient. Allogeneic stem cell transplant is most successful in younger patients. Patients up to about sixty years of age who have a matched donor may be considered. Doctors are studying a type of stem cell transplant called a nonmyeloablative stem cell transplant or mini-transplant. It may be helpful for older patients.

Autologous stem cell infusion: Many patients with lymphoma cannot have an allogeneic stem cell transplant. Doctors are studying the use of a patient's own stem cells in these cases. This is called an autologous stem cell infusion.

High-dose chemotherapy plus autologous stem cell infusion is not a cure. It does give patients longer disease-free periods than standard-dose chemotherapy without stem cell transplant.

Treatment for Slow-Growing NHL

In most cases, a patient begins treatment for NHL right away. But when a patient has NHL that is widespread throughout the body, that is not growing or is slow-growing, the doctor may recommend watch and wait. This allows the patient to avoid side effects of therapy until treatment is needed. Patients in watch and wait need follow-up visits with the doctor. At each office visit the doctor will check for any health changes. The results of exams and lab tests over time will help the doctor advise the patient about when to start treatment and the type of treatment to have. If there are signs the lymphoma is starting to grow, then treatment will begin.

Patients may be treated with one to five drugs. The goal of treatment is a series of remissions—each lasting a number of years. This can be true even when tests show disease remains in some parts of the body. Many patients lead active, good-quality lives.

Patients with some types of slow-growing lymphoma may stay in treatment to keep their remission. This is called "maintenance" treatment.

Relapsed or Refractory Slow-Growing NHL

Slow-growing lymphoma may return after a period of remission (called a "relapse"). Patients can have more treatment and return to remission.

Some patients may not respond to treatment for newly diagnosed or relapsed lymphoma. This is called "refractory" lymphoma. Doctors can change the patient's treatment and use a different drug or drug combination.

Bendamustine (Treanda®) is an example of treatment for slow-growing B-cell NHL. This agent is a recently approved chemotherapy for slow-growing B-cell NHL that has progressed during or within six months of treatment with Rituxan or a Rituxan-containing treatment. Treanda is also approved for the treatment of patients with chronic lymphocytic leukemia.

Bexxar® and Zevalin® are two other monoclonal antibody therapies that are used to treat NHL. These agents are called "radioimmunotherapies." This means that the monoclonal antibodies carry a radioactive substance to the NHL cells, helping to reduce radiation side effects to normal cells. This treatment is approved for relapsed or refractory CD20-positive, low-grade, follicular or transformed B-cell lymphomas. Radioimmunotherapies are being studied as a possible treatment for previously untreated NHL patients.

Patients with refractory disease should talk with the doctor about the risks and benefits of participating in a clinical trial.

Treatment for Fast-Growing Lymphoma

The goal of treatment is cure of the disease.

Many drug combinations are used to treat NHL. The drug choice depends on the type of NHL and the stage of treatment.

Relapsed or Refractory Disease for Fast-Growing Lymphoma

Patients may have a return (relapse) of lymphoma months or years after treatment. Additional treatment restores remission for many patients. In these cases, there are many drug choices and approaches to treatment. If relapse occurs long after treatment, the same drugs that were used for the patient before may be effective. In other cases, new drugs or treatment approaches are used.

Treatment Side Effects

There are many possible side effects of treatment for NHL. Patients react to lymphoma treatment in different ways. Most side effects are mild and last only a short time. Other side effects may be serious or last a long time.

When side effects occur, most:

• can be helped with treatment;

• do not last long;

• clear up when treatment ends.

The number of red cells may decrease in patients (this is called anemia) treated with chemotherapy. Blood transfusions or growth factors to increase red cells may be needed. Darbepoetin alfa (Aranesp®) and epoetin alfa (Procrit®, EPO) are drugs that might be given to increase red cell count.

A severe drop in white cells may lead to an infection. Infections caused by bacteria or fungi are treated with antibiotics. To help a patient's white cell count to improve:

• The amount of chemotherapy drugs may be reduced.

• the time between treatments may be increased.

• Growth factors to increase neutrophils may be given. G-CSF (Neupogen® or Neulasta®) and GM-CSF (Leukine®) are drugs that increase the number of neutrophils.

Some common side effects from treatment for NHL are:

• mouth sores;

• nausea;

• vomiting;

• diarrhea;

• constipation;

• bladder irritation;

• blood in the urine.

Other side effects from treatment may include:

• extreme tiredness;

- fever;

- cough;

- rash;

- hair loss;

- weakness;

- tingling sensation;

- lung, heart, or nerve problems.

Fertility (the ability to conceive a baby) may be affected by lymphoma treatment in both men and women. Patients may want to talk to their doctors about this before treatment begins. For example, men who plan to have children in the future may want to consider banking sperm before starting treatment. If a couple's ability to have children is not affected by treatment, their chance of having a healthy baby is the same as for a healthy couple.

Patients should talk with their health care providers about any long-term effects of treatment. Cancer-related fatigue is one type of long-term effect.

Clinical Trials

Clinical trials are used to study new drugs, new treatments, or new uses for approved drugs or treatments.

There are clinical trials for:

- newly diagnosed NHL patients;

- patients who do not get a good response to treatment;

- patients who relapse after treatment;

- patients who continue treatment after remission (maintenance).

Gene profiling will be used more in the future to design more specific treatments for the different types of lymphoma.

Cytokines are natural substances made by cells. They can also be made in the lab. Cytokines that affect lymphoma cells may one day be used to treat this disease.

Vaccines are being tested as a possible treatment for NHL. These types of vaccines would not prevent NHL. One type of vaccine being studied might be used to help a patient stay in remission.

Stem cell transplants under study: A type of transplant called a mini-transplant is under study. A mini-transplant uses lower doses of chemotherapy in combination with an allogeneic stem cell transplant. This treatment is also called a nonmyeloablative transplant. Older and sicker patients may be able to be helped by this treatment.

Stem cells from umbilical cord blood are also used for some transplants. One cord blood unit provides enough stem cells for a child or small adult. Clinical trials are ongoing using multiple cord blood units from more than one donor to make this stem cell resource available for average-size adults.

Talk to the Doctor

It may be helpful to write down questions to ask your doctor. Then you can write down your doctor's answers and review them later. You may want to bring a family member or friend with you to the doctor. This person can listen, take notes, and offer support. Some patients record information and listen to it at home.

Section 18.3

Waldenström Macroglobulinemia

Reprinted from "Waldenström Macroglobulinemia: Questions and Answers," National Cancer Institute, September 25, 2007.

What is Waldenström macroglobulinemia?

Waldenström macroglobulinemia (WM) is a rare, indolent (slow-growing) non-Hodgkin lymphoma (cancer that begins in the cells of the immune system). WM is also called lymphoplasmacytic lymphoma. It starts in white blood cells called B lymphocytes or B cells.

B cells are an important part of the body's immune system. They form in the lymph nodes, spleen, and other lymphoid tissues, including bone marrow (the soft, spongy tissue inside bones). Some B cells become plasma cells, which make, store, and release antibodies. Antibodies help the body fight viruses, bacteria, and other foreign substances.

Lymphoplasmacytic cells are cells that are in the process of maturing from B cells to plasma cells. In WM, abnormal lymphoplasmacytic cells multiply out of control, producing large amounts of a protein called monoclonal immunoglobulin M (IgM or "macroglobulin") antibody. High levels of IgM in the blood cause hyperviscosity (thickness or gumminess), which leads to many of the symptoms of WM.

How often does Waldenström macroglobulinemia occur?

WM is a rare cancer; about 1,500 new cases occur annually in the United States. The incidence of WM is higher in males and higher in whites than in African Americans. Incidence increases sharply with age. The median age at diagnosis is sixty-three (half of the cases are diagnosed before age sixty-three, and half are diagnosed after age sixty-three).[1]

What are the possible causes of Waldenström macroglobulinemia?

The exact cause of WM is not known. However, scientists believe that genetics may play a role in WM, because the disease has been seen to run in families.[1]

What are the symptoms of Waldenström macroglobulinemia?

Some patients do not have symptoms. For those who do have symptoms, the most common ones are weakness, severe fatigue, bleeding from the nose or gums, weight loss, and bruises or other skin lesions. Severely high levels of IgM can lead to hyperviscosity syndrome, in which the blood becomes abnormally thick. Symptoms of this syndrome include visual problems (e.g., blurring or loss of vision) and neurological problems (e.g., headache, dizziness, vertigo). During a physical exam, a doctor may also find swelling of the lymph nodes, spleen, and/or liver.[2]

How is Waldenström macroglobulinemia diagnosed?

Initial diagnosis of WM is based on blood test and bone marrow biopsy results. Blood tests are used to determine the level of IgM in the blood and the presence of proteins, or tumor markers, that can indicate WM. For the biopsy, a sample of bone marrow (soft, sponge-like tissue in the center of most bones) is removed, usually from the back of the pelvis bone, through a needle for examination under a microscope. The pathologist (a doctor who identifies diseases by studying cells and tissue under a microscope) looks for certain types of lymphocytes (white blood cells) that indicate WM.[1] Flow cytometry (a method of measuring cell properties using a light-sensitive dye and laser or other type of light) is often used to look at markers on the cell surface or inside the lymphocytes.

Additional tests may be recommended to confirm the diagnosis. A computed tomography (CT or CAT) scan uses a computer linked to an x-ray machine to create pictures of areas inside the body. This test may be used to evaluate the chest, abdomen, and pelvis, particularly swelling of the lymph nodes, liver, and/or spleen.[1] A skeletal survey (x-rays of the skeleton) can help distinguish between WM and a similar plasma cell cancer, multiple myeloma.[1]

How is Waldenström macroglobulinemia treated?

At this time, there is no known cure for WM. However, several treatment options are available to prevent or control the symptoms of the disease.

Patients who do not have symptoms of WM are usually monitored without being treated; these patients often live for many years before requiring treatment.[2] Patients with symptoms are usually treated with chemotherapy. Biological therapy (treatment that stimulates the immune system to fight cancer) is also used to treat WM.[3] Promising results have been seen with biological therapy and chemotherapy in combination. An example of combination therapy uses rituximab and fludarabine.[4] Patients with high levels of IgM and hyperviscosity syndrome may undergo plasmapheresis. In this procedure, blood from the patient is removed and circulated through a machine that separates the plasma (which contains the antibody IgM) from other parts of the blood (red blood cells, white blood cells, and platelets). The red and white blood cells and platelets are returned to the patient, along with a plasma substitute.[4] Plasmapheresis is often followed by chemotherapy.

Because WM is rare, some doctors may suggest treatments that have been effective in some cases but are not considered standard treatment and/or are under study in clinical trials (research studies). Some of these treatments include the following[4]:

- **High-dose chemotherapy with autologous stem cell transplantation:** Blood-forming stem cells (cells from which all blood cells develop) are harvested (removed) and stored, then given back to the patient following high-dose chemotherapy. The harvested cells may be treated before transplantation to get rid of cancer cells. The transplanted cells travel to the bone marrow and begin to produce new blood cells.

- **Splenectomy:** Surgery to remove the spleen. This procedure has been used in WM patients who have a significantly enlarged spleen. Occasionally, WM patients who have had this procedure have experienced remissions (decrease in or disappearance of signs or symptoms of cancer) lasting for many years. The remissions are believed to be due to the removal of a major source of IgM production.

- **Thalidomide and bortezomib:** Drugs used to treat multiple myeloma, a disease similar to WM. Side effects of thalidomide include constipation, weakness, and peripheral neuropathy (a problem in nerve function that causes pain, numbness, tingling, swelling, and muscle weakness). Both agents are currently being studied in clinical trials for WM.

Are clinical trials (research studies) available? Where can people get more information about clinical trials?

Yes. The National Cancer Institute (NCI), a component of the National Institutes of Health, is sponsoring clinical trials that are designed to find new treatments and better ways to use current treatments. Before any new treatment can be recommended for general use, doctors conduct clinical trials to find out whether the treatment is safe for patients and effective against the disease. Participation in clinical trials may be a treatment option for patients with WM.

People interested in taking part in a clinical trial should talk with their doctor.

Selected References

1. Munshi NC, Anderson KC. Plasma cell neoplasms. In: DeVita VT Jr., Hellman S, Rosenberg SA, editors. *Cancer: Principles and Practice of Oncology.* Vol. 2. 7th ed. Philadelphia: Lippincott Williams and Wilkins, 2004.

2. Richardson P, Hideshima T, Anderson KC. Multiple myeloma and related disorders. In: Abeloff MD, Armitage JO, Niederhuber JE, Kastan MB, McKenna WG, editors. *Clinical Oncology.* 3rd ed. London: Churchill Livingstone, 2004.

3. Gertz MA, Anagnostopoulos A, Anderson K, et al. Treatment recommendations in Waldenstrom's macroglobulinemia: Consensus panel recommendations from the Second International Workshop on Waldenstrom's Macroglobulinemia. *Seminars in Oncology* 2003; 30(2):121–26.

4. Dimopoulos MA, Kyle RA, Anagnostopoulos A, Treon SP. Diagnosis and management of Waldenstrom's macroglobulinemia. *Journal of Clinical Oncology* 2005; 23(7):1564–77.

Chapter 19

Myeloproliferative Disorders

Chapter Contents

Section 19.1

Idiopathic Myelofibrosis

Excerpted from "Idiopathic Myelofibrosis," © 2009 University of Iowa
Hospitals and Clinics. Reprinted with permission.

Introduction

Blood cells, including red cells, white cells, and platelets, are made
in the bone marrow. The bone marrow is a soft, spongy tissue found
in the center of large bones. In healthy people, millions of new blood
cells are made each hour to carry out body functions. Red blood cells
(erythrocytes) carry oxygen from the lungs to the rest of the body.
White blood cells (leukocytes) fight infections and illness. Platelets
(thrombocytes) cause the blood to clot when there is an injury.

The body carefully controls the bone marrow to make the correct
number of each type of cell. If this process is upset and the marrow
makes too many or too few cells, a blood disorder occurs.

Blood disorders require treatment by a doctor. There may be long
periods of time when you have no symptoms, but you should be alert
to any changes that occur with your disease. If your symptoms start
or get worse, call your doctor right away. Also, feel free to call your
doctor with questions you have about your disease, the treatment you
are getting, or any other concerns you may have.

Idiopathic Myelofibrosis

Idiopathic myelofibrosis (MF) is sometimes called agnogenic myeloid
metaplasia (AMM). It is a disease that causes the gradual replacement of
the bone marrow with fibrous (scar) tissue. This leads to a lower number
of red blood cells made. The cells that are made do not work correctly.
The body knows this, and tries to make up for it by making the spleen
and liver create new blood cells. However, the cells made by this process
do not work properly, and the patient is left with too few blood cells.

Sometimes, patients with MF do not have any symptoms. Some patients will have an enlarged spleen or liver. Patients also may have

symptoms of anemia, including weakness and fatigue. A low platelet count due to MF can cause bleeding. A low number of white blood cells can cause an increased risk of infection. Frequently these blood cell counts are high rather than low, but the cells don't work correctly leading again to possible infection. Varying levels of platelets can also be seen.

Every year, there are two new cases of MF per one hundred thousand people. It usually occurs between the ages of fifty and eighty years old, although it can occur at all ages. It affects both men and women.

Diagnostic Tests

To diagnose MF, your doctor will do a blood test to find out if your bone marrow is making the correct amount of each type of cell. If the results are abnormal, you may be referred to a hematologist, a doctor who diagnoses and treats bone marrow and blood disorders. The doctor may do more tests, including a bone marrow aspiration and biopsy. For this test, the doctor will inject some local anesthetic to make the bone and skin less sensitive. Then a small amount of marrow and a small piece of bone are removed to check for defects.

Treatment Overview

The goal of treatment is to control the swelling of the spleen and to provide the body with enough red blood cells and platelets. The treatment you receive will depend on your age, health, if you have any symptoms, and the results of your blood, bone, and bone marrow tests. It may include:

- monitoring;
- blood transfusions;
- hormonal therapy;
- chemotherapy;
- surgery;
- external beam radiation therapy;
- biological therapy;
- bisphosphates;
- other medicines;
- bone marrow (stem cell) transplant;
- other treatments in clinical trials.

Monitoring. In some patients, the best plan is to watch the disease for any increase in symptoms and do regular blood counts. This may be the only treatment ever needed.

Blood transfusions. To treat symptoms of anemia, you may be given blood transfusions. Your doctor and nurse will discuss risks of blood transfusions with you. Infusions of iron and folate may also be given.

Hormonal therapy. Hormonal therapy uses medicines to increase the number of red blood cells in the body. Androgens are a type of hormonal therapy. Oxymetholone and fluoxymesterone are androgens your doctor might use. Glucocorticoids (like prednisone or Decadron®), another type of hormone, are sometimes given along with the androgens to increase the length of time red blood cells will live.

Chemotherapy. Chemotherapy treatment uses medicines to slow the making of abnormal blood cells in the body. One type of chemotherapy used to treat MF is hydroxyurea.

Surgery. The doctor may take out the spleen if it becomes so swollen that it causes pain, eating, breathing, or heart problems. This surgery is called a splenectomy.

External beam radiation therapy. If the spleen becomes swollen, your doctor may suggest external beam radiation therapy. This treatment uses high-energy x-rays to shrink the spleen.

Biological therapy. Biological therapy, or immunotherapy, uses natural substances to boost your immune system. Interferon-alpha is a medicine used to lower the white blood cell and platelet counts if they are too high.

Bisphosphates. Bisphosphates are medicines that strengthen the bones and reduce bone pain and improve blood cell counts.

Other medicines. Other medicines might be used to control symptoms of MF. Some doctors may give allopurinol to prevent a high uric acid level, which causes gout.

Bone marrow (stem cell) transplant. Some patients may benefit from a transplant from another person, called an allogenic stem cell transplant.

New Treatments. There are several treatments that are being studied in clinical trials:

- Thalidomide (Thalomid®).

- Lenalidomide (Revlimid®) is similar to thalidomide but may have fewer side effects.

- Bortezomib (Velcade®) is a proteosome inhibitor. A proteosome inhibitor attaches to the proteosome and stops it from breaking down proteins in the cell. This can cause the cell to stop growing or die. Cancer cells are more sensitive to this reaction than normal cells.

- A nonmyeloablative stem cell transplant is used in some patients with leukemia, lymphoma, or myeloma. This transplant does not require as much chemotherapy or radiation therapy as an allogenic stem cell transplant. Researchers hope it can be as effective as an allogeneic stem cell transplant with less risk. So far this type of transplant has had good outcomes in a small number of patients with MF. However, those patients need to be watched over several years to find out if the transplant's long-term results are as good as other types of stem cell transplants.

Managing Idiopathic Myelofibrosis

There are steps you can take to help prevent or reduce the symptoms of MF:

- Avoid crowds or people with colds or contagious illnesses if your leukocytes (white blood cells) are low.

- Use good hygiene, wash your hands often.

- Brush your teeth twice a day, bathe daily, and pay special attention to hard-to-clean areas such as skin folds of the rectal area.

- Avoid bruising or bumping yourself.

- Use an electric razor. Be careful when using nail trimmers, knives, etc.

- Wear hard-soled shoes, gloves, and long pants when working outside (i.e. gardening).

- Use a sponge toothbrush if you have problems with gum bleeding. Your doctor or nurse can tell you if you need to use one and where it can be found.

- Avoid aspirin or aspirin-like medicines (for example, Motrin, ibuprofen, or other anti-inflammatory drugs) unless your doctor has told you to take it. These medicines can affect blood clotting. Be sure to tell your doctor of all medicines that you take (including vitamins, herbs, and dietary supplements).

- Eat a well-balanced diet during this time. This helps your body to make new red blood cells.

- Sleep and rest between activities to save energy.

- Try light exercise, such as walking, to help circulation and improve energy levels.

- Tell your dentist and all other health care staff that you have this disease. Some procedures may increase your risk of infection and bleeding.

It is important that you watch for any change or increase in symptoms. If this occurs you should call your doctor right away. These symptoms require prompt attention:

- Swelling of spleen or liver symptoms:

  - Feeling full quickly when eating

  - Abdominal swelling that you see

  - Abdominal fullness or pain that you feel

  - weight loss

- Symptoms:

  - Weakness

  - Shortness of breath

  - Fatigue

  - Pale appearance

  - Rapid heart rate

- Infection symptoms:

  - Fever exceeding 100.4° F (38.0° C)

  - Chills

  - Night sweats

  - Cough

- Sore throat

- Rectal soreness

- Mouth or lip sores

- Pain during urination

- Sores that do not heal, have drainage, or are swollen, red, and warm to the touch

- Stiff neck

- Bleeding symptoms:

  - Easy bruising

  - Heavy or prolonged bleeding

  - Bleeding for no apparent reason

  - Severe headache or changes in vision

  - Stiff neck

  - Joint pain

  - Petechiae, or tiny areas of bright red pinpoint bleeding on the skin of the arms or legs, typically the wrists and ankles

Follow-Up Care and Prognosis

MF requires regular check-ups with your doctor. He or she will want to discuss your symptoms and do regular blood counts to see how you respond to treatment.

Idiopathic myelofibrosis is a disease that cannot be cured, but can be controlled. Some patients may only be watched and need little care. Other patients may need more active treatment. In a very small percentage of patients, MF may change into other chronic disorders or an acute leukemia.

If you have questions or concerns about your treatment and prognosis, be sure to talk with your doctor. It may be helpful to write your questions out before your visit.

Section 19.2

Myelodysplastic Syndrome

What Is Myelodysplastic Syndrome?

Myelodysplastic syndrome (MDS) describes a group of bone marrow disorders that are characterized by a defect in stem cells. The bone marrow is the tissue located in the center of long bones in the body and is responsible for producing most of the cells in the body. Stem cells are the precursor cells that divide and grow to produce each of the particular cell lineages. Hemopoietic stem cells produce cells in the blood of three classes—white blood cells (leukocytes), red blood cells (erythrocytes), and platelets (thrombocytes). In myelodysplastic syndrome (MDS) the stem cells become mutant and are no longer able to divide effectively into each of the blood cells. The normal bone marrow gradually becomes replaced with the mutant cells and there is a fall in each of the different cells within the bloodstream. Patients with this disorder therefore typically have anemia, neutropenia, and thrombocytopenia (low platelets). The latter two can predispose to infection and bleeding. The abnormal cells in the bone marrow can also pose a risk of transformation to acute myeloid leukemia (AML).

Who Gets Myelodysplastic Syndrome?

The true incidence of myelodysplastic syndrome (MDS) is difficult to estimate as it has only recently been regarded as a distinct class of disorders and controversies exist regarding its classification. However, MDS is now considered as common as acute myeloid leukemia (AML) and more cases are beginning to be recognized. MDS is most common in elderly patients as they are more prone to bone marrow damage but it can occur in any age group. The overall incidence is thought to be around 0.5–4 cases per one million people per year.

Predisposing Factors

The risk of MDS increases with age where patients usually older than fifty years get the primary form (no known exposure) of the disorder. The second type of MDS is acquired following drug treatments or radiotherapy that damage the bone marrow. This type accounts for most cases under fifty years of age and arises two to eight years following the damaging treatment. Certain genetic defects (such as Down syndrome), cigarette smoking, benzene exposure, and deoxyribonucleic acid (DNA) repair disorders can also increase your risk of this condition. Males are affected slightly more commonly than females in all age groups.

Progression

The mechanism of development of MDS is not known. The course of the disease is variable, but serious complications of bone marrow failure and transformation into acute myeloblastic leukemia commonly occur. Patients may also get infections (due to reduced neutrophils that normally fight diseases) and bleeding problems (due to reduced platelets). The therapy-related form of the disease is normally much worse and rapidly progresses to cause a fall in red blood cells, neutrophils, and platelets within the bloodstream.

Probable Outcomes

The median survival in primary (non-therapy-related) MDS varies from nine to twenty-nine months, although some individuals in good prognostic groups live for five years or more. Overall, progression to AML occurs in around 30 percent. Other causes of death include bleeding and infection due to the reduction in platelets and neutrophils respectively. Patients with therapy-related MDS have a much worse outlook and most only survive for four to eight months following the diagnosis.

How Will Myelodysplastic Syndrome Affect Me?

The signs and symptoms of this disorder are quite nonspecific and a significant proportion of patients may have no symptoms at all. These patients are sometimes diagnosed by routine blood tests for other disorders that happen to identify abnormal or reduced numbers of certain cells in the peripheral blood. If symptoms do occur, the most common are fatigue, weakness, reduced exercise tolerance, and dizziness, which is caused by the underlying anemia (reduction in oxygen carrying red blood cells in the blood). You may also notice symptoms of infection such as fever, cough, or discomfort urinating as your body is more prone to bacterial and other infections due to reduced neutrophils. Reduced platelets can cause easy bruising and bleeding from the gums or nose. If you have any of the above symptoms you should talk to your doctor. They will ask you a more detailed history about your symptoms and any possible predisposing factors to the disorder (such as certain chemotherapy drugs).

Clinical Examination

Your doctor will carefully examine you and may identify several particular signs that suggest the diagnosis of MDS. Often you will appear pale due to anemia or the doctor may detect a rapid heart rate or signs of heart failure. Signs of infection include fever, rigors, chills, sweating, and increased heart rate. Your doctor will also carefully examine your skin, gums, and nose for signs of bleeding. They may also take a urine or stool sample to determine the presence of blood. In addition, they will gently feel your stomach and may identify a big spleen, which is associated with a particular advanced type of the disease.

How Is Myelodysplastic Syndrome Diagnosed?

The most common test performed is a full blood count that shows low hemoglobin (oxygen-carrying protein), low red cell count, low white cell count, high monocytes, and low platelets. These abnormalities may occur alone or in combination but later stages of disease are characterized by deficiencies in all cell types. The cells also have abnormal shapes and appearances that help the doctor make the diagnosis. In addition, a bone marrow biopsy (sample of bone marrow) is often taken to confirm the diagnosis as this can visualize the actual abnormal precursor cells.

How Is Myelodysplastic Syndrome Treated?

Treatment of MDS largely aims to control the symptoms of the underlying cellular deficiencies and reduce progression of disease without causing severe side effects. Patients with mild disease and less than 5 percent blasts cells (abnormal precursors) in the bone marrow will usually be managed conservatively with red cell and platelet transfusions and antibiotics for infections, as they are needed. Patients with more severe disease and more than 5 percent blast cells in the bone marrow will require more aggressive treatment. A number of options are available, including: supportive care only, low-dose chemotherapy,

258

intensive chemotherapy, and bone marrow transplantation. The choice of treatment will depend on your age, risk of disease, and current performance status. Note that many of the treatments for MDS are fairly new and still under investigation. The mainstay of treatment for all patients is therefore to focus on prompt treatment of infection, bleeding complications, and anemia.

References

Besa E, Woermann U. Myelodysplastic Syndrome, eMedicine, Web MD, 2006. Available [online] at URL: http://www.emedicine.com/med/topic2695.htm

Cotran RS, Kumar V, Collins T. *Robbins Pathological Basis of Disease*, Sixth Ed. WB Saunders Company 1999. p 678.

Doll D, Landaw S. Clinical manifestations and diagnosis of the myelodysplastic syndromes, UpToDate, 2006.

Estey E, Schrier S. Treatment and prognosis of the myelodysplastic syndromes, UpToDate, 2006.

Kumar P, Clark M. *Clinical Medicine*. Fifth Ed. WB Saunders, 2002. p 390.

Longmore, Wilkinson, Rajagopalan. *Oxford Handbook of Clinical Medicine*. 6th Edition. Oxford University Press. 2004.

Murtagh J. *General Practice*, 3rd Ed. McGraw-Hill, Australia, 2003.

Section 19.3

Polycythemia Vera

Excerpted from "Polycythemia Vera," National Heart Lung and Blood
Institute, National Institutes of Health, February 2009.

What Is Polycythemia Vera?

Polycythemia vera, or PV, is a rare blood disease in which your body
makes too many red blood cells.

The extra red blood cells make your blood thicker than normal.
As a result, blood clots can form more easily and block blood flow
through your arteries and veins. This can lead to heart attack and
stroke.

Thicker blood also flows more slowly to all parts of your body, preventing your organs from getting enough oxygen. This can cause other
serious complications, such as angina and heart failure.

Overview

Red blood cells carry oxygen to all parts of your body. They also
remove carbon dioxide (a waste product) from your body's cells and
carry it to the lungs to be exhaled.

Red blood cells are made in your bone marrow—a sponge-like tissue inside the bones. White blood cells and platelets also are made
in your bone marrow. White blood cells help fight infection. Platelets
help your blood clot.

If you have PV, your bone marrow makes too many red blood cells.
It also can make too many white blood cells and platelets.

A mutation, or change, in the body's JAK2 gene is the major cause
of PV. The JAK2 gene makes an important protein that helps the body
produce blood cells. What causes the change in the JAK2 gene isn't
known. PV generally isn't passed from parent to child.

PV develops slowly and may not cause symptoms for years. Thus, the
disease often is found during routine blood tests done for other reasons.

When signs and symptoms do occur, they're the result of the thick
blood that occurs with PV. This thickness slows the flow of oxygen-rich

blood to all parts of your body. Without enough oxygen, many parts of your body won't work normally.

For example, slower blood flow deprives your arms, legs, lungs, and eyes of the oxygen they need. This can cause headaches, dizziness, itching, and vision problems, such as blurred or double vision.

Outlook

PV is a serious, chronic (ongoing) disease that can be fatal if not diagnosed and treated. PV can't be cured, but treatments can help control the disease and its complications.

PV is treated with procedures, medicines, and other methods. You may need one or more treatments to manage the disease.

Other Names for Polycythemia Vera

- Cryptogenic polycythemia
- Erythremia
- Erythrocytosis megalosplenia
- Myelopathic polycythemia
- Myeloproliferative disorder
- Osler disease
- Polycythemia rubra vera
- Polycythemia with chronic cyanosis
- Primary polycythemia
- Splenomegalic polycythemia
- Vaquez disease

What Causes Polycythemia Vera?

Polycythemia vera (PV) also is known as primary polycythemia. A mutation, or change, in the body's JAK2 gene is the main cause of PV. The JAK2 gene makes an important protein that helps the body produce blood cells.

What causes the change in the JAK2 gene isn't known. PV generally isn't passed from parent to child. However, in some families, the JAK2 gene may have a tendency to mutate. Other, unknown genetic factors also may play a role in causing PV.

Secondary Polycythemia

Another type of polycythemia, called secondary polycythemia, isn't related to the JAK2 gene. Long-term exposure to low oxygen levels causes secondary polycythemia.

A lack of oxygen over a long period can cause your body to make more of the hormone erythropoietin (EPO). High levels of EPO can prompt your body to make more red blood cells than normal. This leads to thicker blood, as seen in PV.

People who smoke, spend long hours at high altitudes, or have severe lung or heart disease may develop secondary polycythemia.

Rarely, tumors can make and release EPO, or certain blood problems can cause the body to make more EPO.

Sometimes secondary polycythemia can be cured—it depends on whether the underlying cause can be stopped, controlled, or cured.

What Are the Signs and Symptoms of Polycythemia Vera?

Polycythemia vera (PV) develops slowly. The disease may not cause signs or symptoms for years.

When signs and symptoms do occur, they're the result of the thick blood that occurs with PV. This thickness slows the flow of oxygen-rich blood to all parts of your body. Without enough oxygen, many parts of your body won't work normally.

The most common signs and symptoms of PV include the following:

- Headache, dizziness, and weakness

- Shortness of breath and problems breathing while lying down

- Feelings of pressure or fullness on the left side of the abdomen due to an enlarged spleen

- Double or blurred vision and blind spots

- Itching all over (especially after a warm bath), reddened face, and a burning feeling on your skin (especially your hands and feet)

- Bleeding from your gums and heavy bleeding from small cuts

- Unexplained weight loss

- Fatigue (tiredness)

In rare cases, people who have PV may have pain in their bones.

Polycythemia Vera Complications

If you have PV, the thickness of your blood and the slowed blood flow can cause serious health problems.

Blood clots are the most serious complication of PV. Blood clots can cause heart attack and stroke. They also can cause your liver and spleen to enlarge. Blood clots in the liver and spleen can cause sudden and intense pain.

The lack of oxygen-rich blood to your organs also can lead to angina (chest pain) and heart failure. The high levels of red blood cells that PV causes can lead to stomach ulcers, gout, or kidney stones.

A small number of people who have PV may develop myelofibrosis. This is a condition in which your bone marrow is replaced by scar tissue. Abnormal bone marrow cells may begin to grow out of control. This abnormal growth can lead to acute myelogenous leukemia (AML), a disease that worsens very quickly.

How Is Polycythemia Vera Diagnosed?

Polycythemia vera (PV) may not cause signs or symptoms for years. Thus, the disease often is found during routine blood tests done for other reasons. If the results of your blood tests aren't normal, your doctor may want to do more tests.

Your doctor will diagnose PV based on your signs and symptoms, your age and overall health, your medical history, a physical exam, and the results from tests.

During the physical exam, your doctor will look for signs of PV. He or she will check for an enlarged spleen, red skin on your face, and bleeding from your gums.

If your doctor confirms that you have polycythemia, the next step is to find out whether you have primary polycythemia (polycythemia vera) or secondary polycythemia.

Your medical history and physical exam may confirm which type of polycythemia you have. If not, you may have tests that check the level of the hormone erythropoietin (EPO) in your blood.

People who have PV have very low levels of EPO. People who have secondary polycythemia usually have normal or high levels of EPO.

Diagnostic Tests

You may have a number of different blood tests to diagnose PV. These tests include a complete blood count (CBC) and other tests, if necessary.

Complete Blood Count

Often, the first test used to diagnose PV is a CBC. The CBC measures many different parts of your blood.

This test checks your hemoglobin and hematocrit levels. Hemoglobin is the iron-rich protein in red blood cells that carries oxygen to the body. Hematocrit is a measure of how much space red blood cells take up in your blood. A high level of hemoglobin or hematocrit may be a sign of PV.

The CBC also checks the number of red blood cells, white blood cells, and platelets in your blood. Abnormal results may be a sign of PV, a blood disorder, an infection, or another condition.

Other Blood Tests

Blood smear. For this test, a small sample of blood is drawn from a vein, usually in your arm. The sample of blood is put on a glass slide. A microscope is then used to look at your red blood cells.

A blood smear can show whether you have a higher-than-normal number of red blood cells. The test also can show abnormal types of blood cells that are linked to myelofibrosis and other conditions related to PV.

Erythropoietin level. This blood test measures the level of EPO in your blood. EPO is a hormone that stimulates bone marrow to make new blood cells. People who have PV have very low levels of EPO. People who have secondary polycythemia usually have normal or high levels of EPO.

Bone Marrow Tests

Bone marrow tests are used to check whether your bone marrow is healthy. These tests also show whether your bone marrow is making normal amounts of blood cells.

If the tests show that your bone marrow is making too many blood cells, it may be a sign that you have PV.

How Is Polycythemia Vera Treated?

Polycythemia vera (PV) can't be cured. However, treatments can help control the disease and its complications. PV is treated with procedures, medicines, and other methods. You may need one or more treatments to manage the disease.

Goals of Treatment

The goals of treating PV are to control symptoms and reduce the risk of complications, especially heart attack and stroke. To do this,

PV treatments reduce the number of red blood cells and the level of hemoglobin (an iron-rich protein) in your blood. This brings the thickness of your blood closer to normal.

Blood with normal thickness flows better through the blood vessels. This reduces the chance that blood clots will form and cause a heart attack or stroke.

Blood with normal thickness also ensures that your body gets enough oxygen. This can help reduce some of the signs and symptoms that PV causes, such as headaches, vision problems, and itching.

Studies show that treating PV greatly improves your chances of living longer.

Treatments to Lower Red Blood Cell Levels

Phlebotomy. Phlebotomy is a procedure that removes some blood from your body. A needle is inserted into your vein, and your blood flows through an airtight tube into a sterile container or bag. The process is similar to the process of donating blood.

Phlebotomy reduces the number of red blood cells in your system and starts to bring your blood thickness closer to normal. Typically, a pint (one unit) of blood is removed each week until your hematocrit level approaches normal. (Hematocrit is the measure of how much space red blood cells take up in your blood.)

You may need to have phlebotomy done every few months.

Medicines. Your doctor may prescribe medicines, such as hydroxyurea or interferon-alpha, to keep your bone marrow from making too many red blood cells.

Hydroxyurea is a medicine generally used to treat cancer. This medicine can reduce the number of red blood cells and platelets in your blood. As a result, this medicine helps improve your blood flow and bring the thickness of your blood closer to normal.

Interferon-alpha is a substance that your body normally produces. It also can be used to treat PV. Interferon-alpha can prompt your immune system to fight bone marrow cells that are making too many red blood cells. As a result, this treatment can help lower the number of red blood cells in your body and maintain blood flow and blood thickness that's close to normal.

Radiation treatment. Radiation treatment can help suppress overactive bone marrow cells. This helps reduce the number of red blood cells in your blood. It also helps keep your blood flow and blood thickness close to normal.

265

However, radiation treatment can raise your risk for leukemia (blood cancer) and other blood diseases.

Treatments for Side Effects

Aspirin can relieve bone pain and burning feelings in your hands or feet that you may have as a result of PV. Aspirin also thins your blood, so it reduces the chance of blood clots forming.

Aspirin can have side effects, including bleeding in the stomach and intestines. For this reason, it's important to take aspirin only as your doctor recommends.

If your PV causes itching, your doctor may prescribe medicines to ease the discomfort. Your doctor also may prescribe ultraviolet light treatment to help relieve your itching.

Other ways to reduce itching include the following:

• Avoiding hot baths. Cooler water can limit the irritation to your skin.

• Gently patting yourself dry after bathing. Vigorous rubbing with a towel can irritate your skin.

• Taking starch baths. Add half a box of starch to a tub of lukewarm water. This can help soothe your skin.

Experimental Treatments

Researchers are studying other treatments for PV. An experimental treatment for itching involves taking low doses of selective serotonin reuptake inhibitors (SSRIs). This type of medicine is used to treat depression. In clinical trials, SSRIs reduced itching in people who had PV.

Imatinib mesylate is a medicine that's approved for treating leukemia. In clinical trials, it has helped reduce the need for phlebotomy in people who have PV. It also has helped reduce the size of enlarged spleens.

Researchers also are trying to develop a treatment that can block or limit the effects of an abnormal JAK2 gene. (A mutation, or change, in the JAK2 gene is the major cause of PV.)

How Can Polycythemia Vera Be Prevented?

Primary polycythemia (polycythemia vera) can't be prevented. However, with proper treatment, you can prevent or delay symptoms and complications.

Sometimes you can prevent secondary polycythemia by avoiding things that deprive your body of oxygen for long periods. For example, you can avoid mountain climbing, living at a high altitude, or smoking.

People who have serious lung or heart diseases may develop secondary polycythemia. Treatment for the underlying disease may improve the secondary polycythemia. Following a healthy lifestyle to lower your risk for heart and lung diseases also will help you prevent secondary polycythemia.

Section 19.4

Thrombocythemia and Thrombocytosis

Excerpted from "Thrombocythemia and Thrombocytosis," National Heart Lung and Blood Institute, National Institutes of Health, February 2008.

What Are Thrombocythemia and Thrombocytosis?

Thrombocythemia and thrombocytosis are conditions in which your blood has a high number of blood cell fragments called platelets.

Platelets are made in your bone marrow along with other kinds of blood cells. They travel through your blood vessels and stick together (clot) to stop any bleeding that could happen if a blood vessel is damaged. Platelets also are called thrombocytes, because a clot also is called a thrombus.

A normal platelet count ranges from 150,000 to 450,000 platelets per microliter of blood.

Overview

The term "thrombocythemia" is preferred when the cause of the high platelet count isn't known. The condition is then called primary or essential thrombocythemia.

This condition occurs when faulty cells in the bone marrow make too many platelets. Bone marrow is the sponge-like tissue inside the bones. It contains stem cells that develop into red blood cells, white blood cells, or platelets. What causes the bone marrow to make too many platelets often isn't known.

With primary thrombocythemia, a high platelet count may occur alone or with other blood cell disorders. The platelet count can be as low as 500,000 platelets per microliter of blood or higher than one million platelets per microliter of blood. This condition isn't common.

When another disease or condition causes a high platelet count, the term "thrombocytosis" is preferred. This condition often is called secondary or reactive thrombocytosis.

In this condition, the platelet count usually is less than one million platelets per microliter of blood. Secondary thrombocytosis is more common than primary thrombocythemia.

Most people who have a high platelet count don't have signs or symptoms. Rarely, serious or life-threatening symptoms can develop, such as blood clots and bleeding. These symptoms mostly occur in people who have primary thrombocythemia.

Outlook

People who have primary thrombocythemia but no signs or symptoms don't need treatment, as long as the condition remains stable. Other people who have this condition may need medicines or procedures to treat it. Most people who have primary thrombocythemia will live a normal life span.

Treatment and outlook for secondary thrombocytosis depend on its underlying cause.

Other Names for Thrombocythemia and Thrombocytosis

Primary thrombocythemia also is called by the following names:

- Essential thrombocythemia. This term is used when a high platelet count occurs alone (that is, without other blood cell disorders).

- Idiopathic thrombocythemia.

- Primary or essential thrombocytosis. These are less favored terms.

Secondary thrombocytosis also is known as the following:

- Reactive thrombocytosis.

- Secondary thrombocythemia. This is a less favored term.

What Causes Thrombocythemia and Thrombocytosis?

Primary Thrombocythemia

In this condition, faulty stem cells in the bone marrow make too many platelets. What causes this to happen usually isn't known. When this process occurs without affecting other blood cells, it's called essential thrombocythemia.

A rare form of thrombocythemia is inherited. ("Inherited" means the condition is passed from parents to children.) In some cases, a genetic mutation may cause the condition.

In primary thrombocythemia, the platelets aren't normal. They may form blood clots, or, surprisingly, cause bleeding when they don't work properly.

Bleeding also can occur because of a condition that develops called von Willebrand disease. This condition affects the blood clotting process.

After many years, scarring of the bone marrow can occur.

Secondary Thrombocytosis

This condition occurs when another disease, condition, or outside factor causes the platelet count to rise. For example, 35 percent of people who have high platelet counts also have cancer—mostly lung, gastrointestinal, breast, ovarian, and lymphoma. Sometimes a high platelet count is the first sign of cancer.

Unlike primary thrombocythemia, the platelets in secondary thrombocytosis usually are normal.

Conditions or factors that can cause a high platelet count include the following:

- Iron-deficiency anemia

- Hemolytic anemia

- Absence of a spleen (after surgery to remove this organ)

- Cancer

- Inflammatory or infectious diseases such as connective tissue disorders, inflammatory bowel disease, and tuberculosis

- Reactions to medicines

Some conditions can lead to a high platelet count that lasts for only a short time. These include the following:

- Recovery from serious loss of blood

- Recovery from a very low platelet count caused by excessive alcohol use and lack of vitamin B_{12} or folate

- Acute infection or inflammation

- Response to physical activity

269

Who Is at Risk for Thrombocythemia or Thrombocytosis?

Primary Thrombocythemia

This condition isn't common. The exact number of people who have the condition isn't known. Some estimates suggest that 1 to 2.5 out of every 100,000 people have primary thrombocythemia. This number may be low, because most people who have the condition don't have symptoms. Therefore, they may not know they have it.

Primary thrombocythemia occurs mostly between the ages of fifty and seventy, but it can occur at any age. For unknown reasons, a higher number of women around the age of thirty have primary thrombocythemia than men of the same age.

Secondary Thrombocytosis

You may be at risk for secondary thrombocytosis if you have a disease, condition, or factor that can cause it.

This condition is more common than primary thrombocythemia. In two studies of people with high platelet levels, most people with platelet counts over 500,000 had secondary thrombocytosis.

What Are the Signs and Symptoms of Thrombocythemia and Thrombocytosis?

Most people who have thrombocythemia or thrombocytosis have no signs or symptoms. These conditions often are discovered only after routine blood tests.

People who have primary thrombocythemia are more likely than those who have secondary thrombocytosis to have serious signs and symptoms.

Primary Thrombocythemia

Often, people who have symptoms of primary thrombocythemia only have a mild form of the condition. The most common symptoms are linked to blood clots and bleeding. They are weakness, bleeding, headache, and numbness of the hands and feet.

Blood clots. In primary thrombocythemia, blood clots most often develop in the brain, hands, and feet. But they can happen anywhere in the body, including in the heart and intestines.

Blood clots in the brain cause symptoms in 25 percent of people who have this condition. Common symptoms are chronic (ongoing) headache and dizziness. In extreme cases, stroke may occur.

Blood clots in the tiny blood vessels of the hands and feet leave them numb and red. This may lead to an intense burning and throbbing pain felt mainly on the palms of the hands and the soles of the feet.

Other signs and symptoms of blood clots may include the following:

- Changes in speech or awareness, ranging from confusion to passing out

- Seizures

- Upper body discomfort in one or both arms, the back, neck, jaw, or stomach

- Shortness of breath and nausea (feeling sick to your stomach)

Blood clots in the placenta cause fetal death or miscarriage in half of pregnant women who have primary thrombocythemia.

Blood clots aren't only linked to having thrombocythemia or thrombocytosis, but to other factors as well. Age (being older than sixty), prior blood clots, diabetes, high blood pressure, and smoking also increase your risk for blood clots.

Bleeding. Bleeding most often occurs in people who have platelet counts higher than one million platelets per microliter of blood. Signs of bleeding include nosebleeds, bruising, bleeding from the mouth or gums, or blood in the stools.

Although bleeding usually is linked to having a low platelet count, it also can occur in people who have high platelet counts. Blood clots that develop in thrombocythemia or thrombocytosis may use up your body's platelets. This means that not enough platelets are left in your bloodstream to seal off any cuts and breaks in the blood vessels.

Another cause of bleeding in patients who have very high platelets counts is a condition called von Willebrand disease. This condition affects the blood clotting process.

In rare cases of primary thrombocythemia (less than 2 percent), the faulty bone marrow cells will cause a form of leukemia. Leukemia is a cancer of the blood cells.

Secondary Thrombocytosis

People who have secondary thrombocytosis have a lower risk for bleeding and blood clots. This is because their platelets are generally normal (unlike in primary thrombocythemia) and their platelet counts aren't as high.

However, people who have this condition are at higher risk for blood clots and bleeding if they're on bed rest or have a severe disease of the arteries.

How Are Thrombocythemia and Thrombocytosis Diagnosed?

Your doctor will diagnose thrombocythemia or thrombocytosis based on your medical history, a physical exam, and test results. A hematologist also may be involved in your care. This is a doctor who treats people who have blood diseases.

Medical History

Your doctor may ask you about factors that can affect your platelets, such as the following:

• Any medical procedures or blood transfusions you've had

• Any recent infections or vaccinations you've had

• The medicines you take, including over-the-counter medicines

• Your general eating habits, including the amount of alcohol you normally drink

• Any family history of high platelet counts

Physical Exam

Your doctor will do a physical exam to look for signs and symptoms of bleeding and blood clots. He or she also will check for signs of conditions that can cause secondary thrombocytosis, such as infection.

Primary thrombocythemia is diagnosed only after all other possible causes of a high platelet count are ruled out. For example, your doctor may order tests to check for early, undiagnosed cancer. If another disease, condition, or factor is causing a high platelet count, the diagnosis is secondary thrombocytosis.

Diagnostic Tests

Your doctor may order one or more of the following tests to help diagnose a high platelet count.

Complete blood count. A complete blood count (CBC) measures the levels of red blood cells, white blood cells, and platelets in your blood. For this test, a small amount of blood is drawn from a blood vessel, usually in your arm.

If you have thrombocythemia or thrombocytosis, the test results will show that your platelet count is high.

Blood smear. A blood smear is used to check the condition of your platelets. For this test, a small amount of blood is drawn from a blood vessel, usually in your arm. Your doctor looks at the blood sample under a microscope.

Bone marrow tests. Bone marrow tests check whether your bone marrow is healthy. Blood cells, including platelets, are made in bone marrow. The two bone marrow tests are aspiration and biopsy.

Bone marrow aspiration may be done to find out whether your bone marrow is making too many platelets. For this test, your doctor removes a small amount of fluid bone marrow through a needle. He or she examines the sample under a microscope to check for faulty cells.

A bone marrow biopsy often is done right after an aspiration. For this test, your doctor removes a small amount of bone marrow tissue through a needle. He or she examines the tissue to check the number and types of cells in the bone marrow. With thrombocythemia and thrombocytosis, the bone marrow has a higher than normal number of the very large cells that make platelets.

Other tests. Your doctor may order other blood tests to look for genetic factors that can cause a high platelet count.

How Are Thrombocythemia and Thrombocytosis Treated?

Primary Thrombocythemia

This condition is considered less harmful today than in the past, and its outlook is often good. People who have no signs or symptoms don't need treatment, as long as the condition remains stable.

Taking aspirin may help people who are at risk for blood clots, because aspirin thins the blood. However, you should talk to your doctor about using aspirin, because it can cause bleeding. Doctors prescribe aspirin to most pregnant women who have primary thrombocythemia. This is because it doesn't have a high risk for side effects to the fetus.

Some people who have primary thrombocythemia may need medicines or medical procedures to lower their platelet counts.

Medicines to Lower Platelet Counts

You may need medicines to lower your platelet count if you:

• have a history of blood clots or bleeding;

• have risk factors (such as high blood cholesterol, high blood pressure, and diabetes);

• are older than sixty;

• have a platelet count over one million.

You will need to take these medicines throughout your life.

Hydroxyurea. This is the most common platelet-lowering medicine to treat primary thrombocythemia. Hydroxyurea is used to treat cancers and other life-threatening diseases. It's most often given under the care of doctors who specialize in cancer or blood diseases. Patients on hydroxyurea are closely monitored.

Currently, hydroxyurea plus aspirin is the standard treatment for people who have primary thrombocythemia and are at high risk for blood clots.

Anagrelide. This medicine has been used to treat thrombocythemia. However, it seems less effective than hydroxyurea. Anagrelide also has side effects such as fluid retention, palpitations, arrhythmias, heart failure, and headaches.

Interferon-alpha. This medicine is effective at lowering platelet counts. However, 20 percent of patients can't handle its side effects. These include a flu-like feeling, decreased appetite, nausea (feeling sick to the stomach), diarrhea, seizures, irritability, and sleepiness.

Doctors may prescribe this medicine to pregnant women who have primary thrombocythemia. This is because it's safer for the fetus than hydroxyurea and anagrelide.

Plateletpheresis

Plateletpheresis is a procedure used to rapidly lower your platelet count. This procedure is only used for emergencies. For example, if you're having a stroke due to primary thrombocythemia, you may need plateletpheresis.

During this procedure, an intravenous (IV) needle that's connected to a tube is placed in one of your blood vessels to remove blood. The blood goes through a machine that removes platelets from the blood. The remaining blood is then put back into you through an IV line in one of your blood vessels.

One or two procedures may be enough to reduce your platelet count to a safe level.

Secondary Thrombocytosis

Secondary thrombocytosis is treated by addressing the underlying condition that's causing it.

People who have this condition usually don't need platelet-lowering medicines or procedures. This is because their platelets are generally normal (unlike in primary thrombocythemia). Also, their platelet counts often aren't high enough to put them at risk for blood clots or bleeding.

How Can Thrombocythemia and Thrombocytosis Be Prevented?

You can't prevent primary thrombocythemia. However, you can take steps to reduce your risk for blood clots and prevent related problems.

Age, prior blood clots, diabetes, high blood pressure, high blood cholesterol, and smoking are all risk factors for blood clots. To reduce your risk, stop smoking and work to control the risk factors that you can.

It's not always possible to prevent conditions that lead to secondary thrombocytosis. But if you have regular medical care, your doctor may find these conditions before you develop a high platelet count.

Living with Thrombocythemia or Thrombocytosis

If you have thrombocythemia or thrombocytosis, it's important to do the following things:

- Get regular medical care.
- Stop smoking and control risk factors for blood clots, such as high blood pressure, diabetes, and high blood cholesterol.
- Watch for signs and symptoms of blood clots and bleeding and report them to your doctor right away.
- Take all medicines as prescribed.

If you're taking medicines to lower your platelet count, tell your doctor or dentist about them before any surgical or dental procedures. These medicines thin your blood and may increase bleeding during such procedures.

Medicines that thin the blood also may cause internal bleeding. Signs of internal bleeding include bruises, bloody or tarry-looking stools, pink or bloody urine, increased menstrual bleeding, bleeding gums, and nosebleeds. Contact your doctor right away if you have any of these signs.

Avoid over-the-counter pain medicines such as ibuprofen (except Tylenol®). These medicines may raise your risk for bleeding in the stomach or intestines and may limit the effect of aspirin. Be aware that cold and pain medicines and other over-the-counter remedies may contain ibuprofen.

Chapter 20

Plasma Cell Disorders

Chapter Contents

Section 20.1

Amyloidosis

Amyloidosis is a condition in which too much of a particular protein (amyloid) collects in the organs, so that they are not able to work normally. Amyloidosis can affect the heart, kidneys, liver, spleen, nervous system, stomach, or intestines. The condition is rare (affecting fewer than three thousand people in the United States each year), but it can be fatal.

Amyloidosis sometimes develops when a person has certain forms of cancer, such as multiple myeloma, Hodgkin disease, or familial Mediterranean fever (an intestinal disorder). It also sometimes occurs in people with kidney disease who have undergone dialysis for a long time.

There are three major forms of amyloidosis:

- Primary amyloidosis, which is the most common. It occurs without another associated disease and most often affects the heart, lungs, skin, tongue, nerves, and intestines.

- Secondary or acquired amyloidosis, which is associated with chronic diseases, such as tuberculosis, rheumatoid arthritis, or osteomyelitis. It most often affects the kidneys, spleen, liver, and intestines. If the underlying disease is treated, this form of amyloidosis will go away.

- Hereditary amyloidosis, which runs in families. This type often affects the nervous and digestive systems.

Symptoms

Symptoms vary widely from person to person and depending on which organs are affected. Some people do not even have symptoms, which makes the condition difficult to diagnose.

When amyloidosis is associated with another disease, symptoms may be masked. The underlying disease may be fatal before amyloidosis is found.

Symptoms include:

- an enlarged liver;
- an enlarged tongue (macroglossia);
- an irregular heartbeat;
- diarrhea alternating with constipation;
- difficulty swallowing;
- dizziness or feeling faint;
- loss of weight;
- numbness or tingling in the hands or feet;
- severe fatigue;
- shortness of breath;
- skin changes;
- swelling of the ankles and legs;
- weakness.

The severity of amyloidosis depends on which organs it affects. It can be life threatening if it causes kidney or heart failure.

If the amyloidosis affects the kidneys, their ability to filter the blood becomes impaired. Protein leaks from the blood into the urine. The loss of protein from the blood can cause fluid to leak out of the blood vessels, resulting in swelling in the feet, ankles, and calves. Eventually, there is so much damage to the kidneys that they are not able to remove waste products from the body and they fail.

If amyloidosis affects the heart, the first symptom typically is shortness of breath even with only light activity. Climbing a flight of stairs or walking long distances may be difficult without having to stop. The buildup of amyloid in the heart lessens its ability to fill up with blood between heartbeats. As a result, less blood is pumped with each beat, and the heart is not able to keep up with the body's needs. The buildup of amyloid can also cause problems with the electrical system of the heart, resulting in irregular heartbeats (arrhythmia).

Other effects of amyloidosis include:

- a burning sensation as a result of nerves being irritated by the amyloid;
- alternating bouts of constipation and diarrhea, if the protein deposits affect the nerves that control the bowels;

- bowel obstruction;

- carpal tunnel syndrome, which causes pain, numbness, or tingling in the fingers (approximately four out of ten people with amyloidosis develop this syndrome);

- disruption of the nervous system;

- dizziness or nearly fainting when standing up too quickly (this can happen if the condition affects the nerves that control blood pressure and a sudden drop in blood pressure occurs when standing up);

- numbness or lack of feeling in the toes or feet;

- weakness in the legs, which can be a result of nerves irritated by the amyloid.

Diseases that are associated with amyloidosis include multiple myeloma, Hodgkin disease, some types of tumors, and Mediterranean fever that runs in families. It may also be associated with aging. Amyloid is often found in the pancreas of people who develop diabetes as adults.

Causes and Risk Factors

The cause for amyloid to be produced and to collect in the tissues is not known. The risk of getting amyloidosis is not connected to what a person eats (including how much protein) or does for a living or to the amount of stress in one's life.

The disease starts in the bone marrow. Bone marrow creates red and white blood cells, platelets, and antibodies that protect the body against infection. After the antibodies have done their work, the body breaks them down. When the bone marrow cells produce antibodies that cannot be broken down, amyloidosis develops. The antibodies build up in the blood and eventually get deposited in the tissues as amyloid.

The risk of developing amyloidosis is greater in people who:

- are older than fifty;

- have a chronic infection or inflammatory disease;

- have a family history of amyloidosis;

- have multiple myeloma (between 10 and 15 percent of people who have multiple myeloma develop amyloidosis);

- have a kidney disease that has required dialysis for more than five years.

Diagnosis

Blood and urine tests may reveal an abnormal protein in the body, but the only way to diagnose amyloidosis for certain is to take a sample of tissue for analysis under a microscope. Tissue is usually taken from the fat around the abdomen or the tissues of the rectum, which can be done on an outpatient basis. Samples can also be taken from the skin, nerves, kidneys, liver, or gums—in which case a hospital stay may be required. The samples are stained with a dye that reacts with amyloid and then examined under a microscope.

Treatment

There is no cure for amyloidosis. Treatment of an underlying illness—if there is one—can cause the amyloidosis to go away. Drugs and diet can help manage symptoms and help prevent the production of more of the protein.

Among the drugs that have been helpful in treating amyloidosis are:

- Melphalan (Alkeran®), which is used to treat some types of cancer;

- Prednisone, a corticosteroid that reduces inflammation (swelling and tenderness);

- Pain relievers.

Several drugs (such as thalidomide, which is being used to treat multiple myeloma) are being studied for their ability to treat amyloidosis.

A nutritionally sound diet provides the body with a good energy supply. Diet may also be helpful to treat the many complications that can arise from amyloidosis. Special diets are usually based on symptoms and which organs have been affected by amyloidosis. For example, a doctor may recommend a low-salt diet or diuretics if the kidneys have been affected.

In secondary amyloidosis, the goal is to treat the underlying condition.

In the case of amyloidosis of the kidney, kidney transplantation may be done. Dialysis may be helpful as well. However, amyloid will eventually appear in the donor kidney. Research is underway to study the effect of stem cell transplantation to treat organs with amyloidosis.

In the case of amyloid heart disease, heart transplantation may also be done. Persons who have amyloid heart disease need to be careful if they are taking digitalis because it can precipitate arrhythmias. Myocardial amyloidosis is the most common cause of death. This is usually due to arrhythmias or intractable heart failure.

In some cases of inherited amyloidosis, liver transplantation can help because it removes the source that produces the mutant protein.

Research is underway to find other treatments for amyloidosis. One area under investigation is stem cell transplantation, which involves using chemotherapy and transfusions of immature blood cells (stem cells) that have been collected to replace diseased or damaged bone marrow. The cells may be collected from a patient's own body (autologous transplant) or from a donor (allogeneic transplant).

Section 20.2

Cryoglobulinemia

"Cryoglobulinemia," © 2009 A.D.A.M., Inc. Reprinted with permission.

Cryoglobulinemia is the presence of abnormal proteins in the blood. These abnormal proteins become thick or gel-like in cold temperatures.

Causes

Cryoglobulins are antibodies. It is not yet known why they become solid at low temperatures. When they do thicken or become somewhat gel-like, they can block blood vessels throughout the body. This may lead to complications ranging from skin rashes to kidney failure.

Cryoglobulinemia is part of a group of diseases that cause vasculitis—damage and inflammation of the blood vessels throughout the body. The disorder is grouped into three main types, depending on the type of antibody that is produced:

- Cryoglobulinemia type I
- Cryoglobulinemia type II
- Cryoglobulinemia type III

Types II and III are also referred to as mixed cryoglobulinemia.

Type I cryoglobulinemia is most often related to cancer of the blood or immune systems.

Types II and III are most often found in people who have a chronic (long-lasting) inflammatory condition, such as an autoimmune disease or hepatitis C. Most patients with mixed cryoglobulinemia have a chronic hepatitis C infection.

Other conditions that may be related to cryoglobulinemia include:

- leukemia;
- multiple myeloma;
- mycoplasma pneumonia;
- primary macroglobulinemia;
- rheumatoid arthritis;
- systemic lupus erythematosus.

Symptoms

Symptoms vary depending on the type of cryoglobulinemia and the organs that are affected. In general, symptoms may include:

- difficulty breathing;
- fatigue;
- glomerulonephritis;
- joint pain;
- muscle pain;
- purpura;
- Raynaud phenomenon;
- skin death;
- skin ulceration.

Exams and Tests

The doctor will perform a physical exam. There may be signs of liver and spleen swelling.

Tests for cryoglobulinemia include:

- complete blood count (CBC);
- complement assay—numbers will be low
- cryoglobulin test—may show presence of cryoglobulins;

- liver function tests—may be high;
- rheumatoid factor—positive in types II and III;
- skin biopsy;
- urinalysis—may show blood in the urine if the kidneys are affected.

Other tests may include:

- angiogram;
- chest x-ray;
- erythrocyte sedimentation rate (ESR);
- hepatitis C test;
- nerve conduction tests, if the person has weakness in the arms or legs;
- protein electrophoresis—blood.

Treatment

Treatment of mild or moderate cryoglobulinemia depends on the underlying cause. Treating the cause will often treat the cryoglobulinemia.

Mild cases can be treated by avoiding cold temperatures.

Standard hepatitis C treatments usually work for patients who have hepatitis C and mild or moderate cryoglobulinemia. However, the condition can return when treatment stops.

Severe cryoglobulinemia (involves vital organs or large areas of skin) is treated with corticosteroids and other medications that suppress the immune system.

Treatment may also involve plasmapheresis. Plasmapheresis is a procedure in which blood plasma is removed from the circulation and replaced by fluid, protein, or donated plasma.

Outlook (Prognosis)

Cryoglobulinemia is not usually deadly. However, if the kidneys are affected, the outlook is poor.

Possible Complications

Complications include:

- bleeding in the digestive tract (rare);

- heart disease (rare);
- infections of ulcers;
- kidney failure;
- liver failure;
- skin death;
- death.

When to Contact a Medical Professional

Call your health care provider if:

- you develop symptoms of cryoglobulinemia;
- you have hepatitis C and develop symptoms of cryoglobulinemia;
- you have cryoglobulinemia and develop new or worsening symptoms.

Prevention

There is no known prevention. Avoiding exposure to cold temperatures may prevent some symptoms.

Because so many cases of mixed cryoglobulinemia are associated with hepatitis C, prevention of hepatitis C infection may reduce your risk of cryoglobulinemia.

References

Goldman L, Ausiello D. *Cecil Textbook of Medicine.* 22nd ed. Philadelphia, Pa: WB Saunders; 2004:1193.

Rakel P, ed. *Conn's Current Therapy 2006.* 58th ed. Philadelphia, Pa: WB Saunders; 2006:980, 1164.

Harris ED, Budd RC, Genovese MC, Firestein GS, Sargent JS, Sledge CB. *Kelley's Textbook of Rheumatology.* 7th ed. St. Louis, Mo: WB Saunders; 2005:1392–93.

Section 20.3

Monoclonal Gammopathy of Undetermined Significance

From *The Merck Manual of Medical Information—Second Home Edition*, edited by Robert Porter. Copyright 2008 by Merck & Co., Inc., Whitehouse Station, New Jersey.

A monoclonal gammopathy of undetermined significance is a buildup of monoclonal antibodies produced by abnormal but noncancerous plasma cells.

In general, monoclonal gammopathies of undetermined significance occur in more than 5 percent of people older than seventy, but they do not cause significant health problems. These disorders do not usually cause symptoms, so they are almost always discovered by chance when laboratory tests are done for other purposes, such as to measure protein in the blood. However, the monoclonal antibody can bind to nerves and lead to numbness, tingling, and weakness. People with these disorders also are more likely to have bone loss and fractures.

The M-protein levels in people with a monoclonal gammopathy of undetermined significance often remain stable for years—twenty-five years in some people—and do not require treatment. However, if evaluation shows evidence of significant loss of bone density (osteopenia or osteoporosis), doctors may recommend treatment with bisphosphonates.

For unknown reasons, in about one quarter of people with these disorders, there is a progression to a cancer, such as multiple myeloma, macroglobulinemia, or B-cell lymphoma, often after many years. This progression cannot be prevented. People with a monoclonal gammopathy of undetermined significance are usually monitored with a physical examination and blood and sometimes urine tests about twice a year, to determine if a progression to cancer is beginning to occur. If progression is detected early, symptoms and complications of the cancer may be prevented or treated sooner.

Section 20.4

Multiple Myeloma

What is multiple myeloma?

Multiple myeloma is a blood cancer of the plasma cell. While this
cancer cannot be cured, it can be treated. Multiple myeloma patients
are now living longer, healthier lives. Each year about sixteen thousand
individuals receive a diagnosis of multiple myeloma, which is the second
most prevalent blood cancer after non-Hodgkin lymphoma. About fifty
thousand people in the United States live with multiple myeloma.

Myeloma begins when a plasma cell becomes abnormal. The abnormal cell divides, and the new cells divide again and again, making more
and more abnormal, or myeloma, cells. Over time, the myeloma cells collect in the bone marrow and in the solid part of the bone, crowding out
normal blood cells. This causes extensive destruction within the skeleton
involving multiple bones, resulting in widespread bone pain and many
fractures; this is the reason this disease is called "multiple myeloma." In
addition to making bone tumors, these abnormal plasma cells usually
secrete an abnormal protein known as the monoclonal component or "M
component." The M component in the blood stream and urinary system
can lead to abnormal clotting and kidney failure.

Who is most likely to have multiple myeloma?

The average age at diagnosis is about sixty-eight years. Only 1 percent
of cases occur in individuals under age forty. Multiple myeloma occurs
more frequently in men than women. Myeloma is one of the leading causes
of cancer death among African Americans. Native Pacific Islanders also
have a high incidence of this disease. Genetics play in role in contracting this disease, experts believe, as do factors including age, exposure to
radiation or toxins, a declining immune system, and obesity. Also, a personal history of monoclonal gammopathy of undetermined significance
(MGUS)—a condition in which abnormal plasma cells make a low level
of monoclonal proteins—is associated with multiple myeloma.

What characterizes multiple myeloma?

Multiple myeloma is characterized by excessive abnormal plasma cells in the bone marrow and overproduction of intact monoclonal immunoglobulin or Bence-Jones protein. Signs of multiple myeloma include high calcium counts, anemia, renal damage, susceptibility to bacterial infection, impaired production of normal immunoglobulin, and osteoporosis.

Symptoms and complications include bone pain, usually in the back; broken bones, usually in the spine; weakness; fatigue; thirst; frequent infections and fevers; weight loss; nausea and constipation; and frequent urination. While these symptoms are usually not due to cancer, you should see a doctor if you experience them so that any problems can be diagnosed and treated as early as possible.

How does the pathologist make a diagnosis?

After obtaining a personal and family medical history and performing a physical exam, your primary care physician may order a blood test, urine test, or x-ray.

The pathologist checks the blood for high levels of calcium, the presence of anemia, and/or a monoclonal protein. The urine is examined for Bence Jones protein, a type of monoclonal protein that can cause kidney damage.

In addition, a hematologist (specialist in blood diseases) or pathologist may remove a specimen from your bone marrow for the pathologist to examine for cancer cells. Local anesthesia is used to reduce discomfort.

What else does the pathologist look for?

If abnormal plasma cells are found, your physician will order more tests to determine the stage of the cancer and the best treatment option. These tests may include more blood tests or computed tomography (CT) or magnetic resonance imaging (MRI) scans that allow the pathologist to look closely at your bones. Stage 1 cancers have fewer myeloma cells, and stage 2 and 3 cancers have progressively more.

How do doctors determine what treatment will be necessary?

The pathologist consults with your primary care physician after reviewing the test results. Together, using their combined experience and knowledge, they determine treatment options most appropriate for your condition.

What kinds of treatments are available for multiple myeloma?

The treatment depends on the stage and symptoms of your disease. Treatment options may include anticancer drugs, stem cell transplantation, or radiation therapy.

Anticancer drug treatment kills cancer cells throughout the body. Chemotherapy drugs include melphalan, cyclophosphamide, vincristine, and doxorubicin. Prednisone, a steroid, also is often used. Your doctor also may recommend a combination of drugs or new treatments. You may receive drugs by mouth or intravenously, usually as an outpatient or at home, rather than in a hospital.

Stem cell transplantation allows your physician to provide more aggressive cancer-fighting treatment—higher-than-usual doses of chemotherapy, radiation therapy, or both. This aggressive hospital treatment kills both myeloma cells and normal blood cells in the bone marrow. After these cells have been destroyed, you receive healthy stem cells transplanted through a flexible tube placed in a large vein in your neck or chest area. New, healthy blood cells develop from the transplanted stem cells, which usually come from a healthy part of your body (autologous) or from a donor (allogeneic).

Radiation therapy kills myeloma cells and helps to control pain with high-energy rays. Local radiation is directed at the bone or part of the body where myeloma cells have collected and are causing pain. Total-body radiation is given before stem cell transplantation; these treatments may be given two or three times a day for several days before the transplant. Depending on the kind of complications of multiple myeloma you experience, you may need pain medication or a brace for back pain, dialysis for kidney complications, antibiotics for infections, medications to prevent bone loss, or erythropoietin injections that stimulate red blood cell production for anemia.

Multiple myeloma patients also are encouraged to stay active, follow a healthy diet, and drink fluids to dilute Bence Jones fragments in the urine. Staying positive and proactive and maintaining a strong support network is also important.

Clinical trials of new treatments for multiple myeloma may be found at www.cancer.gov/clinicaltrials. These treatments are highly experimental in nature but may be the best option for advanced cancers.

What kinds of questions should I ask my doctors?

Ask any question you want. There are no questions you should be reluctant to ask. Here are a few to consider:

- Please describe the type of cancer I have and what treatment options are available.

- What stage is the cancer in?

- What are the chances for full remission?

- What treatment options do you recommend? Why do you believe these are the best treatments?

- What are the pros and cons of these treatment options?

- What are the side effects?

- Should I receive a second opinion?

- Is your medical team experienced in treating the type of cancer I have?

- Can you provide me with information about the physicians and others on the medical team?

Chapter 21

Rh Disease

When a mother is pregnant with a baby whose blood type is in-compatible with hers, antibodies in the mother's blood may cross the placenta and attack the baby's red blood cells.

This causes anemia in the baby. If it is severe enough, it can cause the baby to die before birth.

Causes and Risk Factors

This most commonly happens when a woman with Rh-negative blood becomes pregnant by a man with Rh-positive blood and conceives a baby with Rh-positive blood.

Red blood cells from the baby can leak across the placenta into the woman's bloodstream during pregnancy or delivery. This causes the mother's body to make antibodies against the Rh factor.

If the mother becomes pregnant again with an Rh-positive baby, it is possible for her antibodies to cross the placenta and attack the baby's red blood cells.

After birth, an affected newborn may develop kernicterus. This happens when bile pigments are deposited in the cells of the brain and spinal cord and nerve cells are degenerated.

Incompatibilities between ABO blood types can also cause this condition. These are less common than those of the Rh factor and tend to be less severe.

"Rh Disease (Erythroblastosis Fetalis)," © 2008 Cedars-Sinai Medical Center (www.csmc.edu). Reprinted with permission.

Diagnosis

During a pregnant woman's first prenatal doctor's visit, she should be screened for blood and Rh type. If she has Rh-negative blood, the father's blood and Rh type should be tested.

If the father has Rh-positive blood and tests of the mother's blood indicate that she hasn't become sensitive to Rh-positive blood, she should be tested again at eighteen to twenty weeks of pregnancy and at twenty-six to twenty-seven weeks of pregnancy.

Depending on the test results, she may need amniocentesis and other tests to measure the levels of bilirubin (a bile pigment) in the amniotic fluid every two weeks starting at twenty-eight weeks of pregnancy. The amniotic fluid surrounds the baby as it grows inside the mother during pregnancy.

Women who are already sensitive to the Rh factor should have amniocentesis at twenty-six to thirty weeks of pregnancy, depending on how great their apparent sensitivity is.

Prevention

Steps can be taken to assure that antibodies aren't made in the first place. This can be done by giving the mother a shot of anti-Rh antibodies within seventy-two hours of the delivery of the baby. This causes any of the baby's red blood cells that may have crossed into the mother's blood to be destroyed before sensitizing the mother's immune system.

This has to be done with each pregnancy—normal or ectopic—whether it ends in a delivery or an abortion.

If there is much blood loss during delivery, additional injections may be needed. Between 1 and 2 percent of the time this treatment fails. This is apparently because the mother has already become sensitized during pregnancy rather than at delivery.

The treatment can be done preventatively to mothers with Rh-negative blood and no apparent sensitization at about twenty-eight weeks of pregnancy. Any antibodies circulating in the mother's blood are gradually destroyed and the mother remains unsensitized. The treatment should also be given after any bleeding or after amniocentesis or chorionic villus sampling.

Treatment

If monitoring shows that the bilirubin levels in the amniotic fluid are normal, no treatment may be needed as the pregnancy proceeds to delivery.

If the levels are high, showing a threat to the fetus, it may be given transfusions inside the uterus every ten days to two weeks until it has reached the thirty-second to thirty-fourth weeks of pregnancy. Then a delivery should be done. These procedures must be done at a medical center that can care for high-risk pregnancies.

The baby should be delivered with as little trauma as possible. The placenta should not be removed manually to avoid squeezing cells from the baby's blood into the mother's bloodstream. A newborn born with Rh disease should be seen immediately by a pediatrician who can do an exchange transfusion at once if necessary.

Chapter 22

White Blood Cell Disorders

Chapter Contents

Section 22.1

Hypereosinophilic Syndrome

What Is an Eosinophil?

An eosinophil is a type of white blood cell that plays an important role in the human immune system. For example, it helps us fight off certain types of infections like parasites. Many different problems can cause high numbers of eosinophils in the blood, including allergies, asthma, some gastrointestinal disorders, parasitic infection, some blood/bone marrow diseases, certain cancers, and other problems. When eosinophils occur in higher than normal numbers in the blood, without a known cause and for a sustained period of time (more than six months), an innate disorder of eosinophils may be present.

Normally, there are less than 3 percent eosinophils circulating in the blood vessels because they migrate quickly into the tissues and organs of the body. The highest concentration of eosinophils is usually found in the gastrointestinal tract. There is a complex series of chemical events that determines the levels of eosinophils in the blood and tissues. The proper balance and function of these events determine eosinophil production, their activity, and their time to die.

Eosinophil production is governed by several chemicals in blood called cytokines, including interleukin 3 (IL-3), interleukin 5 (IL-5), and granulocyte-macrophage colony-stimulating factor (GM-CSF). Cytokines have many functions. They mediate and regulate immunity, inflammation, and hematopoiesis (production of blood cells) and different cytokines are produced in high amounts in different diseases. IL-5 appears to be the most important and specific cytokine that is responsible for the production and activity of eosinophils. Cytokines bind to specific chemicals on the surface of cells, called membrane receptors, that initiate the cascade of changes in other chemicals inside the cell leading toward the change in cell's behavior, including higher activity and multiplication. Many of the membrane receptors and intracellular chemicals belong to a class of chemicals called tyrosine kinases.

What Is Hypereosinophilic Syndrome (HES)?

HES is a group of disorders in which there are very high numbers of eosinophils found in the blood for a prolonged period of time (more than six months) for which a cause cannot be found. The continuous presence of high numbers of eosinophils in blood can eventually cause multiple organ tissue damage as these eosinophils infiltrate different tissues and cause inflammation. HES can affect any organ in the body, including the stomach and intestines, the heart, lungs, skin, and other organs.

Since many different problems can cause high numbers of eosinophils in the blood, higher then normal blood eosinophil number alone does not mean an individual has, or will develop, HES. Criteria have been developed that must be fulfilled for an individual to be diagnosed with HES.

Criteria for Diagnosis of HES

1. Peripheral blood eosinophilia (high numbers of eosinophils in the blood); more than 1,500 eosinophils/ml, for at least six months' duration

2. End-organ (heart, lungs, gastrointestinal [GI] tract, brain, skin, etc.) involvement with eosinophil tissue infiltration (invasion) and injury

3. Exclusion of known other causes for the eosinophilia such as parasitic infections and certain bone marrow/blood diseases

A bone marrow biopsy may be recommended in a patient fulfilling these criteria and suspected of having HES.

Standard Treatments for HES

Treatment goals include decreasing blood eosinophil numbers, preventing organ damage, and slowing disease progression. Treatments vary based on organs involved and disease severity, as well as on the presence of other medical problems a patient may have.

Systemic steroids are often needed to treat HES with organ involvement or with systemic symptoms, like severe rash, fluid retention, and similar. Steroids are very effective for controlling eosinophil numbers in blood and most patients can be maintained on oral steroid medication (called prednisone) for long periods of time with good control of the disease. However, the blood eosinophils and disease symptoms generally return once steroids have been stopped. Long-term steroid use (especially when used in high doses) has, unfortunately, been associated with side effects.

Interferon alpha (IFNa) is used for a variety of diseases including infections (like hepatitis) and malignancies (like certain types of leukemia). IFNa has been shown to be effective in HES by suppressing the symptoms related to the disease. Toxicity, however, is a major obstacle to the use of this therapy. IFNa is commonly injected into the fatty tissue under the skin three to five times a week. Upon the initiation of therapy most patients experience influenza-like symptoms such as fever, chills, muscle aches, headaches, and joint pain. Other side effects of IFNa are low blood counts and elevated liver enzymes that require careful monitoring. These side effects usually lessen over time, but other toxicities can manifest themselves in various forms after long-term therapy. Overall experience with IFNa in myeloproliferative diseases is that about 25 to 30 percent of patients require discontinuation of therapy due to side effects. New long-acting forms of IFNa (pegylated interferons) have been developed over the last few years and are now approved as therapy for hepatitis. These medications are administered only once a week and may, therefore, be better tolerated.

Cyclosporine is a potent medication that suppresses the immune system and it is used primarily to prevent organ rejection in people who have had organ transplants. In some patients with HES there might be evidence that the immune cells have a role in supporting the disease's existence (so called T cells) and cyclosporine may have a role as therapy in such cases.

Antineoplastic agents provide an alternative approach to therapy of advanced cases of HES. These are chemotherapeutic agents that may control the disease. They are used to treat many malignancies and are not specific for eosinophilic disorders. They are potent medications that kill cells that grow the fastest (eosinophils in HES) but may potentially have harmful side effects and are reserved only for more severe cases. Careful monitoring while taking these medications is essential. Chemotherapeutic agents that have been used in HES include: hydroxyurea, methotrexate, etoposide, cyclophosphamide, vincristine, and cladribine.

New Therapies for HES

As a result of cell growth research, scientists have been able to develop a group of therapeutic agents known as tyrosine kinase inhibitors. By blocking the ability of tyrosine kinases to function, these compounds provide a valuable tool for controlling malignant cell growth.

The novel approach for treating HES is to "target" specific receptors on the eosinophil surface in order to interrupt their unregulated replication. Platelet derived growth factor receptor (PDGF-R) is a receptor that is tyrosine kinase involved with the maintenance of normal blood cell production, skin pigment production, formation of female ova and male sperm, and the growth and activity of certain white blood cells involved in allergy and immune response. Alteration in PDGF-R tyrosine kinase activity is known to be responsible for disease onset and progression in some patients with HES. Therefore, medications (tyrosine kinase inhibitors) were developed to interfere with this process.

Gleevec® (imatinib mesylate) is a tyrosine kinase inhibitor that is known to inhibit PDGF-R. Gleevec was developed for and is currently approved by the Food and Drug Administration for use as a treatment for chronic myelogenous leukemia (CML); in this disease it blocks the activity of one other tyrosine kinase and is very effective therapy. Gleevec may eliminate disease in select HES patients, those having alteration in PDGF-R tyrosine kinase activity. Therefore, it is mandatory that HES patients be tested for this abnormality; there are two ways this can be accomplished, either using polymerase chain reaction (PCR) test for FIP1L1-PDGFRa gene rearrangement, or using fluorescent in situ hybridization (FISH) test for CHIC2 gene deletion. Most HES patients do not have PDGF-R alteration, and some patients without it may still respond to Gleevec therapy, by improving signs and symptoms of the disease. Gleevec is given at a starting dose of 100 mg orally daily, with a dose escalation up to 400 mg after one month if no response is observed. Other tyrosine kinase inhibitors are being evaluated as therapy for HES patients.

Dasatinib is a tyrosine kinase inhibitor that was recently approved for therapy of CML patients failing Gleevec. It may affect many different tyrosine kinases and is being evaluated in a clinical study for HES patients not responding to standard therapies.

Nilotinib is another tyrosine kinase inhibitor that is also being developed for CML patients losing a response to Gleevec, but is not approved yet. This agent too is being evaluated in a clinical study for HES patients not responding to standard therapies.

Mepolizumab is an investigational medication for HES, not yet approved. It is a medication given intravenously monthly that binds to IL-5, which is the primary cytokine responsible for eosinophil growth. This therapy is being evaluated in clinical trials for patients with HES and other eosinophilic diseases and the initial results are encouraging.

Alemtuzumab is a monoclonal antibody reactive with several cell populations carrying a particular molecule termed CD52. Recent reports have shown the usefulness of alemtuzumab (anti-CD52) for the treatment of two female HES patients with cutaneous manifestations, one with a CD3_ CD4+ T-cell population [30_,31_]. Although this medication carries a black box warning because of hematological toxicity, infusion reactions, and opportunistic infections, it may have a place in the treatment of certain HES patients who are resistant to other therapies.

Section 22.2

Histiocytosis

Excerpted from "Histiocytosis," © 2009 A.D.A.M., Inc.
Reprinted with permission.

Alternative Names

Histiocytosis X; Langerhans cell histiocytosis; eosinophilic granuloma; pulmonary histiocytosis X; nonlipid reticuloendotheliosis; pulmonary Langerhans cell granulomatosis; Hand-Schuller-Christian disease; Letterer-Siwe disease

Definition

Histiocytosis is a general name for a group of syndromes that involve an abnormal increase in the number of immune cells called histiocytes.

There are three major classes of histiocytoses:

- Langerhans cell histiocytosis, which is also called histiocytosis X

- Malignant histiocytosis syndrome (now known as T-cell lymphoma)

- Non-Langerhans cell histiocytosis (also known as hemophagocytic syndrome)

This section focuses only on Langerhans cell histiocytosis (histiocytosis X).

Causes

Histiocytosis X has typically been thought of as a cancer-like condition. More recently researchers have begun to suspect that it is actually an autoimmune phenomenon, in which immune cells mistakenly attack the body, rather than fight infections. Extra immune cells may form tumors, which can affect various parts of the body including the bones, skull, and other areas.

Some forms of the disorder are genetic.

Histiocytosis X is thought to affect roughly 1 in 200,000 people each year. It is most often seen in children age one to fifteen. The rate peaks among children age five to ten.

Pulmonary histiocytosis X is a specific type of this disorder that involves swelling of the small airways (bronchioles) and small blood vessels in the lungs. It is most common in adults. The inflammation leads to lung stiffening and damage. The cause is unknown. It most often affects those aged thirty to forty, usually cigarette smokers.

Symptoms

Histiocytosis X often affects the whole body. A disease that affects the whole body is called a systemic disorder.

Symptoms can vary between children and adults, although there can be some overlap. Tumors in weight-bearing bones, such as the legs or spine, may cause the bones to fracture without apparent reason.

Symptoms in children may include:

- abdominal pain;
- bone pain (possibly);
- delayed puberty;
- dizziness;
- ear drainage that continues long-term;
- eyes that appear to stick out (protrude) more and more;
- irritability;
- failure to thrive;
- fever;
- frequent urination;
- headache;
- jaundice;

301

- limping;
- mental deterioration;
- rash (petechiae or purpura);
- seborrheic dermatitis of the scalp;
- seizures;
- short stature;
- swollen lymph glands;
- thirst;
- vomiting;
- weight loss.

Note: Children over five years old often have only bone involvement. Symptoms in adults may include:

- bone pain;
- chest pain;
- cough;
- fever;
- general discomfort, uneasiness, or ill feeling (malaise);
- increased amount of urine;
- rash;
- shortness of breath;
- thirst and increased drinking of fluids;
- weight loss.

Exams and Tests

The tumors produce a "punched-out" look on a bone x-ray. Specific tests vary depending on the age of the patient.

Tests in children may also include:

- biopsy of skin to check for the presence of Langerhans cells;
- bone marrow biopsy to check for the presence of Langerhans cells;
- complete blood count (CBC);
- x-rays of all the bones in the body (skeletal survey) to find out how many bones are affected.

Tests in adults may include:

• bronchoscopy with biopsy;

• chest x-ray;

• pulmonary function tests.

Histiocytosis X is sometimes associated with cancer. Computed tomography (CT) scans and biopsy should be done to rule out possible cancer.

Treatment

This disorder is treated with corticosteroids, which suppress immune function (including the dangerous cells). Smoking may worsen the response to treatment and should be stopped.

Children may be given other medications depending on their estimated outlook. Such medications may include:

• cyclophosphamide;

• etoposide;

• methotrexate;

• vinblastine.

Radiation therapy or surgery may also be used to treat bone lesions.

Other treatments may include:

• antibiotics to fight infections;

• breathing support (with a breathing machine);

• hormone replacement therapy;

• physical therapy;

• special shampoos for scalp problems;

• supportive care to relieve symptoms.

Outlook (Prognosis)

Histiocytosis X affects many organs and can lead to death.

About half of those with pulmonary histiocytosis see improvement, while others eventually have permanent loss of lung function.

In very young patients, the outlook depends on the specific histiocytosis and severity of the disease. Some children can live a normal life with minimal disease involvement, while others may have a poor outcome. Young children, especially infants, are more likely to have body-wide symptoms that lead to death.

Possible Complications

Complications may include:

- diffuse interstitial pulmonary fibrosis;

- spontaneous pneumothorax.

Children may also develop:

- anemia caused by spreading of the tumors to the bone marrow;

- diabetes insipidus;

- lung problems that lead to lung failure;

- problems with the pituitary gland that lead to growth failure.

When to Contact a Medical Professional

Call your health care provider if you or your child have symptoms of this disorder. Go to the emergency room if shortness of breath or chest pain develop.

Prevention

Avoid smoking. Quitting smoking can improve the outcome in people with histiocytosis that affects the lungs.

There is no known prevention for the childhood forms of the disease.

References

Ladisch S. Histiocytosis Syndromes of Childhood. In: Kliegman RM, Behrman RE, Jenson HB, Stanton BF, eds. *Nelson Textbook of Pediatrics*. 18th ed. Philadelphia, Pa: Saunders Elsevier; 2007: chap. 507.

Raghu G. Interstitial Lung Disease. In: Goldman L, Ausiello D, eds. *Cecil Textbook of Medicine*. 23rd ed. Philadelphia, Pa: Saunders Elsevier; 2007: chap. 92.

Section 22.3

Lymphocytopenia

Excerpted from "Lymphocytopenia," National Heart Lung and Blood Institute, National Institutes of Health, February 2009.

What Is Lymphocytopenia?

Lymphocytopenia is a condition in which your blood has a low number of white blood cells called lymphocytes.

These cells are made in the bone marrow along with other kinds of blood cells. Lymphocytes help protect your body from infection. Low numbers of lymphocytes can increase your risk for infection.

Overview

About 20 to 40 percent of all white blood cells are lymphocytes. A normal lymphocyte count for adults usually is between 1,000 and 4,800 lymphocytes per microliter of blood. For children, a normal count usually is between 3,000 and 9,500 lymphocytes per microliter of blood.

"Lymphocytopenia" refers to a count of less than 1,000 lymphocytes per microliter of blood in adults or less than 3,000 lymphocytes per microliter of blood in children.

There are three types of lymphocytes: B lymphocytes, T lymphocytes, and natural killer cells. All of these cells help protect the body from infection. Most people who have lymphocytopenia have low numbers of T lymphocytes. Sometimes they also have low numbers of the other types of lymphocytes.

Outlook

Lymphocytopenia can range from mild to severe. The condition alone may not cause any signs, symptoms, or serious problems.

How long lymphocytopenia lasts depends on its cause. The treatment for this condition also depends on its cause and severity. Mild lymphocytopenia may not require treatment. If an underlying condition is successfully treated, lymphocytopenia will likely improve.

If you get serious infections due to lymphocytopenia, you may need medicines or other treatments.

What Causes Lymphocytopenia?

In general, lymphocytopenia (a low lymphocyte count) occurs because of one or more of the following:

- The body doesn't make enough lymphocytes.

- The body makes enough lymphocytes, but they are destroyed due to an abnormal condition.

- The lymphocytes get stuck in the spleen or lymph nodes.

- A combination of these factors also may cause a low lymphocyte count.

A number of diseases, conditions, and factors can cause the problems that lead to a low lymphocyte count. These conditions can be inherited (passed from parents to children), or they can develop at any age.

Exactly how each disease, condition, or factor affects your lymphocyte count isn't known. Sometimes, people have low lymphocyte counts with no underlying cause.

Acquired Causes

A number of acquired diseases, conditions, and factors can cause lymphocytopenia. Examples include the following:

- Infectious diseases, such as acquired immunodeficiency syndrome (AIDS), viral hepatitis, tuberculosis, and typhoid fever

- Autoimmune disorders, such as lupus

- Steroid therapy

- Blood cancer and other blood diseases, such as Hodgkin disease and aplastic anemia

- Radiation and chemotherapy (treatments for cancer)

Inherited Causes

Certain inherited diseases and conditions can lead to lymphocytopenia. Examples include DiGeorge anomaly, Wiskott-Aldrich syndrome, severe combined immunodeficiency syndrome, and ataxia-telangiectasia. These inherited conditions are rare.

What Are the Signs and Symptoms of Lymphocytopenia?

Lymphocytopenia alone may not cause any signs or symptoms. The condition usually is found when a person is tested for other diseases or conditions, such as AIDS.

If you have unusual infections, repeat infections, and/or infections that won't go away, your doctor may suspect that you have lymphocytopenia. Fever is the most common symptom linked to infections.

How Is Lymphocytopenia Diagnosed?

Your doctor will diagnose lymphocytopenia based on your medical history, a physical exam, and the results from tests.

Lymphocytopenia alone may not cause any signs or symptoms. As a result, the condition often is diagnosed during testing for other diseases or conditions.

Diagnostic Tests

Your doctor may order one or more of the following tests to help diagnose a low lymphocyte count.

Complete blood count with differential. A complete blood count (CBC) measures many different parts of your blood. It checks the number of red blood cells, white blood cells, and platelets in your blood. The CBC shows whether you have a low number of white blood cells.

Lymphocytes account for 20 to 40 percent of all white blood cells. Although a CBC will show an overall low white blood cell count, it won't show whether the number of lymphocytes is low.

You may need a more detailed test, called a CBC with differential, to see whether you have a low lymphocyte count. This test shows whether you have low levels of different types of white blood cells, such as lymphocytes. The results of this test can help your doctor diagnose lymphocytopenia.

Flow cytometry. This test looks at many types of blood cells. It's even more detailed than a CBC with differential.

Flow cytometry can measure the levels of the different types of lymphocytes—T cells, B cells, and natural killer cells. This can help diagnose the underlying cause of lymphocytopenia. Some underlying conditions cause low levels of T cells. Others may cause low levels of B cells or natural killer cells.

Tests for underlying conditions. A number of diseases and conditions can cause lymphocytopenia. Thus, your doctor will want to find out what's causing the condition. You may be tested for human immunodeficiency virus (HIV)/AIDS, tuberculosis, blood diseases, and immune disorders.

Tests for these underlying conditions might include blood tests, bone marrow tests, and lymph node tests.

Lymph nodes are part of the immune system. They're found in many places in your body. During a physical exam, your doctor may find that certain lymph nodes are swollen. In lymphocytopenia, the lymph nodes may hold on to too many lymphocytes and not release them into the bloodstream.

To test a lymph node, you may need to have it removed. This involves a minor surgical procedure.

How Is Lymphocytopenia Treated?

If you have mild lymphocytopenia with no underlying cause, you may not need any treatment. The condition may improve on its own.

If you have unusual infections, repeat infections, and/or infections that won't go away due to lymphocytopenia, you'll need treatment for the infections.

If you have a disease or condition that's causing lymphocytopenia, your doctor will prescribe treatment for that illness. Treating the underlying problem will help treat the lymphocytopenia.

Emerging Treatments

Researchers are looking at ways to increase lymphocyte production in people who have lymphocytopenia with serious underlying conditions.

For example, some studies are looking into blood and marrow stem cell transplants. Conditions that cause the body to not make enough blood cells, including lymphocytes, may cause lymphocytopenia. A blood or marrow stem cell transplant may help treat or cure some of these conditions.

Other studies are looking at medicines and other substances that can help the body make more lymphocytes.

Talk to your doctor about whether a clinical study might benefit you.

Section 22.4

Neutropenia

What Is Neutropenia?

Neutropenia is a disorder of the blood, with low levels of a special type of cell called the neutrophil. There are many types of cells in the blood, but the two main kinds are red blood cells and white blood cells.

A neutrophil is a type of white blood cell, which helps destroy bacteria in the body. Therefore someone who has low levels of neutrophils is more likely to get bacterial infections. There are many causes for neutropenia—sometimes it can occur after an infection, ingestion of a particular drug, or some people can be born with it. If the neutrophil levels fall extremely low, the condition is called agranulocytosis.

Who Gets Neutropenia?

Internationally the incidence of agranulocytosis is 3.4 cases per million persons per year. The incidence of drug-induced neutropenia is 1 case per million persons per year.

Predisposing Factors

Patients can be at increased risk of neutropenia due to congenital (patient is born with the condition) or acquired causes.

Congenital Neutropenias

- **Chronic benign neutropenia:** This group of people can be born with low levels of neutrophils and experience only mild infections.

- **Congenital immune defects:** These patients have abnormal levels of immunoglobulins (part of a group of large proteins secreted by white cells, called plasma cells, that play an important part in our body's immune response) and have a high infection risk.

- **Congenital or chronic neutropenias:** This group includes Kostmann syndrome, which is a severe neutropenia apparent in babies by age three months, with the child experiencing recurrent bacterial infections.

- **Idiopathic chronic severe neutropenia:** Some cases of neutropenia occur when there is no known or apparent cause.

- **Neutropenia associated with phenotypic (observable physical features of an organism, as determined by both genetic makeup and environmental factors) abnormalities:** There are some conditions, such as Shwachman syndrome and Barth syndrome, which are associated with specific physical abnormalities and a moderate to severe neutropenia.

- **Metabolic diseases:** These include glycogen storage diseases. Variable neutrophil counts are observed.

- **Immune mediated neutropenia:** Here, the immune system produces antibodies to immunoglobulins, which results in severe neutropenia.

Acquired Neutropenias

- The most common cause of acquired neutropenia are infections.

- Vitamin B$_{12}$, folate, copper, and low levels of other nutrients can cause neutropenia.

- Many drugs and chemicals can be involved:

  - Medications for the thyroid gland, and certain types of antibiotics are most frequently involved.

  - Antibiotics include cephalosporins, penicillin, gentamicin, clindamycin, trimethoprim, and vancomycin.

  - Anti-inflammatory agents and pain killers such as ibuprofen, acetylsalicylic acid and aminopyrine are involved.

  - Antidepressants and antipsychotics including phenothiazines (chlorpromazine), clozapine, risperidone, imipramine, and desipramine may be seen to produce neutropenia.

  - Drugs for the thyroid gland include carbimazole, thiouracil, propylthiouracil, and methimazole.

  - Drugs involved with the heart—procainamide, propranolol, captopril, aprindine, hydralazine, methyldopa, and nifedipine—may be implicated.

- Heavy metals such as gold and mercury should be considered.

- Drugs used in cancer patients for chemotherapy and radio-therapy. Most chemotherapy agents are myelosuppressive (they suppress bone marrow function and thus production of white blood cells, including neutrophils).

Progression

If you have been diagnosed with neutropenia, your body is more likely to develop bacterial infections. Prolonged neutropenia also increases the risk of widespread infection with fungi. Neutropenia alone does not place you at increased risk of parasitic or viral infections.

Probable Outcomes

It is hard to predict what might happen to the patient with this condition. Infections obtained in people with low levels of neutrophils are usually severe and can be life threatening. Any sick patients with neutropenia should be treated with an antibiotic with a wide range of activity if there are any signs of infection.

How Will Neutropenia Affect Me?

Patients with low levels of neutrophils can have many problems. If you are affected by this condition, there may be signs of infection such as fever (temperature above 101.3° F), aches and pains, shortness of breath, productive coughing, chest pain, ear pain, sore throat, headache, etc. The lower the neutrophil count, the greater the risk of infection. Other symptoms may be a result of low levels of other cells that have been affected. This can produce anemia symptoms such as tiredness, weakness, and shortness of breath. If there are low platelets (cells which help the body's blood to clot) there may be bruising and increased nosebleeds. It is important to remember that every person with neutropenia is unique and will experience different symptoms.

It may be important to tell your doctor what medications you are taking, as these may have an effect on the condition. A family history may reveal that some other people in your family experienced similar problems.

If you have had any tests done, the results of these tests should be obtained and passed on to the doctor. These results can help in telling the doctor how long your neutropenia has been going on for.

311

Clinical Examination

People with neutropenia get many infections. During your examination, the doctor may find some signs of infections. Most infections occur in the mouth, lungs, and skin:

- Examination of the mouth area may reveal some signs of thrush (e.g., white coating on tongue), gum infections, and painful mouth ulcers.

- Abnormal lumps, which may be enlarged glands, may indicate spread of infection or, possibly, malignancy.

- There may be some rashes, ulcers, or abnormal sores on your skin.

- If needed, the area around your buttocks and rectum may be examined for sores, rashes, or enlarged nodes.

How Is Neutropenia Diagnosed?

The following tests may be ordered as the doctor sees appropriate:

- Blood may be taken for a complete blood examination. The severity of neutropenia depends on the absolute neutrophil count (ANC) and is categorized as follows:

  - Mild: ANC of 1000–1500 cells per mm3.

  - Moderate: ANC falls between 500 and 1000 cells per mm3.

  - Severe: ANC falls below 500 per mm3.

- In patients with fevers, the following tests may be obtained:

  - Two sets of blood taken for cultures (a procedure to see if any organisms are grown in the blood)

  - Urine for investigation

  - Chest x-ray, looking for signs of chest infections

  - Sputum analysis, looking for any growths of organisms

- HIV testing may be carried out, if suspected in the patient.

- If low levels of blood and low platelets are present, Vitamin B_{12} and folate levels may be obtained. Obtaining bone marrow from within our bones helps assess for any problems within the marrow.

How Is Neutropenia Treated?

If you are affected by neutropenia, the doctor will provide supportive care such as oxygen, pain or fever relief, and education. Care may vary depending on the cause, severity, and duration of your neutropenia.

Antibacterial (Antibiotic) Therapy

If you have neutropenia, you are more likely to become infected with a wide variety of bacteria. Antibiotic therapy targeting these bacteria should be started immediately if there are any signs of infection. You are susceptible to many bacteria normally found on the skin and in the bowel. There are a few rules that may guide your treatment:

- The doctor should give you antibiotics active against bacteria that could be causing your infection.

- The antibiotics used should target the bacteria commonly found in the hospital you are staying in.

- If you are already receiving antibiotics, the choice of subsequent antibiotics to treat any bacterial infections should target resistant organisms. Organisms known to cause infections in patients being treated with antibiotics already given should also be targeted.

The initial antibiotic treatment should be reviewed on the basis of test results.

Antifungal Therapy

If you are a cancer patient, fungal infections are most often associated with neutropenia. You are predisposed to the development of invasive fungal infections, most commonly those due to *Candida* and *Aspergillus* species.

Conventionally, it has been common clinical practice to add an antifungal drug called Amphotericin B to treatment regimens, if a neutropenic patient continues to have a fever after four to seven days of treatment. This is because it is difficult to grow fungi before the onset of widespread disease, which is associated with a high mortality.

Fluconazole is another antifungal drug which has demonstrated efficacy against infections due to many *Candida* species. However it has no activity against some fungal species like *Aspergillus*. Newer antifungal drugs can target a wider spectrum of fungi (e.g., Voriconazole), thus providing another option for the treatment of fungal infections.

313

Antiviral Therapy

If you are a cancer patient, viral infections can cause large problems. There has been increasing availability of drugs with activity against Herpes group viruses. Serious infections due to herpes viruses and cytomegalovirus have been well documented, and varicella zoster virus (implicated in chicken pox and shingles) infections may be fatal in patients receiving chemotherapy. Acyclovir is an antiviral drug that is well known, which can be used for treatment or prevention of infection.

Other Therapeutic Modalities

Another option in treating your neutropenia is to replenish the amount of neutrophils in the body. Transfusing the cells that neutrophils are produced from helps treat some bacterial infections. However, this treatment is expensive and associated with side effects. This treatment is usually reserved for patients who are unresponsive to antibiotics.

References

Godwin JE, Shin JJ. Neutropenia 2005 E-medicine [serial online]. 2005 [cited 29th April 2006]. Available from URL: www.emedicine. com/MED/topic1640.htm.

Kasper DL. Harrisons *Principles of Internal Medicine*. New York: The McGraw-Hill Companies; 2006.

Kumar V, Abbas A K & Fausto N. *Robbins & Cotran Pathologic Basis of Disease*. China: Elseiver Saunders; 2005.

Kumar P, Clark M. *Clinical Medicine*. United Kingdom: WB Saunders; 2002.

Peakman M, Vergani D. *Basic and Clinical Immunology*. USA: Churchill Livingstone, 2000.

Part Four

Bleeding and Clotting Disorders

Chapter 23

What Are Hereditary Bleeding and Clotting Disorders?

What Is a Bleeding Disorder?

Bleeding disorders is a general term for a wide range of medical problems that lead to poor blood clotting and continuous bleeding. Doctors also call them terms such as coagulopathy, abnormal bleeding, and clotting disorders.

When someone has a bleeding disorder they have a tendency to bleed longer. The disorders can result from defects in the blood vessels or from abnormalities in the blood itself. The abnormalities may be in blood clotting factors or in platelets.

Blood clotting, or coagulation, is the process that controls bleeding. It changes blood from a liquid to a solid. It's a complex process involving as many as twenty different plasma proteins, or blood clotting factors. Normally, a complex chemical process occurs using these clotting factors to form a substance called fibrin that stops bleeding. When certain coagulation factors are deficient or missing, the process doesn't occur normally.

Within seconds of an injury, tiny cells in the blood, called platelets, bunch together around the wound. Blood proteins, platelets, calcium, and other tissue factors react together and form what's called a clot, which acts like a net over the wound. Over the next several days to weeks, the clot strengthens, then dissolves when the wound is healed.

Reprinted from "What Is a Bleeding Disorder?" and "What Are Clotting Disorders?" © 2006 National Hemophilia Foundation (www.hemophilia.org). Reprinted with permission.

In people with bleeding disorders, clotting factors are missing or don't work as they should. This causes them to bleed for a longer time than those whose blood factor levels are normal. It's a myth that persons with bleeding disorders bleed to death from minor injuries or their blood flows faster. Bleeding problems can range from mild to severe.

Symptoms include:

- excessive bleeding;

- excessive bruising;

- easy bleeding;

- nose bleeds;

- abnormal menstrual bleeding.

Bleeding disorder risks include:

- scarring of the joints or joint disease;

- vision loss from bleeding into the eye;

- chronic anemia from blood loss (anemia is a low red blood cell count);

- neurologic or psychiatric problems;

- death, which may occur with large amounts of blood loss or bleeding in critical areas, such as the brain.

Causes

Some bleeding disorders are present at birth and are caused by rare inherited disorders. Others are developed during certain illnesses (such as vitamin K deficiency, severe liver disease) or treatments (such as use of anticoagulant drugs or prolonged use of antibiotics). They can include hemophilia and other very rare blood disorders. There are many causes of bleeding disorders, including:

- von Willebrand disease, which is an inherited blood disorder thought to affect between 1 and 2 percent of the population;

- immune system–related diseases, such as allergic reactions to medications, or reactions to an infection;

- cancer, such as leukemia, which is a blood cancer;

- liver disease;

- bone marrow problems;

- disseminated intravascular coagulation, which is a condition often associated with childbearing, cancer, or infection, in which the body's clotting system functions abnormally;

- pregnancy-associated eclampsia, also known as severe toxicity of pregnancy;

- antibodies, a type of immune system protein, that destroy blood clotting factors;

- medicines, such as aspirin, heparin, warfarin, and drugs used to break up blood clots.

Congenital bleeding disorders are very rare, and with the exception of hemophilia and von Willebrand disease, education about them has not been a priority of the medical community. Most have only been discovered and described in the past few decades.

What Are Clotting Disorders?

Clotting disorders is a term used to describe a group of conditions in which there is an increased tendency, often repeated and over an extended period of time, for excessive clotting.

These disorders include inherited conditions such as factor V Leiden, protein C deficiency, protein S deficiency, anti-thrombin deficiency, and prothrombin 20210A mutations.

Thrombophilia affects a large number of people around the world. Factor V Leiden is the most common inherited abnormality in this class. It affects approximately 5 to 7 percent of the Caucasian population of European descent in the United States.

People who experience episodes of thrombosis, either as an isolated event or as a repeated event, may be affected with a thrombophilic disorder. There are people who have inherited the gene, who have an increased tendency for thrombosis, but may never personally experience a blood clot. Many people can have a known thrombophilic condition and never experience a thrombosis.

The development of a blood clot is called thrombosis. The vascular system includes both the venous system (the veins that deliver blood from the tissues to the heart) and the arterial system (the system that delivers blood from the heart to the tissues). Thrombotic episodes may occur in either system. The symptoms relate to the part of the vascular system in which they occur, the extent of the clot, and whether the clot breaks off and travels to another part of the body (e.g., the lungs—pulmonary embolus, the brain—embolic stroke, etc.). There are different terms used to further define these thrombotic episodes, such as deep vein thrombosis (DVT) or peripheral vascular disease, when the clots are in the arterial system (usually in the extremities). Although we are now able to determine the underlying cause in some patients and families for this tendency to an increased risk of excessive blood clotting, we are still not able to make this determination in all cases. This means that there is still more to be understood about why some persons and families have thrombophilia.

Recent research shows that these disorders contribute significantly to morbidity and mortality in the United States. Each year, more than six hundred thousand Americans die from abnormal blood clots.

Even though men and women can have clotting disorders, these conditions pose added difficulties for women because of their relationship to reproductive issues. Women with these disorders can develop serious complications during pregnancy leading to miscarriage. Pregnancy, oral contraceptives, and postmenopausal hormone replacement therapy are all triggering events for DVT in women with thrombophilia.

What Is Thrombophilia?

Thrombophilia is the reverse side of the process of blood clotting when compared to hemophilia. While people with hemophilia have an increased tendency to bleed, people with thrombophilia have an increased tendency to clot. Just as hemophilia is caused by an abnormality of a blood-clotting factor, some forms of thrombophilia are also caused by an abnormality or deficiency of a blood-clotting factor. In some cases these clotting factors may have an abnormality that leads to an increase in their function (such as factor V Leiden).

Thrombophilia is not a new disease, but it has become a more recognized and more discussed due to an increased ability to test for and identify some of the underlying contributing abnormalities.

Thrombosis is a very common medical problem. It is estimated that approximately two million people experience a DVT each year in the United States. In addition, nearly half of patients with deep vein clots experience long-term health consequences that adversely affect their quality of life and require millions of dollars of treatment. Thrombosis may manifest itself as the formation or presence of a blood clot in a blood vessel or one of the cavities in the heart. In fact, emboli (clots or plugs brought by the blood from another blood vessel and forced into a smaller vessel so as to obstruct the circulation) from deep vein clots are a leading cause of death in hospitalized patients. Annually, two hundred thousand to three hundred thousand patients develop this form of clot for the first time during a hospitalization. Nearly 40 percent of these patients suffer from a complication known as pulmonary embolism (a clot that travels to the lung and obstructs a significant amount of blood flow to the organ). This complication is fatal in 30 percent of the cases.

Both children and adults can have thrombophilia. However, it is more commonly diagnosed in adolescents and adults due to normal changes in the hemostatic balance that occur with growth and aging.

Genetic thrombophilia is an inherited abnormality that leads to an increased risk of thrombosis throughout a person's life. The most common inherited thrombophilic disorder is factor V Leiden, initially described by Dr. B. Dahlback in 1993. Acquired thrombophilia refers to a group of disorders that an individual is not born with, but may develop throughout his or her life due to another circumstance such as illness. An example of acquired thrombophilia is the development of a lupus anticoagulant or antiphospholipid antibody syndrome.

People with thrombophilia may receive medications that affect the coagulation system, just as people with hemophilia do, but not always in the same manner. Some people with thrombophilia may be prescribed products to treat their thrombophilia either on a long-term or an intermittent basis, depending on the underlying cause of their thrombophilia. Some people with thrombophilia are treated with medications that are classified as blood thinners, which decrease a person's ability to form a clot. Examples of these medications include aspirin, heparin, low molecular weight heparin, and Coumadin®. There are also some specific medications (thrombolytic agents) that are given under certain circumstances to dissolve clots. People with hemophilia, who have central venous access devices that have become clotted, may receive small doses of these medications locally. People with thrombosis may receive these agents in larger doses that are either given at the site of thrombosis or systemically. People with thrombophilia may receive medications only during a time of increased risk of thrombosis or for a prolonged period of time (even for a lifetime), depending on their specific diagnosis and clinical circumstances.

Many healthcare professionals take care of people with thrombophilia. For example, primary healthcare providers (pediatricians, internal medicine physicians, family practitioners, obstetricians and gynecologists, emergency physicians, etc.) may all care for patients with this disorder. Subspecialists, such as pulmonologists, vascular surgeons, neurologists, and hematologists, may also care for this patient population. Other specialists, such as pathologists and radiologists, may provide services to these patients including diagnostic and interventional services. There is an increasing need to have these patients seen by a team of medical professionals within one facility.

Similar to hemophilia care and prevention services delivered through hemostasis and thrombosis centers (HTCs), the Centers for Disease Control (CDC) has launched a pilot program to demonstrate the effectiveness of multidisciplinary comprehensive care to people with clotting disorders.

Chapter 24

Hemophilia

What Is Hemophilia?

Hemophilia is a rare, inherited bleeding disorder in which your blood doesn't clot normally. If you have hemophilia, you may bleed for a longer time than others after an injury. You also may bleed internally, especially in your knees, ankles, and elbows. This bleeding can damage your organs or tissues and, sometimes, be fatal.

People born with hemophilia have little to none of a protein needed for normal blood clotting. The protein is called a clotting factor. There are several types of clotting factors, and they work together with platelets to help the blood clot. Platelets are small pieces of blood cells that are formed in the bone marrow. They play a major role in blood clotting.

When blood vessels are injured, clotting factors help the platelets stick together to plug cuts and breaks at the site of the injury to stop the bleeding. Without clotting factors, normal blood clotting can't take place. Sometimes people with hemophilia need injections of a clotting factor or factors to stop bleeding.

There are two main types of hemophilia. If you have hemophilia A, you have little to no clotting factor VIII (8). About nine out of ten people with hemophilia have type A. If you have hemophilia B, you're missing or have low levels of clotting factor IX (9).

Excerpted from "Hemophilia," National Heart Lung and Blood Institute, National Institutes of Health, August 2008.

Hemophilia can be mild, moderate, or severe, depending on how much clotting factor is in the blood. About seven out of ten people who have hemophilia A have the severe form of the disorder. People who don't have hemophilia have a factor VIII activity of 100 percent; people who have severe hemophilia A have a factor VIII activity of less than 1 percent.

In addition to being inherited, hemophilia also can be acquired, which means that you can develop it during your lifetime. It can develop if your body forms antibodies to the clotting factors in your bloodstream. The antibodies can block the clotting factors from working. Only inherited hemophilia is discussed in this chapter.

About eighteen thousand people in the United States have hemophilia. Each year, about four hundred babies are born with the disorder. Hemophilia usually occurs only in males (with very rare exceptions).

Other Names for Hemophilia

Hemophilia A

- Classic hemophilia
- Factor VIII deficiency

Hemophilia B

- Christmas disease
- Factor IX deficiency

What Causes Hemophilia?

If you have inherited hemophilia, you're born with the condition. It's caused by a defect in one of the genes that determine how the body makes blood clotting factors VIII or IX. These genes are located on the X chromosomes.

Chromosomes come in pairs. Females have two X chromosomes, while males have one X and one Y chromosome. Only the X chromosome carries the genes related to clotting factors.

A male who has the abnormal gene on his X chromosome will have hemophilia. A female must have the abnormal gene on both of her X chromosomes to have hemophilia; this is very rare.

A female is a "carrier" of hemophilia if she has the abnormal gene on one of her X chromosomes. Even though she doesn't have the condition, she can pass the gene on to her children.

Females who are carriers usually have enough clotting factors from their one normal X chromosome to prevent serious bleeding problems. Very rarely, a girl is born with hemophilia. This can happen if her father has hemophilia and her mother is a carrier.

Some males with the disorder are born to mothers who aren't carriers. In these cases, a mutation (random change) occurs in the gene as it is passed to the child.

What Are the Signs and Symptoms of Hemophilia?

The major signs and symptoms of hemophilia are excessive bleeding and easy bruising.

Excessive Bleeding

The extent of bleeding depends on the type and severity of the hemophilia. Children with mild hemophilia may not have symptoms until they have excessive bleeding from a dental procedure, an accident, or surgery. Males with severe hemophilia may bleed heavily after circumcision. Bleeding can be obvious (external bleeding) or hidden within the body (internal bleeding).

Signs of excessive external bleeding include the following:

* Bleeding in the mouth from a cut or bite or from cutting or losing a tooth

* Nosebleeds for no obvious reason

* Heavy bleeding from a minor cut

* Bleeding from a cut that resumes after stopping for a short time

Signs of internal bleeding include blood in the urine (from bleeding in the kidneys or bladder) and blood in the stool (from bleeding in the intestines or stomach).

Bleeding in the Joints

Bleeding in the knees, elbows, or other joints is another common form of internal bleeding in people with hemophilia. This can occur without obvious injury. At first, this bleeding causes tightness in the joint with no real pain or any visible signs of bleeding. The joint then becomes swollen, hot to touch, and painful to bend.

Swelling continues as bleeding continues, and eventually movement in the joint is temporarily lost. Pain can be severe. Joint bleeding that isn't quickly treated can permanently damage the joint.

Bleeding in the Brain

Internal bleeding in the brain is a very serious complication of hemophilia that can happen after a simple bump on the head or a more serious injury. The signs and symptoms of bleeding in the brain include the following:

- Long-lasting painful headaches or neck pain or stiffness

- Repeated vomiting

- Changes in behavior or being very sleepy

- Sudden weakness or clumsiness of the arms or legs or difficulty walking

- Double vision

- Convulsions or seizures

How Is Hemophilia Diagnosed?

If hemophilia is suspected or if you appear to have a bleeding problem, your doctor will take a personal and family medical history. This will reveal whether you or anyone in your family has a history of frequent and/or heavy bleeding and bruising. Your doctor also will do a physical exam and order blood tests.

Blood tests are used to determine the following:

- How long it takes for your blood to clot

- Whether your blood has low levels of any of the clotting factors

- Whether one of the factors is completely missing from your blood

The test results will show if you have hemophilia, what type of hemophilia you have, and how severe it is.

Hemophilia A and B are classified as mild, moderate, or severe, depending on the amount of clotting factor VIII or IX in the blood. Mild hemophilia is defined as having 5 to 30 percent of normal clotting factor, moderate hemophilia is defined as having 1 to 5 percent of normal clotting factor, and severe hemophilia is defined as having less than 1 percent of normal clotting factor.

The degree of symptoms can overlap between the categories. For example, some people with mild hemophilia may have bleeding problems almost as often or as problematic as some people with moderate hemophilia.

Severe hemophilia can cause serious bleeding problems in babies. Therefore, children with severe hemophilia are usually diagnosed during the first year of life. People with milder forms of hemophilia may not be diagnosed until they're adults.

The bleeding problems of hemophilia A and hemophilia B are the same. Only special blood tests can tell which type a person has. Knowing which type is important because the treatments are different.

Pregnant women who are known carriers of hemophilia can have the condition diagnosed in their unborn child as early as ten weeks into their pregnancy.

Women who are hemophilia carriers also can have "preimplantation diagnosis" to have a child without hemophilia. For this process, women have their eggs removed and then fertilized by sperm in a laboratory. The embryos that result from this fertilization are then tested for hemophilia. Only embryos that lack the condition will then be implanted in the womb.

How Is Hemophilia Treated?

Treatment with Replacement Therapy

The main treatment for hemophilia is called replacement therapy—giving or replacing the clotting factor that's too low or missing. Concentrates of clotting factor VIII (for hemophilia A) or clotting factor IX (for hemophilia B) are slowly dripped in or injected into a vein.

Clotting factor concentrates can be made from human blood that has been treated to prevent the spread of diseases, such as hepatitis. With the new methods of screening and treating donated blood, the risk of developing an infectious disease from clotting factors taken from human blood is now very small.

To further reduce that risk, you or your child can take clotting factor concentrates that don't use human blood. These are called recombinant clotting factors. Clotting factors are easy to store, mix, and use at home—it takes only about fifteen minutes to receive the factor.

You may have replacement therapy on a regular basis to prevent bleeding. This is called preventive or prophylactic therapy. Or, you may only need replacement therapy to stop bleeding when it occurs. This use of the treatment, on an as-needed basis, is called demand therapy. Therapy that's given as needed is less intensive and less expensive than preventive therapy. However, there is a risk that bleeding will cause damage before the as-needed treatment is given.

Complications of Replacement Therapy

Complications of replacement therapy include the following:

- Developing antibodies, which are proteins that act against the clotting factors

- Developing viral infections from human clotting factors

- Damage to joints, muscles, or other parts of the body resulting from delays in treatment

Antibodies to the clotting factor. Antibodies destroy the clotting factor before it has a chance to work. This is a very serious problem, because it makes the main treatment for hemophilia—replacing clotting factors—no longer effective.

Antibodies to clotting factor develop in about 20 percent of people with severe hemophilia A and 1 percent of people with hemophilia B.

When antibodies develop, doctors may use larger doses of clotting factors or try different sources of the clotting factor. Sometimes, the antibodies go away. Researchers are studying ways to deal with antibodies to clotting factors.

Viruses from human blood factors. The viruses that cause human immunodeficiency virus/acquired immunodeficiency syndrome (HIV/AIDS) and hepatitis can be carried in clotting factors. However, there has been no documented case of these viruses being transmitted during replacement therapy for about a decade.

Transmission of viruses has been prevented by the following measures:

- Careful screening of blood donors

- Testing of donated blood products

- Treating donated blood products with a detergent and heat to destroy viruses

- Vaccinating people with hemophilia for hepatitis A and B

Researchers continue to find ways to make blood products safer.

Home Treatment with Replacement Therapy

Both preventive and as-needed replacement therapy can be done at home. Many people learn to do the infusions at home for their child or for themselves. Home treatment has several advantages:

- You or your child can get treatment quicker when bleeding happens. Early treatment means that fewer complications are likely to occur.

- Fewer visits to the doctor or emergency room are needed.

- Home treatment costs less than treatment in a medical care setting.

- Home treatment helps children accept treatment and take responsibility for their own health.

Discuss options for home treatment with your doctor or your child's doctor. A doctor or other health care provider can teach you the steps and safety procedures for home treatment. Another valuable resource for learning about home treatment is hemophilia treatment centers.

Vein access devices can be surgically implanted to make it easier to get into a vein for treatment with replacement therapy. These devices can be helpful when such treatment occurs often. However, infections can be a problem with these devices. Your doctor can help you decide whether this type of device is right for you or your child.

Other Types of Treatment

Desmopressin. Desmopressin (DDAVP) is a man-made hormone used to treat people with mild to moderate hemophilia A. DDAVP can't be used to treat hemophilia B or severe hemophilia A.

DDAVP stimulates the release of stored factor VIII and von Willebrand factor and increases the level of these proteins in your blood. Von Willebrand factor carries and binds factor VIII, which then can stay in the bloodstream longer.

DDAVP usually is given by injection or in a nasal spray. Because the effect of this medicine wears off when used often, it's given only in certain situations. For example, your doctor may have you take this medicine prior to dental work or before playing certain sports to prevent or reduce bleeding.

Antifibrinolytic medicines. Antifibrinolytic medicines (including tranexamic acid and aminocaproic acid) may be used with replacement therapy. They're usually given as a pill, and they help keep clots from breaking down. They're most often used before dental work, for treating bleeding from the mouth or nose, and for mild intestinal bleeding.

Gene therapy. Researchers are trying to develop ways to correct the defective genes that cause hemophilia to cure the disorder. Such gene therapy hasn't yet developed to the point that it's an accepted treatment. But researchers continue to test gene therapies for hemophilia in clinical trials.

Which Treatment Is Best for You?

The type of treatment you or your child receives depends on several things, including how severe the hemophilia is, what activities you will be doing, and what dental or medical procedures you will be having.

- **Mild hemophilia:** Replacement therapy isn't usually needed for mild hemophilia. But DDAVP is sometimes given to raise the body's levels of factor VIII.

- **Moderate hemophilia:** You may need replacement therapy only when bleeding occurs or to prevent bleeding that could occur when participating in some activity. DDAVP is another treatment option on occasion, prior to having a procedure or doing an activity that increases the risk of bleeding.

- **Severe hemophilia:** You usually need replacement therapy to prevent bleeding that could cause permanent damage to your joints, muscles, or other parts of the body. Typically, replacement therapy is given at home two or three times a week. It may be needed on a long-term basis or just for short periods when you expect to do an activity that might increase your risk of bleeding. However, some people with severe hemophilia receive treatment only when bleeding occurs.

For all types of hemophilia, getting treatment quickly for bleeding to limit damage is important. Learn to recognize signs of bleeding. Family members also should learn to watch for signs of bleeding in a child with hemophilia. Children sometimes ignore signs of bleeding because they want to avoid the discomfort of treatment.

Living with Hemophilia

If you or your child has hemophilia, you can take steps to prevent bleeding problems. Thanks to improvements in treatment, a child with hemophilia today is likely to live a normal lifespan.

Ongoing Health Care Needs

To avoid complications, it's important that people who have hemophilia do the following:

- Continue any treatment prescribed for hemophilia.

- Get regular checkups and vaccinations as recommended. Vaccines for hepatitis A and B are recommended for those who are treated with blood transfusions. There is currently no vaccine for hepatitis C.

- Tell all of your health care providers, such as your doctor, dentist, and pharmacist, that you have hemophilia. You also may want to tell people like your employee health nurse, gym trainer, and sports coach about your condition.

- Get regular dental care. Dentists at the HTCs are experts in providing dental care for people who have hemophilia. If you see another dentist, tell the dentist that you or your child has hemophilia. The dentist can provide medicine that will reduce bleeding during dental work.

- Know the signs and symptoms of bleeding in joints and other parts of the body and when to call the doctor or go to the emergency room.

Contact your doctor or go to the emergency room when any of the following occur:

- Heavy bleeding that can't be stopped or a wound that continues to ooze blood.

- Any signs or symptoms of bleeding in the brain. Such bleeding is life threatening and requires immediate emergency care.

- Limited motion, pain, or swelling of any joint.

It's a good idea to keep a record of all previous treatments. Be sure to take this information with you to medical appointments and to the hospital or emergency room.

When Your Child Is Diagnosed with Hemophilia

Young children with hemophilia need extra protection from things in the home and elsewhere that could cause injuries and lead to bleeding:

- Protect toddlers with kneepads, elbow pads, and protective helmets. All children should wear safety helmets when riding tricycles or bicycles.

- Be sure to use the safety belts and straps in highchairs, car seats, and strollers to protect the child from falls.

331

- Remove furniture with sharp corners or pad them while the child is a toddler.

- Keep out of reach or locked away small and sharp objects and other items that could cause bleeding or harm.

- Check play equipment and outdoor play areas for possible hazards.

You also need to learn how to examine your child for and recognize signs of bleeding as well as prepare for bleeding episodes when they do occur. Keep a cold pack in the freezer ready to use as directed or to take along with you to treat bumps and bruises. Popsicles work fine when there is minor bleeding in the mouth. You also might want to keep a bag ready to go with items you will need if you must take your child to the emergency room or elsewhere.

Be sure that anyone who is responsible for your child knows that he or she has hemophilia. Talk with your child's babysitters, daycare providers, teachers, other school staff, and coaches or leaders of after-school activities about when to contact you or to call 9-1-1 for emergency care.

Consider having your child wear a medical identification (ID) bracelet or necklace. If your child is injured, the ID will alert anyone caring for your child about the condition.

Physical Activity and Hemophilia

Physical activity helps keep muscles flexible, strengthens joints, and helps maintain a healthy weight. Children and adults with hemophilia should get regular physical activity, but they may have limits on what they can do safely.

People with mild hemophilia can participate in a variety of activities. Those with severe hemophilia should avoid contact sports and other activities that are likely to lead to injuries that could cause bleeding.

The physical therapist at the HTC can develop an exercise program tailored to your needs and teach you how to exercise safely. Talk with your doctor or physical therapist about recommended types of physical activity and sports.

To prevent bleeding, you also may be able to take clotting factors prior to exercise or a sporting event.

In general, some safe physical activities are swimming, biking (wear a helmet), walking, and golf.

Activities that aren't usually considered safe for those with bleeding problems include most contact sports, such as football, hockey, and wrestling.

Medicine Precautions

Some medicines increase the chance for bleeding. You should avoid medicines such as the following:

- Aspirin and other drugs that contain salicylates

- Ibuprofen, naproxen, and some other nonsteroidal anti-inflammatory drugs

For more information about medicines to avoid, talk to your doctor or pharmacist.

Treatment at Home and When Traveling

Home treatment with replacement therapy has many benefits. It lets you treat bleeding early before complications are likely to develop. Home treatment also can save you from having to make frequent trips to the doctor's office or hospital. This can give you more independence and a sense of control over your hemophilia.

But if you're treating yourself or your child with clotting factors at home, you should take some precautions:

- Follow instructions for storage, preparation, and use of clotting factors and treatment materials.

- Keep a record of all medical treatment.

- Know the signs and symptoms of bleeding, infection, or an allergic reaction, and how to respond appropriately.

- Have someone with you when you treat yourself.

- Know when to call the doctor or 9-1-1.

When you're traveling, be sure to take enough treatment materials along. You should carry with you a letter from your doctor describing your hemophilia and treatment. It's also a good idea to find out in advance where to go for care when out of town.

Chapter 25

Von Willebrand Disease

If you often have large, lumpy bruises; frequent or difficult-to-stop nosebleeds; bleed a lot after a fairly minor cut; or are a woman who has very heavy or long menstrual periods, you should ask your doctor about an inherited bleeding disorder called von Willebrand disease (VWD). Named for Dr. Erik von Willebrand, a Finnish doctor who first described the condition in 1926, VWD affects your blood's ability to clot and can lead to heavy, hard-to-stop bleeding after an injury. The bleeding from VWD can lead to damage of your internal organs or even be life threatening, but this is rare.

In VWD, you either have low levels of a certain protein in your blood or the protein doesn't work the way it should. The protein is called von Willebrand factor (VWF). It is made in the walls of your blood vessels and released into your blood.

Normally, when one of your blood vessels is injured, you start to bleed. As soon as this happens, small cells in your blood that are called platelets clump together to plug the hole in the blood vessel and stop the bleeding. Von Willebrand factor acts like glue to help the platelets stick together and form a blood clot.

Von Willebrand factor also carries with it clotting factor VIII (8), another important protein that helps your blood clot. Factor VIII is the protein that is inactive or missing in hemophilia, another clotting disorder.

Excerpted from "In Brief: Your Guide to von Willebrand Disease," National Heart Lung and Blood Institute, National Institutes of Health, January 2008.

Von Willebrand disease, like hemophilia, is an inherited bleeding disorder, but VWD is more common and usually milder. In fact, VWD is the most common of all the inherited bleeding disorders. It occurs in about one out of every one hundred to one thousand people. It also affects both males and females, while hemophilia mainly affects males.

There are three major types of von Willebrand disease:

- In type 1 VWD, you have a low level of the von Willebrand factor, and you may have lower levels of factor VIII than normal. This is the mildest and most common form of VWD. About three out of every four people with VWD have type 1 VWD.

- In type 2 VWD, the von Willebrand factor does not work the way it's supposed to. Type 2 VWD is divided into subtypes 2A, 2B, 2M, and 2N. Each type is caused by different gene mutations and treated differently. This makes knowing the exact type of VWD that you have very important.

- In type 3 VWD, you usually have no von Willebrand factor and low levels of factor VIII. Type 3 is the most serious form of VWD, but very rare.

Von Willebrand disease cannot be cured, but it can be treated. Early diagnosis is important, and with the right treatment plan, even people with type 3 VWD can be helped to live active lives.

What Causes von Willebrand disease?

Von Willebrand disease is almost always inherited. Your parents pass the gene for the disease on to you. You can develop types 1 or 2 VWD when only one of your parents carries the gene for it. You usually inherit type 3 VWD only if both of your parents pass the gene on to you. Your symptoms may be different from your parent's.

Some people develop a form of the disease later in life as a result of other medical conditions. This is called acquired von Willebrand syndrome (AVWS).

What Are the Signs and Symptoms of von Willebrand Disease?

The signs and symptoms of VWD depend on the type and severity of the disease. Many people have such mild symptoms that they may not know they have the disorder. Some people have the gene for the disease but don't have any symptoms.

If you have type 1 or type 2 VWD, you may have the following mild to moderate symptoms:

- Frequent large bruises from minor bumps or injuries
- Frequent or difficult-to-stop nosebleeds
- Extended bleeding from the gums after a dental procedure
- Heavy or extended menstrual bleeding in women
- Blood in your stools from bleeding in your intestines or stomach
- Blood in your urine from bleeding in your kidneys or bladder
- Heavy bleeding after a cut or other accident
- Heavy bleeding after surgery

Heavy menstrual bleeding is the most common symptom in women. If it isn't treated, it can lead to iron deficiency and anemia. (Not all heavy menstrual bleeding is due to VWD.)

If you have type 3 VWD, you may have any or all of the symptoms listed above, as well as the following:

- Severe bleeding episodes for no reason. These bleeding episodes can be life threatening if not treated right away.
- Bleeding into soft tissue or joints, causing severe pain and swelling.

How Is von Willebrand Disease Diagnosed?

Von Willebrand disease is sometimes difficult to diagnose. People with type 1 or type 2 VWD may not have major bleeding problems; as a result, they may not be diagnosed until they have heavy bleeding after surgery or some other trauma.

On the other hand, type 3 VWD can cause major bleeding problems during infancy and childhood. As a result, children with type 3 VWD are usually diagnosed during their first year of life.

To find out if you have VWD, your doctor will take a complete medical history and do a physical exam. For the history, he or she will likely want to know about your personal and family history—in particular these areas:

- Any episodes of bleeding from a small wound that lasted more than fifteen minutes or started up again within the first seven days following the injury
- Any episodes of extended, heavy, or repeated bleeding after surgery or dental extractions that required medical attention

- Any episodes of bruising with little or no apparent trauma, especially if you could feel a lump under the bruise

- A nosebleed that occurred for no apparent reason and lasted more than ten minutes despite pressure on the nose or a nosebleed that needed medical attention

- Any episode of blood in your stool for no apparent reason

- Any heavy menstrual bleeding in women (usually with clots or lasting longer than seven to ten days)

- Any history of muscle or joint bleeding

- Any medicines you've taken that might cause bleeding or increase the risk of bleeding—for example, aspirin, other nonsteroidal anti-inflammatory drugs (NSAIDs), clopidogrel (Plavix®), warfarin, or heparin

- Any history of liver or kidney disease, blood or bone marrow disease, or high or low blood platelet counts.

The doctor will also do a physical examination to look for the following:

- Unusual bruising or other signs of recent bleeding

- Evidence of liver disease or anemia

No single test exists for diagnosing VWD. As a result, your doctor will order a combination of blood tests to diagnose the disease. These tests may include the following:

- **Von Willebrand factor antigen:** This test measures the amount of von Willebrand factor in your blood.

- **Von Willebrand factor ristocetin cofactor activity:** This test shows how well the von Willebrand factor works.

- **Test for factor VIII clotting activity:** Some people with von Willebrand disease have low levels of factor VIII activity, while others have normal levels.

- **Von Willebrand factor multimers:** This test is performed if one or more of the three tests above are abnormal. It shows the makeup or structure of the von Willebrand factor. It helps your doctor diagnose what type of VWD you have.

- **Platelet function test:** This test measures how well your platelets are working.

Your doctor may order these tests more than once to confirm the diagnosis. He or she may also refer you to a hematologist (a doctor who specializes in treating blood diseases) to confirm the diagnosis and for follow-up care.

Early diagnosis is important to make sure you are treated effectively and can live a normal, active life.

How Is von Willebrand Disease Treated?

Your doctor will decide what treatment you need, based on the type of VWD you have and how severe it is. Most cases of von Willebrand disease are mild, and you may need treatment only if you have surgery, tooth extraction, or an accident.

Treatments for von Willebrand disease include medicines to do the following:

- Increase release of von Willebrand factor and factor VIII into the bloodstream

- Replace von Willebrand factor

- Prevent breakdown of clots

- Control heavy menstrual bleeding in women

Specific treatments are as follows:

- Desmopressin (DDAVP). This is a synthetic hormone that you usually take by injection or nasal spray. It makes your body release more von Willebrand factor and factor VIII into your bloodstream. DDAVP works for most patients with type 1 and some with type 2 VWD.

- VWF replacement therapy. This involves getting an infusion of a concentrate of von Willebrand factor and factor VIII into a vein in your arm. This treatment can be used if you: can't take DDAVP or need extended treatment, have type 1 VWD that doesn't respond to DDAVP, or have type 2 or type 3 VWD.

- Oral contraceptives, or birth control pills, can help women who have heavy menstrual bleeding. The hormones in the pills can increase the amount of VWF and factor VIII in the bloodstream.

- Antifibrinolytic drugs help prevent the breakdown of blood clots. They are used mostly to stop bleeding after minor surgery, tooth extraction, or an injury. They may be used alone or together with DDAVP and replacement therapy.

- Fibrin glue is medicine that is placed directly on a wound to stop the bleeding.

Tips for Living with von Willebrand Disease

It's important that you try to prevent bleeding and stay healthy. You should do the following things:

- Avoid over-the-counter medicines that can affect blood clotting, including aspirin, ibuprofen, and other nonsteroidal anti-inflammatory drugs (NSAIDs).

- Always check with your doctor before taking any medicines.

- Tell your doctor or dentist that you have von Willebrand disease. Your dentist can talk to your doctor about whether you need medicine before dental work to reduce bleeding.

- Consider wearing a medical identification bracelet or necklace if you have a serious form of VWD (for example, type 3 VWD), so that in case of serious injury or accident the doctors caring for you will know you have VWD.

- Exercise regularly and maintain a healthy weight. Exercise helps keep muscles flexible. It also helps prevent damage to muscles and joints. Always stretch before exercising.

Some safe exercises or activities are swimming, biking, and walking. Football, hockey, wrestling, and lifting heavy weights are not safe activities if you have bleeding problems. Always check with your doctor before starting any exercise program.

Chapter 26

Factor V Leiden

What is factor V Leiden thrombophilia?

Factor V Leiden thrombophilia is an inherited disorder of blood clotting. Factor V Leiden is the name of a specific mutation (genetic alteration) that results in thrombophilia, or an increased tendency to form abnormal blood clots in blood vessels. People who have the factor V Leiden mutation are at somewhat higher than average risk for a type of clot that forms in large veins in the legs (deep venous thrombosis, or DVT) or a clot that travels through the bloodstream and lodges in the lungs (pulmonary embolism, or PE).

Factor V Leiden is the most common inherited form of thrombophilia. Between 3 and 8 percent of the Caucasian (white) U.S. and European populations carry one copy of the factor V Leiden mutation, and about one in five thousand people have two copies of the mutation. The mutation is less common in other populations.

A mutation in the factor V gene (F5) increases the risk of developing factor V Leiden thrombophilia. The protein made by F5 called factor V plays a critical role in the formation of blood clots in response to injury. The factor V protein is involved in a series of chemical reactions that hold blood clots together. A molecule called activated protein C (APC) prevents blood clots from growing too large by inactivating factor V. In people with the factor V Leiden mutation,

"Learning about Factor V Leiden Thrombophilia," National Human Genome Research Institute, February 25, 2009.

APC is unable to inactivate factor V normally. As a result, the clotting process continues longer than usual, increasing the chance of developing abnormal blood clots.

What are the symptoms of factor V Leiden thrombophilia?

The symptoms of factor V Leiden vary among individuals. There are some individuals who have the F5 gene and who never develop thrombosis, while others have recurring thrombosis before the age of thirty years. This variability is influenced by the number of F5 gene mutations a person has, the presence of other gene alterations related to blood clotting, and circumstantial risk factors, such as surgery, use of oral contraceptives, and pregnancy.

Symptoms of Factor V Leiden include the following:

- Having a first DVT or PE before fifty years of age

- Having recurring DVT or PE

- Having venous thrombosis in unusual sites in the body such as the brain or the liver

- Having a DVT or PE during or right after pregnancy

- Having a history of unexplained pregnancy loss in the second or third trimester

- Having a DVT or PE and a strong family history of venous thromboembolism

The use of hormones, such as oral contraceptive pills (OCPs) and hormone replacement therapy (HRT), including estrogen and estrogen-like drugs taken after menopause, increases the risk of developing DVT and PE. Healthy women taking OCPs have a three- to four-fold increased risk of developing a DVT or PE compared with women who do not take OCP. Women with factor V Leiden who take OCPs have about a thirty-five-fold increased risk of developing a DVT or PE compared with women without factor V Leiden and those who do not take OCPs. Likewise, postmenopausal women taking HRT have a two- to three-fold higher risk of developing a DVT or PE than women who do not take HRT, and women with factor V Leiden who take HRT have a fifteen-fold higher risk. Women with heterozygous factor V Leiden who are making decisions about OCP or HRT use should take these statistics into consideration when weighing the risks and benefits of treatment.

Information courtesy of the American Heart Association.

How Is factor V Leiden thrombophilia diagnosed?

Your doctor would suspect a diagnosis of thrombophilia if you have a history of venous thrombosis and/or a family history of venous thrombosis. The diagnosis is made using a screening test called a coagulation screening test or by genetic testing (deoxyribonucleic acid [DNA] analysis) of the F5 gene.

How is factor V Leiden thrombophilia treated?

The management of individuals with factor V Leiden depends on the clinical circumstances. People with factor V Leiden who have had a DVT or PE are usually treated with blood thinners, or anticoagulants. Anticoagulants such as heparin are given for varying amounts of time depending on the person's situation. It is not usually recommended that people with factor V Leiden be treated lifelong with anticoagulants if they have had only one DVT or PE, unless there are additional risk factors present. Having had a DVT or PE in the past increases a person's risk for developing another one in the future, but having factor V Leiden does not seem to add to the risk of having a second clot. In general, individuals who have factor V Leiden but have never had a blood clot are not routinely be treated with an anticoagulant. Rather, these individuals are counseled about reducing or eliminating other factors that may add to one's risk of developing a clot in the future. In addition, these individuals may require temporary treatment with an anticoagulant during periods of particularly high risk, such as major surgery.

Factor V Leiden increases the risk of developing a DVT during pregnancy by about seven-fold. Women with factor V Leiden who are planning pregnancy should discuss this with their obstetrician and/or hematologist. Most women with factor V Leiden have normal pregnancies and only require close follow-up during pregnancy. For those with a history of DVT or PE, treatment with an anticoagulant during a subsequent pregnancy can prevent recurrent problems.

Information courtesy of the American Heart Association.

What do we know about heredity and factor V Leiden thrombophilia?

Factor V Leiden is the most common inherited form of thrombophilia. The risk of developing a clot in a blood vessel depends on whether a person inherits one or two copies of the factor V Leiden mutation. Inheriting one copy of the mutation from a parent increases by four-fold to eight-fold the chance of developing a clot. People who inherit two copies of the mutation, one from each parent, may have up to eighty times the usual risk of developing this type of blood clot. Considering that the risk of developing an abnormal blood clot averages about 1 in 1,000 per year in the general population, the presence of one copy of the factor V Leiden mutation increases that risk to 1 in 125 to 1 in 250. Having two copies of the mutation may raise the risk as high as 1 in 12.

Chapter 27

Factor Deficiencies

Other Factor Deficiencies

There are ten clotting factors that are necessary in forming a blood clot. Deficiencies in factors VIII and IX [hemophilia A and B] are well known to most people, but what of the other factor deficiencies? Not everyone is as familiar with these conditions because they are diagnosed so rarely. To date, deficiencies in eight of the lesser known coagulation factors have been documented in the medical literature. Many of these disorders were only discovered or described within the last forty years.

In most cases, rare factor deficiencies are not genetically sex-linked. They occur in equal frequency among men and women. By and large the gene is passed down in an autosomal recessive fashion. This means that when the factor deficiency is inherited from only one parent, the child will be a carrier of the condition, but usually not have symptoms. It is possible for people to inherit a gene from both parents, but this happens very rarely and usually means a more severe manifestation of the disease.

Obtaining a detailed family history is an important component to diagnosing the condition. Most people with rare factor deficiencies are best seen by hematologists at hemophilia treatment centers. Making

Reprinted from "Other Factor Deficiencies," "Factor I Deficiency," "Factor II Deficiency," "Factor V Deficiency," "Factor VII Deficiency," "Factor X Deficiency," "Factor XI Deficiency," "Factor XII Deficiency," and "Factor XIII Deficiency," © 2006 National Hemophilia Foundation (www.hemophilia.org). Reprinted with permission.

a proper diagnosis for some of these rare conditions requires a quality lab and an experienced hematologist.

Not all factor deficiencies have the same severity. Not everyone with these disorders needs treatment. However for those who do, the treatments available for people with rare factor deficiencies are not optimal. Many people in the United States with rare factor deficiencies need to take fresh frozen plasma, prothrombin complex concentrates (PCCs), or cryoprecipitate.

Since there are such a small number of patients with these conditions, there are few clinical studies regarding the use of products to treat them. Without solid clinical data, obtaining U.S. Food and Drug Administration (FDA) approval for products is extremely difficult. Very few pharmaceutical companies will choose to invest the research dollars needed to produce such products for so few patients.

Factor I Deficiency

(Can also be known as fibrinogen deficiency, afibrinogenemia, dysfibrinogenemia, or hypofibrinogenemia.)

Factor I deficiency is actually a collective term for several rare inherited fibrinogen deficiencies. Fibrinogen may be absent from the blood altogether (afibrinogenemia), present in only very low levels in the blood (hypofibrinogenemia), or measurable in normal quantities but defective (dysfibrinogenemia).

The incidence of Factor I deficiency is estimated at one to two per million. It is inherited in an autosomal recessive fashion, which means it affects men and women equally.

Fibrinogen helps platelets to glue together to form the initial "plug" in response to an injury. Therefore, people with factor I deficiency have a combined bleeding disorder because both platelets and clotting are abnormal. The severity of the disorder is directly related to the amount of fibrinogen present.

Afibrinogenemia and hypofibrinogenemia are usually diagnosed in newborns who can present with head bleeds, bleeding after circumcision, and bleeding from the site of the umbilical cord. Easy bruising, nose and mouth bleeds, and soft tissue bleeds are also common. Joint bleeding is relatively uncommon. Women with afibrinogenemia have an increased risk of spontaneous abortion. Persons with dysfibrinogenemia may have a disposition to thrombosis.

Diagnosis is made by measuring the amount of fibrinogen in the blood, prothrombin time (PT) test, activated partial thromboplastin time (aPTT) test, and thrombin clotting time (TCT) test.

Treatment

For now, cryoprecipitate is the treatment of choice in the United States. FFP may be given, but cryoprecipitate is used more often to avoid volume overload. There are no Factor I concentrates available for use in the United States. However, there are three fibrinogen concentrates being used in Europe and Japan. There have also been some reports of adverse reactions with use of these concentrates.

Factor II Deficiency

(Can also be known as prothrombin deficiency.)

Factor II deficiency is quite rare, with only twenty-six cases reported in the medical literature. The incidence is estimated at one in two million. It is inherited in an autosomal recessive fashion, which means it affects men and women equally.

Prothrombin is a precursor to thrombin, which converts fibrinogen into fibrin, which in turn strengthens a protective clot. Factor II deficiency usually takes the form of an abnormality in the structure of prothrombin rather than a lack of the protein itself. People with a more severe factor II deficiency have severe bruising, bleeding from the nose and mouth, menorrhagia, as well as muscle bleeds, head bleeds, and bleeding after trauma. Joint bleeding is rare.

Diagnosis is made with a prothrombin time (PT) test and an activated partial thromboplastin time (aPTT) test. Levels of prothrombin deficiency can range from 2 to 50 percent of normal. Patients with levels reaching 50 percent of normal have little to no bleeding problems. The inherited condition must be distinguished from the acquired form of Factor II, which is also associated with bleeding. Hereditary Factor II deficiency has also been reported as part of a combined disorder with factor VII, IX, X, and protein C and S.

Treatment

Moderate bleeding can be treated with fresh frozen plasma. Correction of prothrombin can also be achieved with the use of prothrombin complex concentrates (PCCs). However, there are differences in the amount of factor II present in PCCs, depending upon the product. There are reported risks of thromboembolic complications with certain use of PCCs.

Factor V Deficiency

(Can also be known as Owren disease, labile factor deficiency, proaccelerin deficiency, or parahemophilia. Not to be confused with factor V Leiden, which is a type of thrombophilia.)

The deficiency was first described in a Norwegian patient in 1944. The incidence of Factor V deficiency is estimated at one per million. It is usually inherited in an autosomal recessive fashion, which means it affects men and women equally. There are some case reports of a dominant pattern of inheritance in some families.

The role of the factor V protein is to be a catalyst or "accelerator" in the process by which prothrombin is converted to thrombin. Common characteristics of factor V deficiency are bruising, nose and mouth bleeds. Severe deep tissue bleeds are uncommon. Among people with severe forms of factor V deficiency, there can be joint bleeding and risks of head bleeds in newborns. Women can also present with menorrhagia.

Diagnosis is made through activated partial thromboplastin time (aPTT) test, prothrombin time (PT) test, and thrombin clotting time (TCT) test. Diagnosis can be confirmed with a factor V assay. Factor V is found in both plasma and platelets, so platelet function may also be affected. A very rare condition, known as combined factor VIII and Factor V, is characterized by more severe bleeding episodes. The combined FVIII+FV deficiency is a separate disorder that can be mistaken for either mild factor V or mild factor VIII deficiency.

Treatment

There are no available factor V concentrates. Fresh frozen plasma (FFP) is the only treatment available. In acute cases of severe bleeding, the addition of platelet concentrates may be helpful. Depending upon availability, solvent-detergent FFP may contain a more reliable level of factor V than standard FFP.

Factor VII Deficiency

(Can also be known as Alexander disease, stable factor deficiency, or proconvertin deficiency. Not to be confused with acquired factor VII deficiency, which is associated with liver disease.)

Factor VII was first recognized in 1951, and originally named serum prothrombin version accelerator (SPCA) deficiency. Although the published incidence of Factor VII deficiency is estimated at one in five hundred thousand, the disorder may be more common. It is inherited in an autosomal recessive fashion, which means it affects men and women equally.

The factor VII protein is part of the cascade of clotting factors that form the chain leading to a protective blood clot. Factor VII deficiency is usually severe. In fact patients with less than 1 percent factor VII activity experience similar symptoms to hemophilia. People with severe factor VII are prone to joint bleeds. In addition to spontaneous nose-bleeds, people can experience bleeds in the stomach, intestines, and urinary tract. Head bleeds and muscle bleeds have also been reported. Women can have severe menorrhagia.

Diagnosis is made through activated partial thromboplastin time (aPTT) test, prothrombin time (PT) test, and thrombin time (TT) test. Diagnosis can be confirmed with a factor VII assay. There have been instances of combined factor VII deficiencies with cases of factors II, IX, and X.

Treatment

In July 2005, Novo Nordisk received FDA approval for a new usage indication of its recombinant factor VIIa product NovoSeven® to treat bleeding episodes in patients with factor VII deficiency.

Prothrombin complex concentrates (PCCs) can also be used to treat Factor VII deficiency. However, the amount of factor VII contained in these products varies considerably among PCCs. Not only is there a marked difference in factor content between the different commercial preparations, but factor content can also vary between product lots produced by the same manufacturer.

Patients with factor VII deficiency can also be treated with fresh frozen plasma (FFP). However, volume constraints may limit the amount of FFP that can be used. There have been cases of thrombosis reported in people with factor VII deficiency.

Factor X Deficiency

(Can also be known as Stuart-Prower Factor deficiency.)

Factor X deficiency was first discovered in a man with the surname Stuart from North Carolina. While his doctors had originally thought he might have factor VII deficiency, a woman with the surname Prower was determined to have the same clotting abnormality. Researchers realized that this was a new factor and called it the Stuart-Prower factor. It was later renamed factor X deficiency.

The incidence of factor X is estimated at one in five hundred thousand births. It is inherited in an autosomal recessive fashion, which means it affects men and women equally.

The factor X protein activates the enzymes that help to form a clot. Several genetic variations of factor X with varying degrees of severity have been described in the medical literature. People with mild forms of the deficiency usually do not experience bleeding episodes, but do have bleeding after trauma or surgery. Patients with severe forms of the disease commonly have joint bleeding, gastrointestinal bleeds, and hematomas.

Spontaneous head bleeds, spinal cord bleeds, and bleeding at the site of the umbilical cord have also been reported. Women with factor X deficiency may have menorrhagia or be susceptible to first trimester miscarriage.

Diagnosis is made through a bleeding time test, prothrombin time (PT) test, and partial thromboplastin time (PTT) test. Diagnosis can be confirmed by a factor X assay or a ruffle viper venom time assay.

Treatment

There are no factor X concentrates available and fresh frozen plasma is normally used as treatment. Prothrombin complex concentrates (PCCs) have been used in patients, but it is important to know that the amount of factor X in each product is not consistent. There has also been a reported risk of thromboembolic complications with PCC product usage.

Factor XI Deficiency

(Can also be known as hemophilia C, plasma thromboplastin antecedent [PTA] deficiency, Rosenthal syndrome.)

Factor XI was only first recognized in 1953. The incidence of factor XI is estimated at one in one hundred thousand. It is inherited in an autosomal dominant fashion, which means it affects men and women equally. It can occur with greater frequency in people of Ashkenazi Jewish descent because intermarriage among this group has been more prevalent. In Israel, factor XI deficiency has been estimated to be around 8 percent among Ashkenazi Jews, making it one of the most common genetic disorders in this group.

Factor XI is another part of the cascade of clotting factors that form the chain leading to a protective clot. Some people with factor XI deficiency may have milder symptoms than those of hemophilia, but there can be quite a bit of variability with this deficiency. Individuals are not likely to bleed spontaneously, and hemorrhage normally occurs after trauma or surgery. Certain procedures carry an increased risk of bleeding, such as dental extractions, tonsillectomies, surgery in the urinary and genital tracts, and nasal surgery. Joint bleeds are uncommon. Patients are more prone to bruising, nosebleeds, or blood in the urine. Woman may experience menorrhagia and prolonged bleeding after childbirth.

Diagnosis is made through bleeding time test, platelet function tests, and prothrombin time (PT) and activated partial thromboplastin time (aPTT) tests. A specific Factor XI assay is extremely useful in ruling out combined deficiencies.

Treatment

In the United States, there are no factor XI concentrates available and fresh frozen plasma is normally used for treatment. Since factor XI is not concentrated in fresh frozen plasma, considerable amounts of plasma may be required to maintain the factor level. In the case of mouth bleeds, antifibrinolytic products such as Amicar® can be helpful.

Currently there are two factor XI concentrates produced in Europe. One is manufactured through Bioproducts Laboratories (BPL) in the United Kingdom. The other product is produced in France through LFB and only for limited patient use.

Factor XII Deficiency

(Can also be known as Hageman factor deficiency.)

This somewhat mysterious deficiency was first discovered in 1955 and named after John Hageman, the first patient diagnosed with the condition. The incidence of factor XII deficiency is estimated at one in one million. This deficiency is inherited in an autosomal recessive fashion, which means it affects men and women equally. It has been reported that factor XII levels seem to be lower among Asians than any other ethnic group.

The mystery of Factor XII centers on how the protein is a step in the process of forming a clot, but people with the deficiency usually do not experience bleeds and normally do not require treatment. Having a low factor XII level has little to no clinical significance.

Even with major surgery, bleeding manifestations are extremely rare. In fact, most people only get diagnosed by chance, or during pre-screening blood tests for surgery. Since bleeding time is usually normal, diagnosis is made by a prolonged activated partial thromboplastin time (aPTT) test. A specific factor XII assay is necessary to confirm the initial diagnosis.

Treatment

Treatment is usually unnecessary. There is some indication that factor XII deficiency may predispose people to thrombosis, but this has not been clearly established.

Factor XIII Deficiency

(Can also be known as fibrin stabilizing factor deficiency.)

This condition is perhaps the rarest of all factor deficiencies. The incidence of factor XIII deficiency is estimated at one in five million births. It is inherited in an autosomal recessive fashion, which means it affects men and women equally. No racial or ethnic group is disproportionately affected.

Factor XIII is the protein responsible for stabilizing the formation of a blood clot. In the absence of factor XIII, a clot will still develop but it will remain unstable. When someone has a deficiency of factor XIII, the tenuously formed clot will eventually break down and cause recurrent bleeds. The prolonged bleeding that is associated with factor XIII is usually associated with trauma. Among severe patients there is a high risk of head bleeds with or without trauma. Bleeding immediately after surgery is usually not excessive, but can be delayed. Women who go untreated risk spontaneous abortion. Men with the deficiency may show signs of infertility. Common characteristics include soft tissue bleeds, menorrhagia, joint bleeding, and persistent bleeding during circumcision or at the site of the umbilical cord.

Diagnosis is made by normal coagulation screening tests and a detailed family history. Specific factor XIII assays can confirm the diagnosis. The condition can also be defined by a clot solubility test.

Treatment

There are currently two commercially produced factor XIII concentrates produced in Europe. One is manufactured by Bio Products Laboratory (BPL) and is only available in the United Kingdom. The other product is called Fibrogammin-P, produced by Beringwerke of Germany. It is only available under IND [investigatory new drug] or through clinical trial in the United States. Neither of these products is FDA-approved for use in the United States. For the time being, cryoprecipitate or fresh frozen plasma is used to treat factor XIII deficiency.

Chapter 28

Hereditary Hemorrhagic Telangiectasia

What is hereditary hemorrhagic telangiectasia?

Hereditary hemorrhagic telangiectasia (HHT) is a condition where malformations of small blood vessels occur in multiple areas throughout the body. These so-called arteriovenous malformations (AVMs) commonly occur in the nose, causing nosebleeds, which occasionally can be severe.

Hereditary hemorrhagic telangiectasia is rare, occurring in approximately one in five thousand to ten thousand people. As the name suggests, this condition is inherited. A person who has HHT has a 50 percent chance of passing it on to their child. However, the severity of symptoms varies considerably between individuals.

What problems are associated with this condition?

Generally, people with hereditary hemorrhagic telangiectasia, also known as Osler-Weber-Rendu syndrome, have a history of recurrent nosebleeds as a child but are otherwise well.

Small AVMs known as telangiectases also occur in the skin (especially on the fingers, hands, face, and lips), the tongue and lining of the mouth, and the conjunctiva (the thin, transparent membrane that covers your eyes). Typically they appear as small red or purple dots that grow slowly in size, although the size can vary from barely visible to up to 1 cm across. The telangiectases appear progressively from late childhood into middle age. Bleeding from these lesions rarely causes problems.

Larger AVMs may occur in organs such as the lungs, liver, and brain—these AVMs can cause problems if they bleed. People with hereditary hemorrhagic telangiectasia may also have AVMs in the lining of the bowel or the bladder that can also bleed, and may lead to the development of anemia.

How is HHT diagnosed?

The diagnosis of hereditary hemorrhagic telangiectasia is based on the symptoms as well as genetic testing, which is available through specialized centers.

Anyone who has been diagnosed as definitely having this disease should have a brain scan to check for AVMs. This is because there are usually no symptoms associated with an AVM in the brain until it bleeds, possibly having serious consequences. Either a magnetic resonance imaging (MRI) scan or a computed tomography (CT) scan can detect these lesions. People with hereditary hemorrhagic telangiectasia should also have a scan to check for AVMs in the lungs.

What treatment is required?

If scans reveal AVMs in the brain or the lungs, the decision to have them treated depends on a number of factors, such as the site of the lesion, the risks of treatment, and the age of the person.

Most people with this condition will only be mildly affected, but regular medical check-ups twice a year, as well as early treatment for any symptoms that might develop, are recommended.

The material provided by CMPMedica Australia Pty Ltd is intended for Australian residents only, is of a general nature and is provided for information purposes only. The material is not a substitute for independent professional medical advice from a qualified health care professional. It is not intended to be used by anyone to diagnose, treat, cure or prevent any disease or medical condition. No person should act in reliance solely on any statement contained in the material provided, and at all times should obtain specific advice from a qualified healthcare professional.

Chapter 29

Bruises:
When to See a Doctor

Man, does that hurt! You took that hill too quickly on your bike, lost your balance on your blades, or someone on the other soccer team missed the ball completely and kicked you right in the shin. The pain is bad enough, but the bruise left behind is pretty ugly. It's nothing new; you've had a bruise or two before. But what exactly is a bruise?

What Is a Bruise?

A bruise, also called a contusion (pronounced: kun-too-zhen) or an ecchymosis (pronounced: eh-ky-moe-sis), happens when a part of the body is struck and the muscle fibers and connective tissue underneath are crushed but the skin doesn't break. When this occurs, blood from the ruptured capillaries (small blood vessels) near the skin's surface escapes by leaking out under the skin. With no place to go, the blood gets trapped, forming a red or purplish mark that's tender when you touch it—a bruise.

Bruises can happen for many reasons, but most are the result of bumping and banging into things—or having things bump and bang into you. Fortunately, as anyone who's ever sported a shiner knows, the mark isn't permanent.

"Bruises," May 2009, reprinted with permission from www.kidshealth.org. Copyright © 2009 The Nemours Foundation. This information was provided by KidsHealth, one of the largest resources online for medically reviewed health information written for parents, kids, and teens. For more articles like this one, visit www.KidsHealth.org, or www.TeensHealth.org.

How Long Do Bruises Last?

You know how a bruise changes color over time? That's your body fixing the bruise by breaking down and reabsorbing the blood, which causes the bruise to go through many colors of the rainbow before it eventually disappears. You can pretty much guess the age of a bruise just by looking at its color:

- When you first get a bruise, it's kind of reddish as the blood appears under the skin.

- Within one or two days, the hemoglobin (an iron-containing substance that carries oxygen) in the blood changes and your bruise turns bluish-purple or even blackish.

- After five to ten days, the bruise turns greenish or yellowish.

- Then, after ten or fourteen days, it turns yellowish-brown or light brown.

Finally, after about two weeks, your bruise fades away.

Who Gets Bruises?

Anyone can get a bruise. Some people bruise easily, whereas others don't. Why? Bruising depends on several things, such as:

- how tough the skin tissue is;

- whether someone has certain diseases or conditions;

- whether a person's taking certain medications.

Also, blood vessels tend to become fragile as people get older, which is why elderly people tend to bruise more easily.

What Can I Do to Help Myself Feel Better?

It's hard to prevent bruises, but you can help speed the healing process. When you get a bruise, you can use stuff you find right in your freezer to help the bruise go away faster. Applying cold when you first get a bruise helps reduce its size by slowing down the blood that's flowing to the area, which decreases the amount of blood that ends up leaking into the tissues. It also keeps the inflammation and swelling down. All you have to do is apply cold to the bruise for half an hour to an hour at a time for a day or two after the bruise appears.

You don't need to buy a special cold pack, although they're great to keep on hand in the freezer. Just get some ice, put it in a plastic bag, and wrap the bag in a cloth or a towel and place it on the bruise (it isn't such a good idea to apply the ice directly to the skin).

Another trick is to use a bag of frozen vegetables. It doesn't matter what kind—carrots, peas, lima beans, whatever—as long as they're frozen. A bag of frozen vegetables is easy to apply to the bruise because it can form to the shape of the injured area. Also, like a cold pack, it can be used and refrozen again and again (just pick your least-favorite vegetables as it's not a good idea to keep thawing and freezing veggies that you plan to eat!).

Another way to help heal your bruise is to elevate the bruised area above the level of your heart. In other words, if the bruise is on your shin, lie down on a couch or bed and prop up your leg. This will slow the flow of the red blood cells to the bruise because more of the blood in your leg will flow back toward the rest of your body instead of leaking out into the tissues of your leg. If you keep standing, more blood will flow to your bruised shin and the bruise will grow faster.

When to See a Doctor

Minor bruises are easily treated, but it's probably best to talk to a doctor if:

- a bruise doesn't go away after two weeks;
- you bruise often and you haven't been bumping into things;
- bruises seem to develop for no known reasons;
- a bruise is getting more painful;
- your bruise is swelling;
- you can't move a joint;
- the bruise is near your eye.

Can Bruises Be Prevented?

Bruises are kind of hard to avoid completely, but if you're playing sports, riding your bike, inline skating, or doing anything where you might bump, bang, crash, or smash into something—or something might bump, bang, crash, or smash into you—it's smart to wear protective gear like pads, shin guards, and helmets. Taking just a few extra seconds to put on that gear might save you from a couple of weeks of aches and pains (not to mention save your life if the accident's really serious)!

Chapter 30

Antiphospholipid Antibody Syndrome

What Is Antiphospholipid Antibody Syndrome?

Antiphospholipid antibody syndrome (APS) is an autoimmune disorder. Autoimmune disorders occur when the immune system makes antibodies that attack and damage the body's tissues or cells by mistake. Antibodies are a type of protein that the immune system usually makes to defend against infection.

In APS, the body mistakenly makes antibodies that attack phospholipids—a type of fat. Phospholipids are found in all living cells and cell membranes, including blood cells and the lining of blood vessels.

When antibodies attack phospholipids, they damage cells. This causes unwanted blood clots to form in the body's arteries and veins. (These are the vessels that carry blood to your heart and body.)

Usually, blood clotting is a normal bodily process. Blood clots help seal small cuts or breaks and prevent you from losing too much blood. In APS, however, too much blood clotting can block blood flow and damage the body's organs.

Overview

Some people have APS antibodies, but don't ever have signs or symptoms of the disorder. The presence of APS antibodies, by itself, doesn't mean that you have APS. To be diagnosed with APS, you

---

Excerpted from "Antiphospholipid Antibody Syndrome," National Heart Lung and Blood Institute, National Institutes of Health, September 2008.

must have APS antibodies and a history of health problems related to the disorder.

APS can lead to a number of health problems, such as stroke, heart attack, kidney damage, deep vein thrombosis, pulmonary embolism, or pregnancy-related problems.

Pregnancy-related problems may include multiple miscarriages, a miscarriage late in pregnancy, or a premature birth due to eclampsia. (Eclampsia, which follows preeclampsia, is a serious condition that causes seizures in pregnant women.)

Very rarely, some people who have APS develop many blood clots within weeks or months. This condition is called catastrophic antiphospholipid syndrome (CAPS).

People who have APS also are at higher risk for thrombocytopenia. This is a condition in which your blood has a low number of blood cells called platelets. This can lead to mild to serious bleeding.

In APS, thrombocytopenia occurs because the platelets are used up by the clotting process or because antibodies destroy them.

In some cases, APS can be fatal. This may occur due to large blood clots or blood clots in the heart, lungs, or brain.

Outlook

APS can affect people of any age. However, it's more common in women and people who have other autoimmune or rheumatic disorders, such as lupus. ("Rheumatic" refers to disorders that affect the joints, bones, or muscles.)

APS has no cure, but medicines can help prevent its complications. Medicines are used to stop blood clots from forming and keep existing clots from getting larger. Treatment for the disorder is long term.

If you have APS and another autoimmune disorder, it's important to control that condition as well. When the other condition is controlled, APS may cause fewer problems.

Other Names for Antiphospholipid Antibody Syndrome

- Antiphospholipid syndrome
- aPL syndrome
- Anticardiolipin antibody syndrome, or aCL syndrome
- Lupus anticoagulant syndrome
- Hughes syndrome
- Sneddon syndrome

What Causes Antiphospholipid Antibody Syndrome?

Antiphospholipid antibody syndrome (APS) occurs when the body's immune system makes antibodies (proteins) that attack phospholipids. Phospholipids are a type of fat found in all living cells and cell membranes, including blood cells and the lining of blood vessels. What causes the immune system to make antibodies against phospholipids isn't known.

APS causes unwanted blood clots to form in the body's arteries and veins. Usually, blood clotting is a normal bodily process. It helps seal small cuts or breaks and prevents you from losing too much blood. In APS, however, too much blood clotting can block blood flow and damage the body's organs.

Researchers don't know why APS occurs. Some believe that the antibodies damage or affect the inner lining of the blood vessels, causing blood clots to form. Others believe that the immune system makes antibodies in response to blood clots damaging the blood vessels.

Who Is at Risk for Antiphospholipid Antibody Syndrome?

Antiphospholipid antibody syndrome (APS) can affect people of any age. The disorder is more common in women than men, but it affects both sexes.

APS also is more common in people who have other autoimmune or rheumatic disorders, such as lupus. About 10 percent of all people who have lupus also have APS. About half of all people who have APS also have another autoimmune or rheumatic disorder.

What Are the Signs and Symptoms of Antiphospholipid Antibody Syndrome?

The signs and symptoms of antiphospholipid antibody syndrome (APS) are related to abnormal blood clotting. The outcome of a blood clot depends on its size and location.

Blood clots can form in or travel to the arteries or veins in the brain, heart, kidneys, lungs, and limbs. Clots can limit or block blood flow. This can damage the body's organs and may cause death.

Major Signs and Symptoms

Major signs and symptoms of blood clots include the following:

- Chest pain and shortness of breath

- Pain, redness, warmth, and swelling in the limbs
- Ongoing headaches
- Speech changes
- Upper body discomfort in the arms, back, neck, and jaw
- Nausea (feeling sick to your stomach)

Blood clots can lead to stroke, heart attack, kidney damage, pulmonary embolism, and deep vein thrombosis.

Pregnant women who have APS can have successful pregnancies. However, they're at higher risk for miscarriages, stillbirths, and other pregnancy-related problems, such as preeclampsia.

Preeclampsia is high blood pressure that occurs during pregnancy. This condition may progress to eclampsia. Eclampsia is a serious condition that causes seizures in pregnant women.

Some people who have APS also have thrombocytopenia. This is a condition in which your blood has a low number of blood cells called platelets. Mild to serious bleeding causes the main signs and symptoms of thrombocytopenia. Bleeding can occur inside the body (internal bleeding) or on the skin.

Other Signs and Symptoms

Other symptoms of APS include chronic headaches, memory loss, or heart valve disease. Some people who have the disorder also get a lacy-looking red rash on their wrists and knees.

How Is Antiphospholipid Antibody Syndrome Diagnosed?

Your doctor will diagnose antiphospholipid antibody syndrome (APS) based on your medical history and the results from blood tests.

Medical History

Some people have APS antibodies, but don't ever have signs or symptoms of the disorder. The presence of APS antibodies, by itself, doesn't mean that you have APS.

To be diagnosed with APS, you must have APS antibodies and a history of health problems related to the disorder. These health problems may include stroke, heart attack, kidney damage, deep vein thrombosis, pulmonary embolism, or pregnancy-related problems.

Pregnancy-related problems may include multiple miscarriages, a miscarriage late in pregnancy, or a premature birth due to eclampsia. (Eclampsia, which follows preeclampsia, is a serious condition that causes seizures in pregnant women.)

Blood Tests

Your doctor can use blood tests to confirm a diagnosis of APS. These tests check your blood for any of the three APS antibodies: anticardiolipin, B2 glycoprotein I, and lupus anticoagulant.

The term "anticoagulant" refers to a substance that prevents blood clotting. It may seem odd that one of the APS antibodies is called lupus anticoagulant. This is because the antibody slows clotting in lab tests. However, in the human body, it increases the risk for blood clots.

To test for the APS antibodies, a small amount of blood is taken from your body. It's often drawn from a vein in your arm using a small needle. The procedure usually is quick and easy, but it may cause some short-term discomfort, such as a slight bruise.

You may need a second blood test to confirm positive results. This is because a single positive test can result from a short-term infection. The second blood test often is done twelve weeks or more after the first one.

Some healthy people may test positive for APS antibodies but have no signs or symptoms of the disorder. The presence of the APS antibodies, by itself, doesn't mean that you have APS.

How Is Antiphospholipid Antibody Syndrome Treated?

Antiphospholipid antibody syndrome (APS) has no cure, but some medicines can help prevent complications. The goals of treatment are to prevent blood clots from forming and keep existing clots from getting larger.

If you have APS and another autoimmune disorder, such as lupus, it's important to control that condition as well. When the other condition is controlled, APS may cause fewer problems.

Research is ongoing for new ways to treat APS.

Medicines

Anticoagulants, or "blood thinners," are used to stop blood clots from forming. They also keep existing blood clots from getting larger. These medicines are taken as either a pill, an injection under the skin, or through a needle or tube inserted into a vein (called intravenous, or IV, injection).

Warfarin and heparin are two blood thinners used to treat people who have APS. Warfarin is given in pill form. (Coumadin® is a common brand name for warfarin.) Heparin is given as an injection or through an IV tube. There are different types of heparin. Your doctor will discuss the options with you.

Your doctor may treat you with both heparin and warfarin at the same time. Heparin acts quickly. Warfarin takes two to three days before it starts to work. Once the warfarin starts to work, the heparin is stopped.

Sometimes aspirin is used with warfarin. In other cases, aspirin may be used alone. Aspirin also thins the blood and helps prevent blood clots.

Blood thinners don't prevent or treat APS. They simply reduce the risk of further blood clotting. Treatment with these medicines is long term. Discuss all treatment options with your doctor.

Treatment during Pregnancy

Pregnant women who have APS can have successful pregnancies. With proper treatment, women who have APS are more likely to carry their babies to term.

Pregnant women who have APS usually are treated with heparin or heparin and low-dose aspirin.

Babies whose mothers have APS are at higher risk for slowed growth while in the womb. If you're pregnant and have APS, you may need to have extra ultrasound tests (sonograms) to check the fetus's growth. This test uses sound waves to look at organs and structures inside your body.

Living with Antiphospholipid Antibody Syndrome

Antiphospholipid antibody syndrome (APS) has no cure. However, you can take steps to control the disorder and prevent complications.

Take all medicines as your doctor prescribes, get ongoing medical care, and talk to your doctor about healthy lifestyle changes and other concerns.

Chapter 31

Disseminated Intravascular Coagulation

What Is Disseminated Intravascular Coagulation?

Disseminated intravascular coagulation (DIC) is a disorder that affects the blood clotting cascade. This disorder occurs when your body's clotting mechanisms are activated inappropriately. DIC can occur in the short or long term, and is the end complication of a variety of diseases such as cancers and some infections. Clots form throughout the whole body, instead of localizing only to the site of injury. Eventually, all the blood clotting factors are used up and unavailable to be used when needed at actual sites of injury.

Who Gets Disseminated Intravascular Coagulation?

Disseminated intravascular coagulation often presents with a subacute thrombotic picture in cancer patients, and is associated with high mortality rates when this acutely develops into the hemorrhagic form.

Disseminated intravascular coagulation occurs in 7 to 10 percent of patients with malignant disease. Adenocarcinomas and leukemias are the most common cancer associations.

Predisposing Factors

About 50 percent of individuals with disseminated intravascular coagulation are patients with complications from pregnancy. Widespread infection and trauma are responsible for the majority of the remaining cases.

There are many causes of disseminated intravascular coagulation. These can be classified as acute or chronic, systemic or localized. The disorder may be the result of single or multiple conditions.

Acute DIC

- Infectious:

  - Bacterial (e.g., gram-negative infections, meningococcal disease)

  - Viral (e.g., human immunodeficiency virus (HIV), cytomegalovirus (CMV), varicella)

  - Fungal (e.g., histoplasma)

  - Parasitic (e.g., malaria)

- Malignant disease:

  - Those originating in cells of the bloodstream (e.g., acute myelocytic leukemias)

  - Spread of cancers

- Obstetric:

  - Placental abruption (early separation of a normal placenta from the wall of the uterus)

  - Eclampsia (a serious complication of pregnancy characterized by convulsions)

- Trauma

- Burns

- Surgery

- Acute liver failure

- Snake bites

- Transfusion reactions of blood

Chronic DIC

- Malignancies:
  - Leukemia
- Obstetric:
  - Retained products of conception (e.g., dead fetus, post-miscarriage)
- Vascular:
  - Rheumatoid arthritis
- Inflammatory:
  - Ulcerative colitis, Crohn disease (inflammatory conditions affecting the bowels)

Progression

Disseminated intravascular coagulation begins with overactivation of your body's coagulation system and excessive clotting. The excessive clotting is usually stimulated by a substance that enters the blood, with possible causes as listed above. As the clotting factors and platelets are consumed, there are less clotting factors available to be used at real sites of bleeding and excessive bleeding occurs. The results of this process (i.e., abnormal small clots [microthrombi] and/or bleeding) are found in many organs and tissues. Significant changes may occur in some of your body's organs such as the kidney, lungs, brain, adrenals, or placenta.

Probable Outcomes

The prognosis for disseminated intravascular coagulation varies according to each individual patient. It depends on the cause of your disseminated intravascular coagulation.

How Will Disseminated Intravascular Coagulation Affect Me?

If you are affected by disseminated intravascular coagulation, some of the following symptoms may be experienced:

- Symptoms of infection: fevers, cough, shortness of breath, pain, rash, behavior changes, sick contacts, and recent travel.

If you are young and affected by disseminated intravascular coagulation, a birth history may be relevant:

- Events occurring just before, around, and after birth—i.e., course of pregnancy, prenatal testing, any neonatal illnesses may be important

- Risk factors for infection around the time of your birth (fever in your mother, premature rupture of the membranes, your mother's status for a particular bacteria called group B streptococcus, and antibiotics given around the time of birth)

Depending on your condition, age, and many other factors, your doctor may ask about symptoms such as:

- abnormal or increased bruising;

- lethargy (tiredness);

- recent illness, infections;

- loss of weight;

- drug use;

- pregnancy history;

- family history suggestive of an inherited clotting disorder or cancers;

- ongoing medical problems including cancers, problems with blood vessels, and inherited or acquired problems affecting the immune system.

Clinical Examination

When your doctor examines you, he or she may find the following signs. There may be no bleeding at all, to widespread bleeding at different sites of the body:

- Bleeding may occur from the mouth, nose, sites of injections, or from virtually any site.

- There may be widespread bruising.

- Abnormal clots may block off vessels to vital organs. Any organ may be involved but the skin, brain, and kidney are most commonly affected. Respiratory symptoms such as shortness of breath or extreme respiratory difficulty may occur if the lungs are involved.

- Neurologic signs such as convulsions (due to abnormal electrical activity in the brain causing things such as abnormal movements, spasms, or changes in behavior) and coma (a state of unconsciousness) may be present.

How Is Disseminated Intravascular Coagulation Diagnosed?

The doctor may decide to do some of the following tests, to help determine the reason for and the severity of your disseminated intravascular coagulation.

In severe cases with increased bleeding, some of these tests may be performed:

- **Blood film:** This is a smear of the blood taken, which may show broken, fragmented red blood cells.

- **Decreased platelets:** Platelets are a type of blood cell which have a key role in normal blood clotting. They clump together during clotting processes, to plug holes in damaged blood vessels.

- **Increased prothrombin time (PT):** This test measures the clotting time of plasma (the liquid portion of the blood).

- **Increased activated partial thromboplastin time (APTT):** This measures the time it takes for clots to form by various pathways in the body.

- **High levels of fibrin degradation products (FDPs):** These are proteins that are produced when clots are broken up by the body.

- **Decreased fibrinogen:** A protein produced by the liver which helps stop bleeding by helping blood clots form.

- **Decreased amounts of factors that help the blood clot:** Factors V, VIII, X, XIII; Protein C.

In mild cases without bleeding, the following test results may be present:

- Increased synthesis of clotting factors and platelets may result in a normal PT, APTT, TT, and platelet counts, although FDPs will be raised.

There is no single diagnostic test for disseminated intravascular coagulation. This condition is suggested by the following combination: a clinical picture consistent with disseminated intravascular coagulation, low levels of platelets, prolonged PT and APTT, and presence of FDPs.

How Is Disseminated Intravascular Coagulation Treated?

If you are affected by disseminated intravascular coagulation, the doctor's first step is to treat the underlying cause of your disease, where possible. For example, if infection is the underlying cause, you may be given appropriate antibiotics.

You may also be given supportive treatment like fluids and your urine output monitored with a urinary catheter.

The next step is to replace missing blood components. If your platelet levels are low, platelet transfusions are appropriate. If plasma coagulation factors are decreased, they may be replaced with fresh frozen plasma. If fibrinogen levels are low, the doctor might consider transfusion with cryoprecipitate, which is a substance rich in fibrinogen.

Doctors might consider heparin therapy in your treatment, which is a controversial issue. Heparin helps stop clotting, working by stopping enzymes that potentiate clotting. However, in some patients, bleeding can be accelerated.

Thus heparin therapy is probably is best reserved for patients with evidence of ischemia (insufficient blood supply) of the digits and cyanosis.

Surgical treatment is limited to treating certain underlying causes—e.g., removal of a cancer.

References

Furlong MA, Furlong BR. Disseminated Intravascular Coagulation 2005 E-medicine [serial online]. 2005 [cited 24th April 2006]. Available from URL: http://www.emedicine.com/emerg/topic150.htm.

Longmore M, Wilkinson I, Torok E. *Oxford Handbook of Clinical Medicine*. New York; Oxford University Press, 2001.

Kumar V, Abbas A K & Fausto N. *Robbins & Cotran Pathologic Basis of Disease*. China: Elseiver Saunders; 2005.

Kumar P, Clark M. *Clinical Medicine* United Kingdom: WB Saunders; 2002.

Chapter 32

Hypercoagulation

Chapter Contents

Section 32.1

Excessive Blood Clotting

What is hypercoagulation?

When you get a cut, your body stops the bleeding by forming a blood clot (a thickened mass of blood tissue). Substances in your blood (called proteins) work with tiny particles (called platelets) to form the clot. Forming a clot is called coagulation. Coagulation helps when you are injured because it slows blood loss. However, your blood shouldn't clot when it's moving through your body in your blood vessels. The tendency to clot too much is called hypercoagulation. It can be very dangerous.

Why is hypercoagulation dangerous?

A clot inside a blood vessel is called a thrombus. Sometimes the thrombus can travel in the bloodstream and get stuck in your lungs. This kind of clot (called a pulmonary embolus) keeps blood from getting to your lungs. A pulmonary embolus can be life-threatening.

A clot that blocks a blood vessel in the brain can cause a stroke. A clot in a blood vessel in the heart can cause a heart attack. Blood clots can cause some women to have miscarriages. All of these conditions can also be life-threatening.

What causes hypercoagulation?

There are proteins in your body that are supposed to keep your blood from clotting too much. Some people do not make enough of these proteins. In other people, these proteins are not doing their job properly, or a person may have extra proteins in their blood that cause too much clotting.

Some people are born with a tendency to develop clots. This tendency is inherited (which means it runs in your family).

Certain situations or risk factors can make it easier for your blood to clot too much. These situations include the following:

- Sitting on an airplane or in a car for a long time

- Prolonged bed rest (several days or weeks at a time), such as after surgery or during a long hospital stay

- Surgery (which can slow blood flow)

- Cancer (some types of cancer increase the proteins that clot your blood)

- Pregnancy (which increases the pressure in your pelvis and legs and can cause blood clots to form)

- Using birth control pills or receiving hormone replacement therapy (which can slow blood flow)

- Smoking (which affects clotting)

How does my doctor know I have a problem with hypercoagulation?

Your doctor might think that you have a problem with hypercoagulation if any of the following are true:

- You have relatives with abnormal or excessive clotting

- You had an abnormal clot at a young age

- You got clots when you were pregnant, were using birth control pills, or were being treated with hormone replacement therapy

- You have had several unexplained miscarriages

If your doctor suspects you have hypercoagulation, tests can check the protein levels in your blood. The tests will also show if your proteins are working the way they should to properly clot your blood.

Can hypercoagulation be treated?

Yes. Several medicines can thin your blood and make it less likely to clot. Some people with hypercoagulation only need to take blood thinners when they're in a situation that makes them more likely to form clots (such as when they are in the hospital recovering from surgery, when they are in a car or airplane for a long time, or when they are pregnant). Other people need to take medicine on an ongoing basis for the rest of their lives. Your doctor will decide what treatment is right for you.

What medicines are used to treat hypercoagulation?

The two most common blood thinners are called heparin and warfarin (brand name: Coumadin®). Your doctor will probably give you heparin first, because heparin works right away. Heparin must be injected with a small needle under the skin. Once the heparin begins to work, your doctor will probably have you start taking oral warfarin. Warfarin takes longer to begin working.

What are the side effects of these medicines?

Both medicines can cause you to bleed more easily. If you cut yourself, you might notice that the blood takes longer to clot than usual. You might also bruise more easily. Call your doctor if you have any unusual or heavy bleeding.

Warfarin has a stronger effect on some people than on others. If you take warfarin, your doctor will want to check you often with a blood test that shows how well the warfarin is working. Some other medicines can increase or decrease the strength of warfarin. Ask your doctor before you take a new medicine, including over-the-counter medicines, vitamins, and herbal supplements. Also, talk to your doctor about foods you should avoid while taking warfarin.

If you're pregnant, you should not take warfarin. Warfarin can cause birth defects. Instead, you must use heparin until you deliver your baby. If you want to get pregnant and you're already taking warfarin, talk with your doctor about changing to heparin. Sexually active women who take warfarin should use birth control.

Section 32.2

Deep Vein Thrombosis

Excerpted from "Deep Vein Thrombosis," National Heart Lung and Blood
Institute, National Institutes of Health, November 2007.

What Is Deep Vein Thrombosis?

Deep vein thrombosis, or DVT, is a blood clot that forms in a vein deep
in the body. Blood clots occur when blood thickens and clumps together.

Most deep vein blood clots occur in the lower leg or thigh. They also
can occur in other parts of the body.

A blood clot in a deep vein can break off and travel through the
bloodstream. The loose clot is called an embolus. When the clot travels
to the lungs and blocks blood flow, the condition is called pulmonary
embolism, or PE.

PE is a very serious condition. It can damage the lungs and other
organs in the body and cause death.

Blood clots in the thigh are more likely to break off and cause PE
than blood clots in the lower leg or other parts of the body.

Blood clots also can form in the veins closer to the skin's surface.
However, these clots won't break off and cause PE.

Other Names for Deep Vein Thrombosis

• Blood clot in the legs.

• Venous thrombosis.

• Venous thromboembolism (VTE). This term is used for both deep
  vein thrombosis and pulmonary embolism.

What Causes Deep Vein Thrombosis?

Blood clots can form in your body's deep veins when the following
conditions occur:

• **Damage occurs to a vein's inner lining.** This damage may
  result from injuries caused by physical, chemical, and biological
  factors. Such factors include surgery, serious injury, inflammation, or an immune response.

375

- **Blood flow is sluggish or slow.** Lack of motion can cause sluggish or slowed blood flow. This may occur after surgery, if you're ill and in bed for a long time, or if you're traveling for a long time.

- **Your blood is thicker or more likely to clot than usual.** Certain inherited conditions (such as factor V Leiden) increase blood's tendency to clot. This also is true of treatment with hormone replacement therapy or birth control pills.

Who Is at Risk for Deep Vein Thrombosis?

Many factors increase your risk for deep vein thrombosis (DVT). They include the following:

- A history of DVT.

- Disorders or factors that make your blood thicker or more likely to clot than normal. Certain inherited blood disorders (such as factor V Leiden) will do this. This also is true of treatment with hormone replacement therapy or using birth control pills.

- Injury to a deep vein from surgery, a broken bone, or other trauma.

- Slow blood flow in a deep vein from lack of movement. This may occur after surgery, if you're ill and in bed for a long time, or if you're traveling for a long time.

- Pregnancy and the first six weeks after giving birth.

- Recent or ongoing treatment for cancer.

- A central venous catheter. This is a tube placed in a vein to allow easy access to the bloodstream for medical treatment.

- Being older than sixty (although DVT can occur in any age group).

- Being overweight or obese.

Your risk for DVT increases if you have more than one of the risk factors listed above.

What Are the Signs and Symptoms of Deep Vein Thrombosis?

The signs and symptoms of deep vein thrombosis (DVT) may be related to DVT itself or to pulmonary embolism (PE). See your doctor right away if you have symptoms of either. Both DVT and PE can cause serious, possibly life-threatening complications if not treated.

Deep Vein Thrombosis

Only about half of the people with DVT have symptoms. These symptoms occur in the leg affected by the deep vein clot. They include the following:

- Swelling of the leg or along a vein in the leg
- Pain or tenderness in the leg, which you may feel only when standing or walking
- Increased warmth in the area of the leg that's swollen or in pain
- Red or discolored skin on the leg

Pulmonary Embolism

Some people don't know they have DVT until they have signs or symptoms of PE. Symptoms of PE include the following:

- Unexplained shortness of breath
- Pain with deep breathing
- Coughing up blood

Rapid breathing and a fast heart rate also may be signs of PE.

How Is Deep Vein Thrombosis Diagnosed?

Your doctor will diagnose deep vein thrombosis (DVT) based on your medical history, a physical exam, and the results from tests. He or she will identify your risk factors and rule out other causes for your symptoms. The most common tests used to diagnose DVT are as follows:

- **Ultrasound.** This is the most common test for diagnosing deep vein blood clots. It uses sound waves to create pictures of blood flowing through the arteries and veins in the affected leg.

- **A D-dimer test.** This test measures a substance in the blood that's released when a blood clot dissolves. If the test shows high levels of the substance, you may have a deep vein blood clot. If your test is normal and you have few risk factors, DVT isn't likely.

- **Venography.** This test is used if ultrasound doesn't provide a clear diagnosis. Dye is injected into a vein, and then an x-ray is taken of the leg. The dye makes the vein visible on the x-ray. The x-ray will show whether blood flow is slow in the vein. This may indicate a blood clot.

Other less common tests used to diagnose DVT include magnetic resonance imaging (MRI) and computed tomography (CT) scanning. These tests provide pictures of the inside of the body.

You may need blood tests to check whether you have an inherited blood clotting disorder that can cause DVT. You may have this type of disorder if you have repeated blood clots that can't be linked to another cause, or if you develop a blood clot in an unusual location, such as a vein in the liver, kidney, or brain.

If your doctor thinks that you have pulmonary embolism (PE), he or she may order extra tests, such as a ventilation perfusion scan (V/Q scan). The V/Q scan uses a radioactive material to show how well oxygen and blood are flowing to all areas of the lungs.

How Is Deep Vein Thrombosis Treated?

Medicines

Medicines are used to prevent and treat DVT.

Anticoagulants. Anticoagulants are the most common medicines for treating DVT. They're also known as blood thinners.

These medicines decrease your blood's ability to clot. They also stop existing blood clots from getting bigger. However, blood thinners can't break up blood clots that have already formed. (The body dissolves most blood clots with time.)

Blood thinners can be taken as either a pill, an injection under the skin, or through a needle or tube inserted into a vein (called intravenous, or IV, injection).

Warfarin and heparin are two blood thinners used to treat DVT. Warfarin is given in pill form. (Coumadin® is a common brand name for warfarin.) Heparin is given as an injection or through an IV tube. There are different types of heparin. Your doctor will discuss the options with you.

Your doctor may treat you with both heparin and warfarin at the same time. Heparin acts quickly. Warfarin takes two to three days before it starts to work. Once the warfarin starts to work, the heparin is stopped.

Pregnant women usually are treated with heparin only, because warfarin is dangerous during pregnancy.

Treatment for DVT with blood thinners usually lasts from three to six months.

Thrombin inhibitors. These medicines interfere with the blood clotting process. They're used to treat blood clots in patients who can't take heparin.

Thrombolytics. These medicines are given to quickly dissolve a blood clot. They're used to treat large blood clots that cause severe symptoms.

Because thrombolytics can cause sudden bleeding, they're used only in life-threatening situations.

Other Types of Treatment

Vena cava filter. A vena cava filter is used if you can't take blood thinners or if you're taking blood thinners and still developing blood clots.

The filter is inserted inside a large vein called the vena cava. The filter catches blood clots that break off in a vein before they move to the lungs. This prevents pulmonary embolism. However, it doesn't stop new blood clots from forming.

Graduated compression stockings. These stockings can reduce the swelling that may occur after a blood clot has developed in your leg. Graduated compression stockings are worn on the legs from the arch of the foot to just above or below the knee.

These stockings are tight at the ankle and become looser as they go up the leg. This creates gentle pressure up the leg. The pressure keeps blood from pooling and clotting.

These stockings should be worn for at least a year after DVT is diagnosed.

Section 32.3

Pulmonary Embolism

"Pulmonary Embolus," © 2009 A.D.A.M., Inc. Reprinted with permission.

Alternative Names

Venous thromboembolism; lung blood clot; blood clot—lung; embolus; tumor embolus

Definition

A pulmonary embolus is a blockage of an artery in the lungs by fat, air, a blood clot, or tumor cells.

Causes

A pulmonary embolus is most often caused by a blood clot in a vein, especially a vein in the leg or in the pelvis (hip area). The most common cause is a blood clot in one of the deep veins of the legs. This type of clot is called a deep vein thrombosis (DVT).

Less common causes include air bubbles, fat droplets, amniotic fluid, or clumps of parasites or tumor cells, all of which may lead to a pulmonary embolus.

Risk factors for a pulmonary embolus include:

- burns;

- cancer;

- childbirth;

- family history of blood clots;

- fractures of the hips or femur;

- heart attack;

- heart surgery;

- long-term bed rest or staying in one position for a long time, such as a long plane or car ride;

- severe injury;

- stroke;

- surgery (especially orthopedic or neurological surgery);

- use of birth control pills or estrogen therapy.

People with certain clotting disorders may also have a higher risk.

Symptoms

- Chest pain

  - Under the breastbone or on one side

  - Especially sharp or stabbing; also may be a burning, aching, or dull, heavy sensation

  - May get worse with deep breathing, coughing, eating, bending, or stooping (person may bend over or hold his or her chest in response to the pain)

- Cough

  - Begins suddenly

  - May cough up blood or blood-streaked sputum

- Rapid breathing

- Rapid heart rate

- Shortness of breath

  - May occur at rest or during activity

  - Starts suddenly

Other symptoms that may occur:

- anxiety;

- bluish skin discoloration;

- clammy skin;

- dizziness;

- leg pain in one or both legs;

- lightheadedness or fainting;

- low blood pressure;

- lump associated with a vein near the surface of the body, may be painful;

- nasal flaring;

- pelvis pain;

- sweating;

- swelling in the legs;

- weak or absent pulse;

- wheezing.

Exams and Tests

The following lab tests may be done to see how well your lungs are working:

- Arterial blood gases

- Pulse oximetry

The following imaging tests can help determine where the blood clot is located:

- Chest x-ray

- Computed tomography (CT) angiogram of the chest

- Pulmonary ventilation/perfusion scan

- Pulmonary angiogram

Other tests that may be done include:

- chest CT scan;

- chest magnetic resonance imaging (MRI) scan;

- D-dimer level;

- Doppler ultrasound exam of an extremity;

- electrocardiogram (ECG);

- echocardiogram;

- plethysmography of the legs;

- venography of the legs.

Treatment

Emergency treatment and a hospital stay are often necessary. The aim is to prevent new clots from forming. Oxygen therapy may be required to maintain normal oxygen levels.

In cases of severe, life-threatening pulmonary embolism, treatment may involve dissolving the clot and preventing new clots from forming.

Treatment to dissolve clots is called thrombolytic therapy. Clot-dissolving medications include:

- streptokinase;

- tissue plasminogen activator (t-PA).

Treatment to prevent clots is called anticoagulation therapy. Such drugs are commonly called blood thinners. Clot-prevention medicines include heparin and warfarin (Coumadin®). Heparin or heparin-type drugs can be given intravenously (by IV, directly into a vein), or as injections under the skin. These are usually the first medications given, and are then transitioned over to warfarin given in pill form.

When you first start taking warfarin you will need frequent lab tests to check the thickness of your blood. This will help your doctor properly adjust your dose.

Patients who have reactions to heparin or related medications may need other medications.

Patients who cannot tolerate blood thinners may need a device called an inferior vena cava filter (IVC filter). This device is placed in the main central vein in the belly area. It keeps large clots from traveling into the blood vessels of the lungs. Sometimes a temporary filter can be placed and removed later.

Outlook (Prognosis)

It is difficult to predict how well a patient will do. Often, the outlook is related to what put the person at risk for pulmonary embolism (for example, cancer, major surgery, trauma). In cases of severe pulmonary embolism, where shock and heart failure occur, the death rate may be greater than 50 percent.

Possible Complications

- Heart failure or shock

- Heart palpitations

383

- Pulmonary hypertension
- Severe breathing difficulty
- Severe bleeding (usually a complication of treatment)
- Sudden death

When to Contact a Medical Professional

Go to the emergency room or call the local emergency number (such as 911) if you have symptoms of pulmonary embolus.

Prevention

Preventing deep venous thrombosis (DVT) is very important, especially in people at high risk. To help prevent DVT, move your legs often or take a stroll during long plane trips, car trips, and other situations in which you are sitting or lying down for long periods of time. Walking and staying active as soon as possible after surgery or during a long-term medical illness can also reduce your risk.

Heparin therapy (low doses of heparin injected under the skin) may be prescribed for those on prolonged bed rest.

Sometimes patients in the hospital wear special soft boots that automatically (and gently) squeeze the calves periodically. This is called intermittent pneumatic compression. It helps keep blood moving and prevents blood clotting.

References

Anderson DR, Kahn SR, Rodger MA, et al. Computed tomographic pulmonary angiography vs ventilation-perfusion lung scanning in patients with suspected pulmonary embolism: a randomized controlled trial. *JAMA*. 2007;298(23):2743–53.

Righini M, Le Gal G, Aujesky D, et al. Diagnosis of pulmonary embolism by multidetector CT alone or combined with venous ultrasonography of the leg: a randomised non-inferiority trial. *Lancet*. 2008;371(9621):1343–52.

Snow V, Qaseem A, Barry P, et al. Management of venous thromboembolism: a clinical practice guideline from the American College of Physicians and the American Academy of Family Physicians. *Ann Intern Med*. 2007;146(3):204–10. Epub 2007 Jan 29.

Tapson VF. Pulmonary embolism. In: Goldman L, Ausiello D, eds. *Cecil Medicine*. 23rd ed. Philadelphia, Pa: Saunders Elsevier; 2007: chap 99.

Section 32.4

Preventing and Treating Blood Clots

Reprinted from "Your Guide to Preventing and Treating Blood Clots,"
Agency for Healthcare Research and Quality, AHRQ Publication No. 09-
0067-C, May 2009.

Blood clots (also called deep vein thrombosis) most often occur in
people who can't move around well or who have had recent surgery
or an injury. Blood clots are serious. It is important to know the signs
and get treated right away.

Causes of Blood Clots

Blood clots can form if you don't move around a lot. You may also
get a blood clot if you:

- have had recent surgery;

- are sixty-five or older;

- take hormones, especially for birth control (ask your doctor
  about this);

- have had cancer or are being treated for it;

- have broken a bone (hip, pelvis, or leg);

- have a bad bump or bruise;

- are obese;

- are confined to bed or a chair much of the time;

- have had a stroke or are paralyzed;

- have a special port the doctor put in your body to give you medicine;

- have varicose or bad veins;

- have heart trouble;

- have had a blood clot before;

- have a family member who has had a blood clot;

- have taken a long trip (more than an hour) in a car, airplane, bus, or train.

Are you at risk?

Some people are more likely to get blood clots. Talk with your doctor to see if you are at risk.

Symptoms of a Blood Clot

You may have a blood clot if you see or feel any of the following:

- New swelling in your arm or leg
- Skin redness
- Soreness or pain in your arm or leg
- A warm spot on your leg

Important: If you think you have a blood clot, call your doctor or go to the emergency room right away!

Blood clots can be dangerous. Blood clots that form in the veins in your legs, arms, and groin can break loose and move to other parts of your body, including your lungs. A blood clot in your lungs is called a pulmonary embolism. If this happens, your life can be in danger. Go to the emergency room or call 911.

A blood clot may have gone to your lungs if you suddenly have:

- a hard time breathing;
- chest pain;
- a fast heartbeat;
- fainting spells;
- a mild fever;
- a cough, with or without blood.

Preventing Blood Clots

You can help prevent blood clots if you do the following:

- Wear loose-fitting clothes, socks, or stockings.
- Raise your legs six inches above your heart from time to time.
- Wear special stockings (called compression stockings) if your doctor prescribes them.

- Do exercises your doctor gives you.
- Change your position often, especially during a long trip.
- Do not stand or sit for more than one hour at a time.
- Eat less salt.
- Try not to bump or hurt your legs and try not to cross them.
- Do not use pillows under your knees.
- Raise the bottom of your bed four to six inches with blocks or books.
- Take all medicines the doctor prescribes you.

Stay active: Staying active and moving around may help prevent blood clots.

Treatment for Blood Clots

If you have been told you have a blood clot, your doctor may give you medicine to treat it. This type of medicine is called a blood thinner (also called an anticoagulant). In most cases, your doctor will tell you to follow this treatment plan:

- For the first week you will receive medicine called heparin that works quickly.

- This medicine is injected under the skin. You will learn how to give yourself these shots, or a family member or friend may do it for you.

- You will also start taking Coumadin®—generic name: warfarin—pills by mouth. After about a week of taking both the shots and the pills, you will stop taking the shots. You will continue to take the Coumadin®/warfarin pills for about three to six months or longer.

Side Effects of Blood Thinners

Blood thinners can cause side effects. Bleeding is the most common problem. Your doctor will watch you closely. If you notice something wrong that you think may be caused by your medication, call your doctor.

If you think you are bleeding too much, call your doctor or go to the nearest emergency room. Tell them you are being treated for blood clots. Tell them the medicines you are taking.

Chapter 33

Thrombocytopenia

What Is Thrombocytopenia?

Thrombocytopenia is a condition in which your blood has a low number of blood cell fragments called platelets.

Platelets are made in your bone marrow along with other kinds of blood cells. They travel through your blood vessels and stick together (clot) to stop any bleeding that could happen if a blood vessel is damaged. Platelets also are called thrombocytes, because a clot also is called a thrombus.

Overview

When your blood has a low number of platelets, mild to serious bleeding can occur. This bleeding can happen inside the body (internal bleeding) or on the skin.

A normal platelet count is 150,000 to 450,000 platelets per microliter of blood. A count of less than 150,000 platelets per microliter is lower than normal. But the risk for serious bleeding doesn't occur until the count becomes very low—less than 10,000 or 20,000 platelets per microliter. Milder bleeding sometimes occurs when the count is less than 50,000 platelets per microliter.

Several factors can cause a low platelet count, such as the following:

- The body's bone marrow doesn't make enough platelets.

Excerpted from "Thrombocytopenia," National Heart Lung and Blood Institute, National Institutes of Health, January 2008.

- The bone marrow makes enough platelets, but the body destroys them or uses them up.

- The spleen holds on to too many platelets. The spleen is an organ that normally stores about one-third of the body's platelets. It also helps your body fight infection and remove unwanted cell material.

- A combination of the above factors.

How long thrombocytopenia lasts depends on its cause. It can range from days to years.

The treatment for this condition also depends on its cause and severity. Mild thrombocytopenia most often doesn't need treatment. If the condition is causing serious bleeding, or if you're at risk for serious bleeding, you may need medicines or blood or platelet transfusions. Rarely, the spleen may need to be removed.

Outlook

Thrombocytopenia can be fatal, especially if the bleeding is severe or occurs in the brain. However, the overall outlook is good, especially if the cause of the low platelet count is found and treated.

What Causes Thrombocytopenia?

A number of factors can cause thrombocytopenia (a low platelet count). The condition can be inherited (passed from parents to children), or it can develop at any age. Sometimes the cause isn't known.

In general, a low platelet count occurs because one of the following occurs:

- The body's bone marrow doesn't make enough platelets.

- The bone marrow makes enough platelets, but the body destroys them or uses them up.

- The spleen holds onto too many platelets.

A combination of the above factors also may cause a low platelet count.

The Bone Marrow Doesn't Make Enough Platelets

Bone marrow is the sponge-like tissue inside the bones. It contains stem cells that develop into red blood cells, white blood cells, and platelets. When stem cells are damaged, they don't grow into healthy blood cells.

Several conditions or factors can damage stem cells.

Cancer. Cancer, such as leukemia or lymphoma, can damage the bone marrow and destroy blood stem cells. Cancer treatments, such as radiation and chemotherapy, also destroy the stem cells.

Aplastic anemia. Aplastic anemia is a rare, serious blood disorder in which the bone marrow stops making enough new blood cells. This lowers the number of platelets in your blood.

Toxic chemicals. Exposure to toxic chemicals, such as pesticides, arsenic, and benzene, can slow the production of platelets.

Medicines. Some medicines, such as diuretics and chloramphenicol, can slow the production of platelets. Chloramphenicol (an antibiotic) is rarely used in the United States.

Common over-the-counter medicines, such as aspirin or ibuprofen, also can affect platelets.

Alcohol. Alcohol also slows the production of platelets. A temporary drop in platelets is common among heavy drinkers, especially if they're eating foods that are low in iron, vitamin B_{12}, or folate.

Viruses. Chickenpox, mumps, rubella, Epstein-Barr virus, or parvovirus can decrease your platelet count for a while. People who have autoimmune deficiency syndrome (AIDS) often develop thrombocytopenia.

Genetic conditions. Some genetic conditions, such as Wiskott-Aldrich and May-Hegglin syndromes, can cause low numbers of platelets in the blood.

The Body Destroys Its Own Platelets

A low platelet count can occur even if the bone marrow makes enough platelets. The body may destroy its own platelets due to autoimmune diseases, certain medicines, infections, surgery, pregnancy, and some conditions that cause too much blood clotting.

Autoimmune diseases. With autoimmune diseases, the body's immune system destroys its own platelets. One example of this type of disease is called idiopathic thrombocytopenic purpura, or ITP.

In most cases, the body's immune system is thought to cause ITP. Normally, your immune system helps your body fight off infections and diseases. But if you have ITP, your immune system attacks and destroys its own platelets—for an unknown reason.

Other autoimmune diseases that destroy platelets include lupus and rheumatoid arthritis.

Medicines. A reaction to some medicines can confuse your body and cause it to destroy its platelets. Any medicine can cause this reaction, but it happens most often with quinine, antibiotics that contain sulfa, and some medicines for seizures, such as Dilantin,® vancomycin, and rifampin.

Heparin is a medicine commonly used to prevent blood clots. But an immune reaction may trigger the medicine to cause blood clots and thrombocytopenia. This condition is called heparin-induced thrombocytopenia (HIT). HIT rarely occurs outside of a hospital.

In HIT, the body's immune system attacks a substance formed by heparin and a protein on the surface of the platelets. This attack activates the platelets and they start to form blood clots. Blood clots can form deep in the legs, or a clot can break loose and travel to the lungs.

Infection. A low platelet count can occur after blood poisoning from a widespread bacterial infection. A virus, such as mononucleosis or cytomegalovirus, also can cause a low platelet count.

Surgery. Platelets can be destroyed when they pass through man-made heart valves, blood vessel grafts, or machines and tubing used for blood transfusions or bypass surgery.

Pregnancy. About 5 percent of pregnant women develop mild thrombocytopenia when they're close to delivery. The exact cause isn't known for sure.

Rare and serious conditions that cause blood clots. Some diseases can cause a low platelet count. Two examples are thrombotic thrombocytopenic purpura (TTP) and disseminated intravascular clotting (DIC).

TTP is a rare blood condition. It causes blood clots to form in the body's small blood vessels, including vessels in the brains, kidneys, and heart.

DIC is a rare complication of pregnancy, severe infections, or severe trauma. Tiny blood clots form suddenly throughout the body.

In both conditions, the blood clots use up many of the blood's platelets.

The Spleen Holds on to Too Many Platelets

Usually, one-third of the body's platelets are held in the spleen. If the spleen is enlarged, it will hold on to too many platelets. This means that not enough platelets will circulate in the blood.

An enlarged spleen is often due to severe liver disease—such as cirrhosis or cancer. Cirrhosis is a disease in which the liver is scarred. This prevents it from working properly.

An enlarged spleen also may be due to a bone marrow condition, such as myelofibrosis. With this condition, the bone marrow is scarred and isn't able to make blood cells.

What Are the Signs and Symptoms of Thrombocytopenia?

Mild to serious bleeding causes the main signs and symptoms of thrombocytopenia. Bleeding can occur inside the body (internal bleeding) or on the skin.

Signs and symptoms can appear suddenly or over time. Mild thrombocytopenia often has no signs or symptoms. Many times, it's found during a routine blood test.

Check with your doctor if you have any signs of bleeding. Severe thrombocytopenia can cause bleeding in almost any part of the body. This can lead to a medical emergency and should be treated right away.

Bleeding on the skin is usually the first sign of a low platelet count. This may appear as any of the following:

- Small red or purple spots on the skin called petechiae. These spots often occur on the lower legs.

- Purple, brown, and red bruises called purpura. Bruising may happen easily and often.

- Prolonged bleeding, even from minor cuts.

- Bleeding or oozing from the mouth or nose, especially nosebleeds or bleeding from brushing your teeth.

A bleeding problem also can appear as abnormal vaginal bleeding (especially heavy menstrual flow). A lot of bleeding after surgery or dental work also may mean you have a bleeding problem.

Heavy bleeding into the intestines or the brain is serious and can be fatal. Signs and symptoms include the following:

- Blood in the urine or stool or bleeding from the rectum. Blood in the stool can appear as red blood or as a dark, tarry color. (Taking iron supplements also can cause dark, tarry stools.)

- Headaches and other neurological symptoms. These are very rare, but you should discuss them with your doctor.

How Is Thrombocytopenia Diagnosed?

Your doctor will diagnose thrombocytopenia based on your medical history, a physical exam, and test results.

Diagnostic Tests

Your doctor may order one or more of the following tests to help diagnose a low platelet count.

Complete blood count. A complete blood count (CBC) measures the levels of red blood cells, white blood cells, and platelets in your blood. For this test, a small amount of blood is drawn from a blood vessel, usually in your arm.

If you have thrombocytopenia, the results of this test will show that your platelet count is low.

Blood smear. A blood smear is used to check the appearance of your platelets under a microscope. For this test, a small amount of blood is drawn from a blood vessel, usually in your arm.

Bone marrow tests. Bone marrow tests check whether your bone marrow is healthy. Blood cells, including platelets, are made in bone marrow. The two bone marrow tests are aspiration and biopsy.

Bone marrow aspiration may be done to find out why your bone marrow isn't making enough blood cells. For this test, your doctor removes a small amount of fluid bone marrow through a needle. He or she examines the sample under a microscope to check for abnormal cells.

A bone marrow biopsy often is done right after an aspiration. For this test, your doctor removes a small amount of bone marrow tissue through a needle. Your doctor examines the tissue to check the number and types of cells in the bone marrow.

Other tests. If a bleeding problem is suspected, you may need other blood tests as well. For example, tests called prothrombin time (PT) and partial thromboplastin time (PTT) may be done to see whether your blood is clotting properly.

Your doctor may order an ultrasound to check your spleen. An ultrasound uses sound waves to create pictures of your spleen. This will allow your doctor to see whether your spleen is enlarged.

How Is Thrombocytopenia Treated?

Treatment for thrombocytopenia depends on its cause and how severe the condition is. The primary goal of treatment is to prevent death and disability caused by bleeding.

If your condition is mild, you may not need treatment. Your doctor should reassure you that a fully normal platelet count isn't necessary to prevent bleeding, even with severe cuts or accidents.

Thrombocytopenia often improves when its underlying cause is treated. People who inherit the condition usually don't need treatment.

If a reaction to medicine is causing a low platelet count, your doctor may prescribe other medicine. Most people recover after the offending medicine has been stopped. For heparin-induced thrombocytopenia (HIT), stopping the heparin isn't enough. Often, you'll need another medicine to prevent blood clotting.

If your immune system is causing a low platelet count, your doctor may prescribe medicines to suppress the immune system. When the condition is severe, treatments may include the following:

- **Medicines.** You may be given steroids. This medicine can be given through a vein or by mouth. One example of this type of medicine is prednisone. You also may be given immunoglobulin. This medicine is given through a vein.

- **Blood or platelet transfusions.** This type of treatment is reserved for people who have active bleeding or are at a high risk for bleeding.

- **Splenectomy.** This is surgery to remove the spleen. This treatment is most often used for adults who have idiopathic thrombocytopenic purpura.

How Can Thrombocytopenia Be Prevented?

Whether you can prevent thrombocytopenia depends on its specific cause. Most cases of the condition can't be prevented. However, you can take steps to prevent its complications.

- Avoid heavy drinking. Alcohol slows the production of platelets.

- Avoid medicines that have decreased your platelet count in the past.

- Be aware of medicines that may affect your platelets and raise your risk for bleeding. Two examples of such medicines are aspirin and ibuprofen. These medicines may thin your blood too much.

- Talk with your doctor about getting vaccinated for viruses that can affect your platelets. You may need vaccines for mumps, measles, rubella, and chickenpox. You may want to have your child vaccinated for these viruses as well. Talk to you child's doctor about these vaccines.

Living with Thrombocytopenia

If you have thrombocytopenia, watch for any signs and symptoms of bleeding. Report these signs and symptoms to your doctor right away.

Symptoms can appear suddenly or over time. Severe thrombocytopenia can cause bleeding in almost any part of the body. This can lead to a medical emergency and should be treated right away.

You can take steps to avoid complications of thrombocytopenia. Watch what medicines you take, avoid injury, and contact your doctor if you have fever or other signs or symptoms of an infection.

Chapter 34

Idiopathic Thrombocytopenic Purpura

Introduction

Blood Cells

Blood cells, including red cells, white cells, and platelets, are made in the bone marrow. The bone marrow is a soft, spongy tissue found in the center of large bones. In healthy people, millions of new blood cells are made each hour to carry out body functions. Red blood cells (erythrocytes) carry oxygen from the lungs to the rest of the body. White blood cells (leukocytes) fight infections and illness. Platelets (thrombocytes) cause the blood to clot when you are hurt.

The body carefully controls the bone marrow to make the right number of each type of cell. If this process is upset and the marrow makes too many or too few cells, a blood disorder occurs.

Blood disorders require treatment by a doctor. There may be long periods of time when you have no symptoms, but you should be alert to any changes that occur with your disease. If your symptoms get worse, call your doctor right away.

Idiopathic Thrombocytopenic Purpura (or Autoimmune Thrombocytopenia)

In a healthy person, antibodies are used by the immune system to fight bacteria, viruses, or other harmful organisms. In idiopathic

Excerpted from "Idiopathic Thrombocytopenic Purpura," © 2009 University of Iowa Hospitals and Clinics. Reprinted with permission.

thrombocytopenic purpura (ITP) the body makes extra antibodies that are not working right. The antibodies attack the platelets, making them die early. Fewer new platelets are made. The result is easy bruising or bleeding with no visible injury.

In the United States each year sixty-six adults per one million people develop ITP. In children, there are fifty cases per one million. It develops most in women over age sixty, but can occur at any age. Children may develop ITP after an illness like mumps or measles. In most children, ITP will disappear on its own.

Diagnostic Tests

To diagnose ITP, your doctor will do a blood test to count the number of platelets in your blood. If the results are abnormal, you may be referred to a hematologist, a doctor who diagnoses and treats bone marrow and blood disorders. The hematologist may run more tests like a bone marrow aspiration and biopsy. For this test, the doctor will inject some local anesthetic to make the bone and skin numb. Then a small amount of marrow and a small piece of bone are removed to check for defects.

Treatment Overview

The goal of treatment is to increase the number of platelets in the blood. The treatment you receive will depend on your age, health, if you have any symptoms, and the results of your blood test and biopsy. It may include:

- monitoring;
- corticosteroids;
- surgery;
- chemotherapy;
- androgens;
- plasmapheresis;
- intravenous immune globulin;
- WinRho® immune globulin IV (also called IV Anti-(Rh)D or IV Rh immune globulin);
- rituximab (Rituxan®);
- Amicar® (aminocaproic acid).

Monitoring. In some patients, the best treatment is to watch the disorder for any increase in symptoms and do regular blood counts. This may be the only treatment ever needed.

Corticosteroids. Corticosteroids are hormones made by the body to control the immune system. Extra steroids can slow down the death of platelets by decreasing the number of lymphocytes and the making of the wrong antibodies. The drug often used for this is prednisone.

Surgery. The spleen is a major site where platelets are destroyed and the antibodies are made. The doctor may suggest a surgery to remove your spleen. This is called a splenectomy.

Chemotherapy. Chemotherapy can slow the formation of the cells making the wrong antibodies. Some types of medicines used include azathioprine, vincristine, cyclophosphamide, cyclosporine, or vinblastine.

Androgens. Androgens are natural hormones that are sometimes helpful in ITP. One androgen used is Danazol®.

Plasmapheresis. Plasmapheresis can reduce the amount of antibodies in the blood. During this procedure, blood is filtered through a machine that takes out the plasma with antibodies and puts in a substitute.

Intravenous immune globulin. Intravenous immune globulin (IVIG) is a special globulin with good antibodies that is given into the vein.

WinRho® immune globulin IV (also called IV Anti-(Rh)D or IV Rh immune globulin). WinRho® immune globulin IV is a special antibody that can slow platelet destruction. It can be used once if the patient is Rh positive and has not had the spleen removed.

Rituximab (Rituxan®). Rituximab is a medicine that is a monoclonal antibody. It can decrease the number of cells making improper antibodies.

Amicar® (aminocaproic acid). Prevents clots from being dissolved so there is decreased bleeding.

Managing Idiopathic Thrombocytopenic Purpura

There are steps you can take to help prevent or reduce the symptoms of ITP:

- Avoid bruising or bumping yourself, especially your head.

- Use an electric razor. Be careful when using nail trimmers, knives, etc.

- Blow your nose gently and keep room air moist to prevent nosebleeds.

- Wear hard-soled shoes, gloves, and long pants when working outside (i.e. gardening).

- Use a sponge toothbrush if you have problems with gum bleeding. Your doctor or nurse can tell you if you need to use one and where to get it.

- Avoid aspirin or aspirin-like medicines (for example, Motrin®, ibuprofen, or other anti-inflammatory drugs) unless your doctor has told you to take it. These medicines can affect blood clotting. Be sure to tell your doctor about all medicines that you take (including vitamins, herbs, and dietary supplements).

It is important to watch for any change or increase in symptoms. If this occurs you should call your doctor right away. These symptoms require prompt attention.

Bleeding symptoms:

- easy bruising;

- bleeding for no apparent reason;

- heavy or prolonged bleeding;

- petechiae, or tiny areas of pinpoint bleeding on the skin of the arms or legs;

- blood in the urine or stools;

- bleeding from the nose or gums;

- headaches;

- confusion;

- severe headache or visual changes;

- stiff neck.

Follow-Up Care and Prognosis

ITP requires regular check-ups with your doctor. He or she will want to discuss your symptoms and do regular blood counts to see how you respond to treatment.

How well you do depends upon the symptoms you have, your age, and the treatment you receive. Some patients may only be watched and need little care. Other patients may need more active treatment.

If you have questions or concerns about your treatment and prognosis, be sure to talk with your doctor. It may help to write your questions out before your visit.

Chapter 35

Thrombotic Thrombocytopenic Purpura

Introduction

Blood Cells

Blood cells, including red cells, white cells, and platelets, are made in the bone marrow. The bone marrow is a soft, spongy tissue found in the center of large bones. In healthy people, millions of new blood cells are made each hour to carry out body functions. Red blood cells (erythrocytes) carry oxygen from the lungs to the rest of the body. White blood cells (leukocytes) fight infections and illness. Platelets (thrombocytes) cause the blood to clot when there is an injury.

The body carefully controls the bone marrow to make the right number of each type of cell. If this process is upset and the marrow makes too many or too few cells, a blood disorder occurs.

Blood disorders require treatment by a doctor. There may be long periods of time when you have no symptoms, but you should be alert to any changes that occur with your disease. If your symptoms start or get worse, call your doctor right away. Also, feel free to call your doctor with questions about your disease, the treatment you are getting, or any other concerns you may have.

Thrombotic Thrombocytopenic Purpura (TTP)

Thrombotic Thrombocytopenic Purpura (TTP) is a rare disorder that causes clotting in the small blood vessels of many organs (microangiopathy). As a result, you may have a low platelet count, anemia, and damage to the organs. Patients with this disorder may have easy bruising and more than usual bleeding. If this occurs in the kidneys they may stop working. In the brain it can result in confusion, stroke, or even coma.

Acquired TTP is most common in adults; inherited TTP is seen in babies and children. Around 1,200 people develop acquired TTP each year in the United States. It is most common in adults from twenty to fifty years old, and it affects women slightly more than men.

Diagnostic Tests

To diagnose TTP, your doctor will order a series of tests:

* Complete blood count.

* Blood smear to look at how the red blood cells look.

* Bilirubin test that shows if red blood cells are breaking apart faster than normal.

* Kidney function and urine tests.

* Coombs Test to see if TTP is causing hemolytic anemia. Hemolytic anemia is when red blood cells break apart faster than they are replaced.

* Lactate dehydrogenase test measures the level of the protein lactate dehydrogenase. The protein is released when hemolytic anemia is happening or blood clots have formed because of TTP.

* ADAMTS13 Assay—ADAMTS13 is an enzyme that causes TTP when it is not active enough. This test checks the activity of the enzyme.

If the results are abnormal, you may be referred to a hematologist, a doctor who diagnoses and treats bone marrow and blood disorders.

Treatment Overview

Your treatment will be based on your age, overall health, if you have any symptoms, and the results of your blood tests. Your treatment may include:

* plasma exchange;

* infusion of new plasma;

- corticosteroids;

- other treatments.

Plasma exchange. In plasma exchange, also called plasmapheresis, the blood is filtered through a machine that removes plasma and replaces it with plasma from healthy blood donors.

Infusion of new plasma. In this treatment, plasma from healthy donors is given to slow down clotting in small vessels.

Corticosteroids. Corticosteroids are hormones made naturally by the body to control the immune system. You may be given more corticosteroids. One type of drug often used is prednisone.

Other treatments. Although rare, chemotherapy or removing the spleen may be necessary.

Managing Thrombotic Thrombocytopenic Purpura

There are steps you can take to help prevent or reduce the symptoms of TTP:

- Avoid bumping or bruising yourself.

- Use an electric razor. Be careful when using nail trimmers, knives, etc.

- Wear hard-soled shoes, gloves, and long pants when working outside (i.e. gardening).

- Use a sponge toothbrush if you have problems with gum bleeding. Your doctor or nurse can tell you if you need to use one and where it can be found.

- Avoid aspirin or aspirin-like medicines (for example, Motrin®, ibuprofen, or other anti-inflammatory drugs) unless your doctor has told you to take it. These medicines can affect blood clotting. Also, be sure to tell your doctor of all medicines that you take (including vitamins, herbs, and dietary supplements).

It is important that you be alert for any change or increase in symptoms. If this occurs you should call your doctor right away. These symptoms require prompt attention.
Bleeding symptoms:

- heavy or prolonged bleeding;

- bleeding for no apparent reason;
- frequent bruising;
- nose or gum bleeding;
- black, tarry, or bloody stools;
- blood in the urine;
- purpura, or purplish spots (like bruises) on skin or mucous membranes such as gums.

Small blood vessel clotting symptoms:

- jaundice or yellowing of the skin or eyes;
- headaches;
- dizziness;
- confusion of speech or changes in speech;
- confusion;
- strokes or seizures.

Anemia symptoms:

- pale color;
- shortness of breath, especially during activity;
- weakness or fatigue.

Other symptoms:

- fever;
- fast heart rate.

Follow-Up Care and Prognosis

TTP requires regular check-ups with your doctor. He or she will want to talk about your symptoms and do regular blood counts to check your response to treatment.

How well you do depends upon the symptoms you may have, your age, and the treatment you receive. Some patients may need little care, while others require more active treatment.

If you have questions or concerns about your treatment and prognosis, be sure to talk with your doctor. It may be helpful to write your questions out before your visit.

Chapter 36

Thrombophilia

What is thrombophilia?

Thrombophilias can be defined as a group of inherited or acquired disorders that increase a person's risk of developing thrombosis (abnormal "blood clotting") in the veins or arteries.

The human body is equipped with a sophisticated and well-balanced blood coagulation (or clotting) system, in which platelets (the "clotting" blood cells) and multiple coagulation proteins mingle in order to avoid both excessive bleeding and excessive clotting. Thrombus (blood clot) formation is a good thing after injuries to blood vessels, regardless of whether the injury results from an accidental cut, major trauma, a broken bone, or surgery. If blood clotting did not occur, you would experience unstoppable (and even life threatening) bleeding. This normal blood clot formation should be localized to the area where blood vessel injury occurred and should be stopped as soon as the leak of blood from the vessels is contained and/or the vessel injury is healed or repaired. In the presence of thrombophilias, the well-balanced coagulation system has a predisposition toward thrombosis, which is also referred to as "hypercoagulability" or "hypercoagulable state."

Thrombophilias can be inherited (hereditary), acquired (not inherited), or both. Inherited thrombophilias are abnormalities of the genes that are responsible for making the coagulation proteins (known as genetic mutations). Acquired thrombophilias are due to increased levels of certain clotting substances in the blood or special proteins called antibodies which may also lead to clotting. The most common inherited thrombophilias include Factor V Leiden (a symptom-free condition that increases the risk of deep vein thrombosis), and the prothrombin gene mutations, as well as the uncommon but well-known deficiencies of protein C, protein S, or antithrombin. Individuals who are born with an inherited thrombophilia are also referred to as "carriers" of that particular genetic mutation. The most common acquired thrombophilias are commonly encountered during surgery, injury, or medical conditions including congestive heart failure and certain respiratory conditions, and these are called antiphospholipid antibodies (APLA). These represent a family of several different individual antibodies which may, as a group or independently, lead both to clotting events and also recurrent miscarriages. Some thrombophilias can both have a genetic predisposition and be acquired. Research studies have estimated that nearly 10 percent of the world population has an underlying thrombophilia, the most common being the Factor V Leiden and the prothrombin gene mutations.

Both inherited and acquired thrombophilias appear to "tilt" the well-balanced coagulation system toward clotting (thrombosis). Such an imbalance in the coagulation system results in a greater risk of clotting events, such as deep venous thrombosis (DVT) or pulmonary embolism (PE). However, the simple fact that a person has a thrombophilia and a greater chance of developing abnormal clotting than a person without thrombophilia does not mean that the former individual will ever have a clotting event. Fortunately, not all people with thrombophilia will have a blood clot in their lifetime, whereas unfortunately many patients who do experience thrombotic events (such as DVT) may not have any detectable thrombophilia at all.

What are the symptoms of thrombophilia?

Thrombophilias cause no specific symptoms other than those related to clotting events. The most common clotting events related to thrombophilias are acute DVT (a blood clot within large veins) and acute pulmonary embolism (PE; pieces of blood clots which form in the veins of the body, then dislodge and travel to the arteries of the heart and lungs), as well as recurrent superficial venous thromboses or clots of the superficial veins of the arms and legs. While most research studies suggest that inherited thrombophilias increase the risk of vein clots only (i.e., DVT and PE), some acquired thrombophilias are also believed to cause arterial clotting events, such as acute strokes, acute limb ischemia (sudden loss of blood flow to the legs or arms), and even acute myocardial infarction (heart attack).

What are the risk factors for thrombophilia?

It has been estimated that 50 to 70 percent of the DVT and PE events that occur in patients with an underlying inherited thrombophilia are triggered by risk factors. These are known as "situational" or "provoked" clotting events. Even though patients with thrombophilias may suffer from "idiopathic" or "unprovoked" ("out-of-the-blue") clotting events, most of the time they occur during or immediately after the person is considered to be high-risk for DVT and PE. Such high-risk situations include orthopedic or other major surgery, bed rest during hospitalization for a medical problem, immobilization in a plaster cast for a broken leg, use of birth control pills or hormone replacement therapy, cancer, obesity, pregnancy, and very long airline flights.

How is thrombophilia diagnosed?

The diagnosis of thrombophilia is made by blood tests; specific blood tests for each known thrombophilia are available. Testing should be offered only to patients for whom the results will have an impact on their care. Thrombophilia testing in individuals without any personal history or family history of DVT or PE is not appropriate.

While there are no formal guidelines as to who should be tested, suggested candidates for testing include:

- young (age less than forty-five years) patients with "idiopathic" or "unprovoked" DVT/PE;

- patients who have had more than one DVT/PE;

- patients who have suffered from blood clots in unusual locations, such as the veins of the abdomen or brain, when there is no triggering event;

- patients with DVT/PE and a strong family history of the same;

- women with multiple miscarriages with no clear explanation.

Even in the circumstances listed above, specific thrombophilia testing should not be viewed as "mandatory," and an in-depth evaluation and discussion with a knowledgeable physician are of utmost importance prior to determining the goals of testing. And even if testing is deemed indicated or appropriate, not all thrombophilias may need to be screened.

The timing of thrombophilia testing is as important as the decision to proceed with testing or not. Testing should be avoided during hospitalization, during periods of severe illness, as well as during pregnancy, because of the potential for false-positive results. The use of certain medications, such as blood thinners and birth control pills or hormone replacement pills or patches, may also lead to false-positive results.

How is thrombophilia treated?

There is no specific treatment for most thrombophilias, except for treatment with anticoagulants ("blood thinners") if there has been a clotting event. Anticoagulants that are used to treat blood clots include heparin, low-molecular-weight heparin, fondaparinux (a newer agent), and warfarin (or Coumadin®). The length of anticoagulation treatment depends upon the type of blood clot and the nature of the thrombophilia and is decided by the patient's physician after reviewing all of the clinical information. If a person without any history of DVT or PE is found to have a thrombophilia, use of blood thinners is rarely recommended.

Part Five

Circulatory Disorders

Chapter 37

Aneurysm

What Is an Aneurysm?

An aneurysm is a balloon-like bulge in an artery. Arteries are blood vessels that carry oxygen-rich blood from your heart to your body.

Arteries have thick walls to withstand normal blood pressure. However, certain medical problems, genetic conditions, and trauma can damage or injure artery walls. The force of blood pushing against the weakened or injured walls can cause an aneurysm.

An aneurysm can grow large and burst (rupture) or cause a dissection. Rupture causes dangerous bleeding inside the body. A dissection is a split in one or more layers of the artery wall. The split causes bleeding into and along the layers of the artery wall.

Both conditions are often fatal.

Overview

Most aneurysms occur in the aorta—the main artery that carries blood from the heart to the rest of the body. The aorta goes through the chest and abdomen.

An aneurysm that occurs in the part of the aorta that's in the chest is called a thoracic aortic aneurysm. An aneurysm that occurs in the part of the aorta that's in the abdomen is called an abdominal aortic aneurysm.

Excerpted from "Aneurysm," National Heart Lung and Blood Institute, National Institutes of Health, April 2009.

Aneurysms also can occur in other arteries, but these types of aneurysm are less common. This chapter will focus on aortic aneurysms.

About fourteen thousand Americans die each year from aortic aneurysms. Most of the deaths result from rupture or dissection.

Early diagnosis and medical treatment can help prevent many cases of rupture and dissection. However, aneurysms can develop and become large before causing any symptoms. Thus, people who are at high risk for aneurysms can benefit from early, routine screening.

Outlook

When found in time, aortic aneurysms often can be successfully treated with medicines or surgery. Medicines may be given to lower blood pressure, relax blood vessels, and reduce the risk of rupture.

Large aortic aneurysms often can be repaired with surgery. During surgery, the weak or damaged portion of the aorta is replaced or reinforced.

Types of Aneurysm

Aortic Aneurysms

The two types of aortic aneurysm are abdominal aortic aneurysm (AAA) and thoracic aortic aneurysm (TAA).

Abdominal aortic aneurysms. An aneurysm that occurs in the part of the aorta that's located in the abdomen is called an abdominal aortic aneurysm. AAAs account for three in four aortic aneurysms. They're found more often now than in the past because of computed tomography, or CT, scans done for other medical problems.

Small AAAs rarely rupture. However, an AAA can grow very large without causing symptoms. Thus, routine checkups and treatment for an AAA are important to prevent growth and rupture.

Thoracic aortic aneurysms. An aneurysm that occurs in the part of the aorta that's located in the chest and above the diaphragm is called a thoracic aortic aneurysm. TAAs account for one in four aortic aneurysms.

TAAs don't always cause symptoms, even when they're large. Only half of all people who have TAAs notice any symptoms. TAAs are found more often now than in the past because of chest CT scans done for other medical problems.

With a common type of TAA, the walls of the aorta weaken, and a section close to the heart enlarges. As a result, the valve between the heart and the aorta can't close properly. This allows blood to leak back into the heart.

A less common type of TAA can develop in the upper back, away from the heart. A TAA in this location may result from an injury to the chest, such as from a car crash.

Other Types of Aneurysms

Brain Aneurysms

When an aneurysm occurs in an artery in the brain, it's called a cerebral aneurysm or brain aneurysm. Brain aneurysms also are sometimes called berry aneurysms because they're often the size of a small berry.

Most brain aneurysms cause no symptoms until they become large, begin to leak blood, or rupture. A ruptured brain aneurysm causes a stroke.

Peripheral Aneurysms

Aneurysms that occur in arteries other than the aorta and the brain arteries are called peripheral aneurysms. Common locations for peripheral aneurysms include the popliteal, femoral, and carotid arteries.

The popliteal arteries run down the back of the thighs, behind the knees. The femoral arteries are the main arteries in the groin. The carotid arteries are the two main arteries on each side of your neck.

Peripheral aneurysms aren't as likely to rupture or dissect as aortic aneurysms. However, blood clots can form in peripheral aneurysms. If a blood clot breaks away from the aneurysm, it can block blood flow through the artery.

If a peripheral aneurysm is large, it can press on a nearby nerve or vein and cause pain, numbness, or swelling.

What Causes an Aneurysm?

The force of blood pushing against the walls of an artery combined with damage or injury to the artery's walls can cause an aneurysm.

A number of factors can damage and weaken the walls of the aorta and cause aortic aneurysms.

Aging, smoking, high blood pressure, and atherosclerosis are all factors that can damage or weaken the walls of the aorta. Atherosclerosis is the hardening and narrowing of the arteries due to the buildup of a fatty material called plaque.

Rarely, infections, such as untreated syphilis (a sexually transmitted infection), can cause aortic aneurysms. Aortic aneurysms also can occur as a result of diseases that inflame the blood vessels, such as vasculitis.

Family history also may play a role in causing aortic aneurysms.

In addition to the factors above, certain genetic conditions may cause thoracic aortic aneurysms (TAAs). Examples include Marfan syndrome, Loeys-Dietz syndrome, and Ehlers-Danlos syndrome (the vascular type).

These conditions can weaken the body's connective tissues and damage the aorta. People who have these conditions tend to develop aneurysms at a younger age and are at higher risk for rupture or dissection.

Trauma, such as a car accident, also can damage the aorta walls and lead to TAAs.

Researchers continue to look for other causes of aortic aneurysms. For example, they're looking for genetic mutations that may contribute to or cause aneurysms.

Who Is at Risk for an Aneurysm?

Certain factors put you at higher risk for an aortic aneurysm. These include the following:

- **Male gender.** Men are more likely than women to have abdominal aortic aneurysms (AAAs)—the most common type of aneurysm.

- **Age.** The risk for AAAs increases as you get older. These aneurysms are more likely to occur in people who are sixty-five or older.

- **Smoking.** Smoking can damage and weaken the walls of the aorta.

- **Family history of aortic aneurysm.** People who have family histories of aortic aneurysm are at higher risk of having one, and they may have aneurysms before the age of sixty-five.

- **Certain diseases and conditions that weaken the walls of the aorta.**

Car accidents or trauma also can injure the arteries and increase your risk for an aneurysm.

If you have any of these risk factors, talk with your doctor about whether you need to be screened for aneurysms.

What Are the Signs and Symptoms of an Aneurysm?

The signs and symptoms of an aortic aneurysm depend on the type of aneurysm, its location, and whether it has ruptured or is affecting other parts of the body.

Aneurysms can develop and grow for years without causing any signs or symptoms. They often don't cause signs or symptoms until they rupture, grow large enough to press on nearby parts of the body, or block blood flow.

Abdominal Aortic Aneurysms

Most abdominal aortic aneurysms (AAAs) develop slowly over years. They often don't have signs or symptoms unless they rupture. If you have an AAA, your doctor may feel a throbbing mass while checking your abdomen.

When symptoms are present, they can include the following:

- A throbbing feeling in the abdomen

- Deep pain in your back or the side of your abdomen

- Steady, gnawing pain in your abdomen that lasts for hours or days

If an AAA ruptures, symptoms can include sudden, severe pain in your lower abdomen and back; nausea (feeling sick to your stomach) and vomiting; clammy, sweaty skin; lightheadedness; and a rapid heart rate when standing up.

Internal bleeding from a ruptured AAA can send you into shock. This is a life-threatening situation that requires emergency treatment.

Thoracic Aortic Aneurysms

A thoracic aortic aneurysm (TAA) may not cause symptoms until it dissects or grows large. Then, symptoms may include the following:

- Pain in your jaw, neck, back, or chest

- Coughing, hoarseness, or trouble breathing or swallowing

A dissection is a split in one or more layers of the artery wall. The split causes bleeding into and along the layers of the artery wall.

If a TAA ruptures or dissects, you may feel sudden, severe pain starting in your upper back and moving down into your abdomen. You may have pain in your chest and arms, and you can quickly go into shock. Shock is a life-threatening condition in which the body's organs don't get enough blood flow.

If you have any symptoms of TAA or aortic dissection, call 9-1-1. If left untreated, these conditions may lead to organ damage or death.

How Is an Aneurysm Diagnosed?

If you have aortic aneurysm, but no symptoms, your doctor may find it by chance during a routine physical exam. More often, doctors find aneurysms during tests done for other reasons, such as chest or abdominal pain.

If you have an abdominal aortic aneurysm (AAA), your doctor may feel a throbbing mass in your abdomen. A rapidly growing aneurysm about to rupture can be tender and very painful when pressed. If you're overweight or obese, it may be hard for your doctor to feel even a large AAA.

If you have an AAA, your doctor may hear rushing blood flow instead of the normal whooshing sound when listening to your abdomen with a stethoscope.

Diagnostic Tests and Procedures

To diagnose and evaluate an aneurysm, your doctor may recommend one or more of the following tests.

Ultrasound. This simple, painless test uses sound waves to create pictures of the structures inside your body. Ultrasound shows the size of an aneurysm, if one is found.

Computed tomography scan. A computed tomography (CT) scan is a painless test that uses x-rays to take clear, detailed pictures of your internal organs.

During the test, your doctor will inject a special dye into a vein in your arm. This dye highlights the aorta on the CT scan images.

Your doctor may recommend this test if he or she thinks you have an AAA or a thoracic aortic aneurysm (TAA). A CT scan can show the size and shape of an aneurysm. This test provides more detailed images than an ultrasound.

Magnetic resonance imaging. Magnetic resonance imaging (MRI) uses magnets and radio waves to create images of the organs and structures in your body. This test is very accurate at detecting aneurysms and pinpointing their size and exact location.

Angiography. Angiography uses a special dye injected into the bloodstream to highlight the insides of arteries on x-ray pictures. An angiogram shows the amount of damage and blockage in blood vessels.

An angiogram of the aorta is called an aortogram. An aortogram may show the location and size of an aortic aneurysm.

How Is an Aneurysm Treated?

Aortic aneurysms are treated with medicines and surgery. A small aneurysm that's found early and isn't causing symptoms may not need treatment. Other aneurysms need to be treated.

The goals of treatment are as follows:

• To prevent the aneurysm from growing

• To prevent or reverse damage to other body structures

• To prevent or treat a rupture or dissection

• To allow you to continue to do your normal daily activities

Treatment for aortic aneurysms is based on the size of the aneurysm. Your doctor may recommend routine testing to make sure an aneurysm isn't getting bigger. This method usually is used for aneurysms that are smaller than five centimeters (about two inches) across.

How often you need testing (for example, every few months or every year) will be based on the size of the aneurysm and how fast it's growing. The larger it is and the faster it's growing, the more often you may need to be checked.

Medicines

If you have an aortic aneurysm, your doctor may prescribe medicines before surgery or instead of surgery. Medicines are used to lower blood pressure, relax blood vessels, and reduce the risk of rupture. Beta blockers and calcium channel blockers are the medicines most commonly used.

Surgery

Your doctor may recommend surgery if your aneurysm is growing quickly or if it reaches a size linked with an increased risk of rupture or dissection.

The two main types of surgery to repair aortic aneurysms are open abdominal or open chest repair and endovascular repair.

Open abdominal or open chest repair. The standard and most common type of surgery for aortic aneurysms is open abdominal or open chest repair. It involves a major incision (cut) in the abdomen or chest. General anesthesia is used for this procedure—that is, you will be temporarily put to sleep so you don't feel pain during the surgery.

The aneurysm is removed, and the section of aorta is replaced with a graft made of material such as Dacron® or Teflon.® The surgery takes three to six hours, and you will remain in the hospital for five to eight days.

It often takes a month to recover from open abdominal or open chest surgery and return to full activity. Most patients make a full recovery.

Endovascular repair. In endovascular repair, the aneurysm isn't removed. Instead, a graft is inserted into the aorta to strengthen it. This type of surgery is done using catheters (tubes) inserted into the arteries; it doesn't require surgically opening the chest or abdomen.

The surgeon first inserts a catheter into an artery in the groin (upper thigh) and threads it to the aneurysm. Then, using an x-ray to see the artery, the surgeon threads the graft (also called a stent graft) into the aorta to the aneurysm.

The graft is then expanded inside the aorta and fastened in place to form a stable channel for blood flow. The graft reinforces the weakened section of the aorta to prevent the aneurysm from rupturing.

Endovascular repair reduces recovery time to a few days and greatly reduces time in the hospital. However, doctors can't repair all aortic aneurysms with this procedure. The location or size of the aneurysm may prevent a stent graft from being safely or reliably placed inside the aneurysm.

Chapter 38

Aortic Dissection

Alternative Names

Aortic aneurysm—dissecting

Definition

Aortic dissection is a potentially life-threatening condition in which there is bleeding into and along the wall of the aorta, the major artery leaving the heart.

Causes

Aortic dissection most often occurs because of a tear or damage to the inner wall of the aorta. This usually occurs in the thoracic (chest) portion of the artery, but may also occur in the abdominal portion.

The aorta has different branches through which blood flows. An aortic dissection is classified as type A or B depending on where it begins and ends.

Type A begins in the first (ascending) part of the aorta and typically moves to another part of the chest.

Type B begins in the last (descending) part of the aorta and moves down the abdomen.

When a tear occurs, it creates two channels: One in which blood continues to travel and another where blood remains still. As the aortic dissection grows bigger, the channel with nontraveling blood can get bigger and push on other branches of the aorta.

An aortic dissection may also involve abnormal widening or ballooning of the aorta (aneurysm).

The exact cause is unknown, but risks include atherosclerosis (hardening of the arteries) and high blood pressure. Traumatic injury is a major cause of aortic dissection, especially blunt trauma to the chest as can be caused by hitting the steering wheel of a car during an accident.

Other risk factors and conditions associated with the development of aortic dissection include:

- bicuspid aortic valve;

- coarctation (narrowing) of the aorta;

- connective tissue disorders;

- Ehlers-Danlos syndrome;

- heart surgery or procedures;

- Marfan syndrome;

- pregnancy;

- pseudoxanthoma elasticum;

- vascular inflammation due to conditions such as arteritis and syphilis.

Aortic dissection occurs in approximately two out of every ten thousand people. It can affect anyone, but is most often seen in men aged forty to seventy.

Symptoms

The symptoms usually begin suddenly, and include severe chest pain. The pain may:

- be described as sharp, stabbing, tearing, or ripping;

- be felt below the chest bone, then moves under the shoulder blades or to the back;

- move to shoulder, neck, arm, jaw, abdomen, or hips;

- change position—pain typically moves to the arms and legs as the aortic dissection gets worse.

Other symptoms may include:

- changes in thought ability, confusion, disorientation;
- decreased movement, any part of the body;
- decreased sensation, any part of the body;
- dizziness;
- dry mouth;
- dry skin;
- fainting;
- intense anxiety, anguish;
- nausea and vomiting;
- pallor;
- profuse sweating (clammy skin);
- rapid, weak pulse;
- shortness of breath—difficulty breathing when lying flat (orthopnea);
- thirst.

Exams and Tests

The healthcare provider will take your family history and listen to your heart, lungs, and abdomen with a stethoscope. A "blowing" murmur over the aorta, a heart murmur, or other abnormal sound may be heard.

There may be a difference in blood pressure between the right and left arms, or between the arms and the legs.

There may be low blood pressure, bulging neck veins, or signs resembling a heart attack. There may be signs of shock, but with normal blood pressure.

Aortic dissection or aortic aneurysm may be seen on:

- aortic angiography;
- chest x-ray—may show chest widening or fluid in the lining of the lung (pleural effusion);
- chest magnetic resonance imaging (MRI);
- computed tomography (CT) scan of chest with dye;
- Doppler ultrasonography (occasionally performed);

- echocardiogram;
- transesophageal echocardiogram (TEE).

Treatment

The goal of treatment is to prevent complications. Hospitalization is required.

Type A aortic dissections require surgery to repair the aorta. Type B aortic dissections may be treated with medication.

Drugs that lower blood pressure may be prescribed. These drugs may be given through a vein (intravenously). Strong pain relievers are usually needed. Heart medications such as beta-blockers may reduce some of the symptoms.

Surgery to repair or replace the damaged section of aorta can cure the condition in some cases. If the aortic valve is damaged, valve replacement is necessary. If the heart arteries are involved, a coronary bypass is also performed.

Outlook (Prognosis)

Aortic dissection is life threatening. The condition can be cured with surgery if it is done before the aorta ruptures. Less than half of patients with ruptured aorta survive.

Possible Complications

- Aortic rupture causing rapid blood loss, shock
- Bleeding from the aorta
- Blood clots
- Cardiac tamponade
- Heart attack
- Not enough blood flow past the dissection
- Permanent kidney failure
- Stroke

When to Contact a Medical Professional

If you have symptoms of aortic dissection or severe chest pain, call 911 or your local emergency number, or go to the emergency room as quickly as possible.

Prevention

Proper treatment and control of atherosclerosis (hardening of the arteries) and high blood pressure may reduce your risk of aortic dissection. Tight control of blood pressure in patients at risk of dissection is very important. Drugs such as angiotensin receptor blockers, angiotensin-converting enzyme (ACE) inhibitors, and beta-blockers may reduce the likelihood of dissection.

Take safety precautions to prevent injuries, which can cause dissections.

Many cases of aortic dissection cannot be prevented.

Chapter 39

Arteritis

Chapter Contents

Section 39.1

Takayasu Arteritis

"Takayasu's Arteritis," © 2008 Cedars-Sinai Medical Center (www.csmc.edu). Reprinted with permission.

Takayasu arteritis is a rheumatic disease that causes the aorta and its branches to become inflamed (swollen and tender).

Symptoms of Takayasu Arteritis

About half the people who have Takayasu arteritis develop a general feeling of being unwell, a fever, night sweats, tiredness, weight loss, and joint pain. This phase gradually goes away and is replaced by chronic inflammation and damaging changes to the aorta and its branches.

The other half of the people who have this disease have symptoms only of chronic inflammation and damage to the aorta.

In advanced stages of the disease, the walls of the arteries may become weak and develop aneurysms. These are weak spots that bulge out from the artery walls due to the pressure of the blood flowing through the artery. If they aren't discovered, they can burst and cause bleeding inside the body.

The blood vessels that branch off of the aorta are particularly at risk. Any or all of them may become blocked. Fainting and temporary interruptions of the blood flow to the brain and head may occur along with weakness of the jaws when chewing or speaking or the arms.

The face and arms may lose muscle mass. Disturbances in a person's ability to see are common. Sometimes the portion of the aorta that runs through the abdomen may be affected. This can cause serious increases in the blood pressure of the kidneys.

The involvement of the coronary arteries, severe high blood pressure, or changes in the aorta's ability to work efficiently can lead to heart failure. Much less often, blockages in the arteries of the lungs can cause high blood pressure in the lungs.

Causes and Risk Factors for Takayasu Arteritis

Takayasu arteritis occurs throughout the world. However, persons with the following characteristics have a higher risk of developing Takayasu arteritis:

- Being between the ages of fifteen and thirty

- Being a woman (women are about eight times more likely than men to develop this condition)

- Being a young Asian woman

Diagnosing Takayasu Arteritis

During a physical examination, the doctor will check for the blood pressure rate in the involved arteries arising from the aorta. In Takayasu arteritis, pulses and blood pressure will be low or impossible to find. By contrast, there will be generally brisk pulses in the legs. Bruits may be heard over partially narrowed arteries.

Treating Takayasu Arteritis

In many patients, Takayasu arteritis goes away without major complications. Such patients may do well for years. In other cases, complications such as stroke, severe high blood pressure, heart attack, heart failure, or aneurysms may occur.

During the acute stage of the symptoms, corticosteroids such as prednisone may be used. Once the symptoms start to go away, the amount of prednisone is tapered off, although treatment may be needed for several months. In cases where a person can't take corticosteroids or where they are not effective, cyclophosphamide may be given. Some studies show that vigorous treatment with corticosteroids and cyclophosphamide when the condition is acute may reduce long-term complications of the blood vessels.

Aspirin or drugs that prevent the blood from clotting such as warfarin may be recommended for ischemia. Hypertension should be treated aggressively. Angiotensin-converting enzyme (ACE) inhibitors may be particularly effective because hypertension is frequently of renovascular origin.

In the later stages of the disease, surgery may be needed to reestablish blood flow in blocked arteries. Balloon angioplasty may provide temporary improvement in selected cases. Arterial and aortic aneurysms may require surgery as well.

Section 39.2

Temporal Arteritis

"Temporal Arteritis (Giant Cell Arteritis)," © St. Luke's Cataract and Laser Institute (www.stlukeseye.com). Reprinted with permission. This document is available online at http://www.stlukeseye.com/conditions/temporalarteritis .asp; accessed on May 6, 2009.

Overview

Temporal arteritis, also known as giant cell arteritis, is an inflammatory condition affecting the medium-sized blood vessels that supply the head, eyes, and optic nerves. The disease usually affects those over sixty years of age and causes the vessels in the temple and scalp to become swollen and tender. Women are approximately four times more likely to suffer from this disease then men.

The major concern with temporal arteritis is vision loss, although if allowed to progress, it may affect arteries in other areas of the body. This condition is potentially vision threatening, however, if treated promptly, permanent vision loss can be prevented. Vision is threatened when the inflamed arteries obstruct blood flow to the eyes and optic nerves. If untreated, permanent vision loss can occur from oxygen deprivation to the retina and optic nerve.

Signs and Symptoms

Patients with temporal arteritis usually notice visual symptoms in one eye at first, but as many as 50 percent may notice symptoms in the fellow eye within days if the condition is untreated.

- Headache
- Tenderness of scalp (combing hair may be painful)
- Pain in temple area (may be excruciating)
- Transient blurred vision
- Loss of appetite
- Fever

- Fatigue

- Depression

- Drooping lid

- Double vision

- Sore neck

- Jaw soreness, especially when chewing food

Detection and Diagnosis

When temporal arteritis is suspected, the doctor will order blood tests including a erythrocyte (red blood cell) sedimentation rate (ESR) and C-reactive protein test. The ESR test measures the time it takes for the erythrocytes to collect in the bottom of a test tube. The sediment layer of erythrocytes is measured in millimeters and recorded. An abnormally high ESR is indicative of active inflammation.

C-reactive protein is produced in the liver. This protein is released when the body responds to an injury or any other event that signals inflammation. C-reactive protein is measured with a blood test.

A biopsy of the temporal artery is usually recommended. The procedure is performed with local anesthesia. A small section of the temporal artery is removed and examined under magnification for inflammatory cells. This test allows doctors to definitively diagnose temporal arteritis.

Treatment

The ophthalmologist often works in conjunction with the patient's internist to treat this disease. The primary treatment for the disease is oral steroid medication to reduce the inflammatory process. Most patients notice an improvement in their symptoms within several days. In some cases, a long-term maintenance dosage of the steroid is required.

Chapter 40

Atherosclerosis

What Is Atherosclerosis?

Atherosclerosis is a disease in which plaque builds up on the insides of your arteries. Arteries are blood vessels that carry oxygen-rich blood to your heart and other parts of your body.

Plaque is made up of fat, cholesterol, calcium, and other substances found in the blood. Over time, plaque hardens and narrows your arteries. The flow of oxygen-rich blood to your organs and other parts of your body is reduced. This can lead to serious problems, including heart attack, stroke, or even death.

Other Names for Atherosclerosis

- Arteriosclerosis

- Hardening of the arteries

What Causes Atherosclerosis?

The exact cause of atherosclerosis isn't known. However, studies show that atherosclerosis is a slow, complex disease that may start in childhood. It develops faster as you age.

Atherosclerosis may start when certain factors damage the inner layers of the arteries. These factors include the following:

Excerpted from "Atherosclerosis," National Heart Lung and Blood Institute, National Institutes of Health, November 2007.

- Smoking

- High amounts of certain fats and cholesterol in the blood

- High blood pressure

- High amounts of sugar in the blood due to insulin resistance or diabetes

When damage occurs, your body starts a healing process. Fatty tissues release compounds that promote this process. This healing causes plaque to build up where the arteries are damaged.

Over time, the plaque may crack. Blood cells called platelets clump together to form blood clots where the cracks are. This narrows the arteries more and worsens angina (chest pain) or causes a heart attack.

Who Is at Risk for Atherosclerosis?

Coronary artery disease (atherosclerosis of the coronary arteries) is the leading cause of death in the United States.

The exact cause of atherosclerosis isn't known. However, certain traits, conditions, or habits may raise your chance of developing it. These conditions are known as risk factors. Your chances of developing atherosclerosis increase with the number of risk factors you have.

You can control most risk factors and help prevent or delay atherosclerosis. Other risk factors can't be controlled.

Major Risk Factors

- **Unhealthy blood cholesterol levels.** This includes high low-density lipoprotein (LDL) cholesterol (sometimes called bad cholesterol) and low high-density lipoprotein (HDL) cholesterol (sometimes called good cholesterol).

- **High blood pressure.** Blood pressure is considered high if it stays at or above 140/90 mmHg over a period of time.

- **Smoking.** This can damage and tighten blood vessels, raise cholesterol levels, and raise blood pressure. Smoking also doesn't allow enough oxygen to reach the body's tissues.

- **Insulin resistance.** This condition occurs when the body can't use its own insulin properly. Insulin is a hormone that helps move blood sugar into cells where it's used.

- **Diabetes.** This is a disease in which the body's blood sugar level is high because the body doesn't make enough insulin or doesn't use its insulin properly.

- **Overweight or obesity.** Overweight is having extra body weight from muscle, bone, fat, and/or water. Obesity is having a high amount of extra body fat.

- **Lack of physical activity.** Lack of activity can worsen other risk factors for atherosclerosis.

- **Age.** As you get older, your risk for atherosclerosis increases. Genetic or lifestyle factors cause plaque to build in your arteries as you age. By the time you're middle-aged or older, enough plaque has built up to cause signs or symptoms. In men, the risk increases after age forty-five. In women, the risk increases after age fifty-five.

- **Family history of early heart disease.** Your risk for atherosclerosis increases if your father or a brother was diagnosed with heart disease before fifty-five years of age, or if your mother or a sister was diagnosed with heart disease before sixty-five years of age.

Although age and a family history of early heart disease are risk factors, it doesn't mean that you will develop atherosclerosis if you have one or both.

Making lifestyle changes and/or taking medicines to treat other risk factors can often lessen genetic influences and prevent atherosclerosis from developing, even in older adults.

Emerging Risk Factors

Scientists continue to study other possible risk factors for atherosclerosis.

High levels of a protein called C-reactive protein (CRP) in the blood may raise the risk for atherosclerosis and heart attack. High levels of CRP are proof of inflammation in the body. Inflammation is the body's response to injury or infection. Damage to the arteries' inner walls seems to trigger inflammation and help plaque grow.

People with low CRP levels may get atherosclerosis at a slower rate than people with high CRP levels. Research is under way to find out whether reducing inflammation and lowering CRP levels also can reduce the risk of atherosclerosis.

High levels of fats called triglycerides in the blood also may raise the risk of atherosclerosis, particularly in women.

Other Factors That Affect Atherosclerosis

Other risk factors also may raise your risk for developing atherosclerosis. These include the following:

• Sleep apnea. Sleep apnea is a disorder in which your breathing stops or gets very shallow while you're sleeping. Untreated sleep apnea can raise your chances of having high blood pressure, diabetes, and even a heart attack or stroke.

• Stress. Research shows that the most commonly reported "trigger" for a heart attack is an emotionally upsetting event—particularly one involving anger.

• Alcohol. Heavy drinking can damage the heart muscle and worsen other risk factors for atherosclerosis. Men should have no more than two drinks containing alcohol a day. Women should have no more than one drink containing alcohol a day.

What Are the Signs and Symptoms of Atherosclerosis?

Atherosclerosis usually doesn't cause signs and symptoms until it severely narrows or totally blocks an artery. Many people don't know they have the disease until they have a medical emergency, such as a heart attack or stroke.

Some people may have other signs and symptoms of the disease. These depend on which arteries are severely narrowed or blocked.

The coronary arteries supply oxygen-rich blood to your heart. When plaque narrows or blocks these arteries (a condition called coronary artery disease, or CAD), a common symptom is angina.

Angina is chest pain or discomfort that occurs when your heart muscle doesn't get enough oxygen-rich blood. Angina may feel like pressure or a squeezing pain in your chest. You also may feel it in your shoulders, arms, neck, jaw, or back.

This pain tends to get worse with activity and go away when you rest. Emotional stress also can trigger the pain.

Other symptoms of CAD are shortness of breath and arrhythmias (irregular heartbeats).

The carotid arteries supply oxygen-rich blood to your brain. When plaque narrows or blocks these arteries (a condition called carotid artery disease), you may have symptoms of a stroke. These symptoms include sudden numbness, weakness, and dizziness.

Plaque also can build up in the major arteries that supply oxygen-rich blood to the legs, arms, and pelvis (a condition called peripheral arterial disease). When these arteries are narrowed or blocked, it can lead to numbness, pain, and sometimes dangerous infections.

How Is Atherosclerosis Diagnosed?

Your doctor will diagnose atherosclerosis based on the following things:

- Your medical and family histories
- Your risk factors
- The results of a physical exam and diagnostic tests

Physical Exam

During the physical exam, your doctor may listen to your arteries for an abnormal whooshing sound called a bruit. Your doctor can hear a bruit when placing a stethoscope over an affected artery. A bruit may indicate poor blood flow due to plaque.

Your doctor also may check to see whether any of your pulses (for example, in the leg or foot) are weak or absent. A weak or absent pulse can be a sign of a blocked artery.

Diagnostic Tests and Procedures

Your doctor may order one or more tests to diagnose atherosclerosis. These tests also can help your doctor learn the extent of your disease and plan the best treatment.

Blood tests. Blood tests check the levels of certain fats, cholesterol, sugar, and proteins in your blood. Abnormal levels may show that you have risk factors for atherosclerosis.

Electrocardiogram (EKG). An EKG is a simple test that detects and records the electrical activity of your heart. An EKG shows how fast your heart is beating and whether it has a regular rhythm. It also shows the strength and timing of electrical signals as they pass through each part of your heart.

Certain electrical patterns that the EKG detects can suggest whether CAD is likely. An EKG also can show signs of a previous or current heart attack.

Chest x-ray. A chest x-ray takes a picture of the organs and structures inside the chest, including your heart, lungs, and blood vessels. A chest x-ray can reveal signs of heart failure.

Ankle/brachial index. This test compares the blood pressure in your ankle with the blood pressure in your arm to see how well your blood is flowing. This test can help diagnose peripheral arterial disease (PAD).

Echocardiography. This test uses sound waves to create a moving picture of your heart. Echocardiography provides information about the size and shape of your heart and how well your heart chambers and valves are working.

The test also can identify areas of poor blood flow to the heart, areas of heart muscle that aren't contracting normally, and previous injury to the heart muscle caused by poor blood flow.

Computed tomography scan. A computed tomography, or CT, scan creates computer-generated images of the heart, brain, or other areas of the body. The test can often show hardening and narrowing of large arteries.

Stress testing. During stress testing, you exercise to make your heart work hard and beat fast while heart tests are performed. If you can't exercise, you're given medicine to speed up your heart rate.

When your heart is beating fast and working hard, it needs more blood and oxygen. Arteries narrowed by plaque can't supply enough oxygen-rich blood to meet your heart's needs. A stress test can show possible signs of CAD, such as the following:

- Abnormal changes in your heart rate or blood pressure

- Symptoms such as shortness of breath or chest pain

- Abnormal changes in your heart rhythm or your heart's electrical activity

During the stress test, if you can't exercise for as long as what's considered normal for someone your age, it may be a sign that not enough blood is flowing to your heart. But other factors besides CAD can prevent you from exercising long enough (for example, lung diseases, anemia, or poor general fitness).

Some stress tests use a radioactive dye, sound waves, positron emission tomography (PET), or cardiac magnetic resonance imaging (MRI) to take pictures of your heart when it's working hard and when it's at rest.

These imaging stress tests can show how well blood is flowing in the different parts of your heart. They also can show how well your heart pumps blood when it beats.

Angiography. Angiography is a test that uses dye and special x-rays to show the insides of your arteries. This test can show whether plaque is blocking your arteries and how severe the plaque is.

A thin, flexible tube called a catheter is put into a blood vessel in your arm, groin (upper thigh), or neck. A dye that can be seen on x-ray is then injected into the arteries. By looking at the x-ray picture, your doctor can see the flow of blood through your arteries.

How Is Atherosclerosis Treated?

Treatments for atherosclerosis may include lifestyle changes, medicines, and medical procedures or surgery.

Lifestyle Changes

Making lifestyle changes can often help prevent or treat atherosclerosis. For some people, these changes may be the only treatment needed:

- Follow a healthy eating plan to prevent or reduce high blood pressure and high blood cholesterol and to maintain a healthy weight.

- Increase your physical activity. Check with your doctor first to find out how much and what kinds of activity are safe for you.

- Lose weight, if you're overweight or obese.

- Quit smoking, if you smoke. Avoid exposure to secondhand smoke.

- Reduce stress.

Medicines

To help slow or reverse atherosclerosis, your doctor may prescribe medicines to help lower your cholesterol or blood pressure or prevent blood clots from forming.

For successful treatment, take all medicines as your doctor prescribes.

Medical Procedures and Surgery

If you have severe atherosclerosis, your doctor may recommend one of several procedures or surgeries.

Angioplasty is a procedure to open blocked or narrowed coronary (heart) arteries. Angioplasty can improve blood flow to the heart, relieve chest pain, and possibly prevent a heart attack. Sometimes a small mesh tube called a stent is placed in the artery to keep it open after the procedure.

Coronary artery bypass grafting (CABG) is a type of surgery. In CABG, arteries or veins from other areas in your body are used to bypass (that is, go around) your narrowed coronary arteries. CABG can improve blood flow to your heart, relieve chest pain, and possibly prevent a heart attack.

Bypass grafting also can be used for leg arteries. In this surgery, a healthy blood vessel is used to bypass a narrowed or blocked blood vessel in one of your legs. The healthy blood vessel redirects blood around the artery, improving blood flow to the leg.

Carotid artery surgery removes plaque buildup from the carotid arteries in the neck. This opens the arteries and improves blood flow to the brain. Carotid artery surgery can help prevent a stroke.

How Can Atherosclerosis Be Prevented or Delayed?

Taking action to control your risk factors can help prevent or delay atherosclerosis and its related diseases. Your chance of developing atherosclerosis goes up with the number of risk factors you have.

Making lifestyle changes and taking prescribed medicines are important steps.

Know your family history of health problems related to atherosclerosis. If you or someone in your family has this disease, be sure to tell your doctor. Also, let your doctor know if you smoke.

Chapter 41

Blood Pressure Disorders

Chapter Contents

Section 41.1

Hypertension (High Blood Pressure)

"High Blood Pressure," National Institute on Aging, National Institutes of Health, September 2007.

You can have high blood pressure, or hypertension, and still feel just fine. That's because high blood pressure does not cause signs of illness that you can see or feel. But, high blood pressure, sometimes called "the silent killer," is a major health problem. If high blood pressure isn't controlled with lifestyle changes and medicine, it can lead to stroke, heart disease, eye problems, or kidney failure.

What Is Blood Pressure?

Blood pressure is the force of blood pushing against the walls of arteries. When the doctor measures your blood pressure the results are given in two numbers. The first number, called systolic pressure, measures the pressure when your heart beats. The second number, called diastolic pressure, measures the pressure while your heart relaxes between beats. Normal blood pressure is a systolic pressure of less than 120 and a diastolic pressure of less than 80.

Do You Have High Blood Pressure?

One reason to have regular visits to the doctor is to have your blood pressure checked. The doctor will say your blood pressure is high when it measures 140/90 or higher at two or more checkups. He or she may ask you to check your blood pressure at home at different times of the day. If the pressure stays high, the doctor may suggest medicine, changes in your diet, and exercise.

Table 41.1. What Do The Numbers Mean?

	Systolic	Diastolic
Normal blood pressure	Less than 120	Less than 80
High blood pressure	140 or more	90 or more
Prehypertension	Between 120 and 139	Between 80 and 89
Isolated systolic hypertension	140 or more	Less than 90

You could have prehypertension if your blood pressure is only slightly higher than normal—for example, the first number (systolic) is between 120 and 139 or the second number (diastolic) is between 80 and 89. Prehypertension can put you at risk for developing high blood pressure. Your doctor will probably want you to make changes in your day-to-day habits to try and lower your blood pressure.

What If Just the First Number Is High?

For older people, the first number (systolic) often is 140 or greater, but the second number (diastolic) is less than 90. This problem is called isolated systolic hypertension. Isolated systolic hypertension is the most common form of high blood pressure in older people, and it can lead to serious health problems. It is treated in the same way as regular high blood pressure. If your systolic pressure is 140 or higher, ask your doctor how you can lower it.

Some Risks You Can't Change

Anyone can get high blood pressure. But some people have a greater chance of having it because of things they can't change. These include the following:

- **Age.** The chance of having high blood pressure increases as you get older.

- **Gender.** Before age fifty-five, men have a greater chance of having high blood pressure. Women are more likely to have high blood pressure after menopause.

- **Family history.** High blood pressure tends to run in some families.

- **Race.** African Americans are at increased risk for high blood pressure.

How Can I Control My Blood Pressure?

More than half of Americans over age sixty and about three-fourths of those seventy years of age and older have high blood pressure. The good news is blood pressure can be controlled in most people. To start, there are many lifestyle changes you can make to lower your risk of high blood pressure, including the following:

- **Keep a healthy weight.** Being overweight adds to your risk of high blood pressure. Ask your doctor if you need to lose weight.

- **Exercise every day.** Moderate exercise can lower your risk of high blood pressure. Try to exercise at least thirty minutes a day most days of the week. Check with your doctor before starting an exercise plan if you have a long-term health problem or are over fifty and have been inactive.

- **Eat a healthy diet.** A diet rich in fruits, vegetables, whole grains, and low-fat dairy products may help to lower blood pressure. Ask your doctor about following a healthy diet.

- **Cut down on salt.** Many Americans eat more salt (sodium) than they need. Most of the salt comes from processed food (for example, soup and baked goods). A low-salt diet might help lower your blood pressure. Talk with your doctor about eating less salt.

- **Drink less alcohol.** Drinking alcohol can affect your blood pressure. Most men shouldn't have more than two drinks a day; most women should not drink more than one drink a day.

- **Don't smoke.** Smoking increases your risk for high blood pressure and heart disease. If you smoke, quit.

- **Manage stress.** People react to stress in different ways. For some, stress can cause their blood pressure to go up. Talk to your doctor about how you can lower stress. Exercise and getting a good night's sleep can help.

If these lifestyle changes don't control your high blood pressure, your doctor will prescribe medicine. You may try several kinds before finding the one that works best for you. Medicine can control your blood pressure, but it can't cure it. You may need to take medicine for the rest of your life. You and your doctor can plan together how to manage your blood pressure.

High Blood Pressure Facts

High blood pressure is serious because it can lead to major health problems. If you have high blood pressure, remember the following things:

- High blood pressure may not make you feel sick, but it is serious. See a doctor to treat it.

- You can lower your blood pressure by changing your day-to-day habits and by taking medicine, if needed.

- If you take high blood pressure medicine, making some lifestyle changes may help lower the dose you need.

- If you are already taking blood pressure medicine and your blood pressure is less than 120/80, that's good. It means medicine and lifestyles changes are working. If another doctor asks if you have high blood pressure, the answer is, "Yes, but it is being treated."

- Tell your doctor about all the drugs you take. Don't forget to mention over-the-counter drugs, vitamins, and dietary supplements. They may affect your blood pressure. They also can change how well your blood pressure medicine works.

- Blood pressure pills should be taken at the same time each day. For example, take your medicine in the morning with breakfast or in the evening after brushing your teeth. If you miss a dose, do not double the dose the next day.

- Know what your blood pressure should be. Don't take more of your blood pressure medicine than your doctor prescribes. Very low blood pressure is not good, either.

- Do not stop taking your high blood pressure medicine unless your doctor tells you to stop. Do not skip a day or take half a pill. Remember to refill your medicine before you run out of pills.

- Taking your blood pressure at home:

  - There are many blood pressure home monitors for sale. Ask your doctor, nurse, or pharmacist to see what monitor you need and show you how to use it.

  - Avoid smoking, exercise, and caffeine thirty minutes before taking your blood pressure.

  - Make sure you are sitting with your feet on the floor and your back is against something.

  - Relax quietly for five minutes before checking your blood pressure.

  - Keep a list of your blood pressure numbers to share with your doctor, physician's assistant, or nurse. Take your home monitor to the doctor's office to make sure your monitor is working right.

Section 41.2

Portal Hypertension

Portal hypertension is high blood pressure of the portal vein. The portal vein, a major vein in the abdomen, collects nutrient-rich blood from the intestines and delivers it to the liver to nourish it, where it is purified for our body to use.

Like other organs, the liver needs oxygen and nutrients to function, which it receives from the portal vein. After the oxygen-rich and nutrient-rich blood passes through the liver, it flows into the hepatic veins and on into the inferior vena cava, which takes it back to the heart. Blocked or reduced blood flow at any point of this process will result in increased pressure inside the portal vein. When this occurs, blood is detoured into other smaller veins that ultimately allow blood to flow back to the heart. However, these smaller veins can enlarge and form varices (varicose or dilated veins).

The most common cause of portal hypertension is cirrhosis, which refers to the "hardening" of the liver because of scar tissue. The other primary cause of portal hypertension is due to clots which narrow or block blood flow through the veins to and from the liver. Portal hypertension is fairly uncommon, but when it occurs, it most often happens in older adults and may result in death, if untreated.

Causes of portal hypertension:

- cirrhosis of the liver (may be due to alcohol use or hepatitis);

- clotting of the portal vein;

- clotting of the hepatic veins.

Symptoms of Portal Hypertension

Symptoms of portal hypertension (not all are present all of the time):

- ascites (fluid buildup in the abdomen);

- weight loss (malnutrition);

- enlarged liver (at times);

- internal hemorrhoids—with possible bleeding;

- varicose veins of the esophagus (varices)—with possible bleeding;

- jaundice (yellowing of the skin).

Varices can rupture or burst, especially where the esophagus and the stomach join. Bleeding from varices can be massive, causing patients to vomit blood, which is a major cause of death in patients with portal hypertension.

Blood may also be detoured through the veins along the rectum, the lowest portion of the large intestine (colon), causing them to enlarge. Enlarged veins along the rectum are called internal hemorrhoids, which can rupture and result in massive bleeding from the rectum and anus. Another symptom of portal hypertension is ascites, the collection of large amounts of fluid in the abdomen. Ascites can lead to early sensations of being full when eating, resulting in malnutrition. People with ascites often have a harder time being active because of the weight of the fluid and the large size of their abdomen. Someone with massive ascites will have a protruding or swollen abdomen, often with thin legs and arms, due to muscle loss because of liver disease and malnutrition.

Ascites can cause the kidneys to fail. Urgent steps must be taken to drain the ascites and to monitor the kidneys and liver. Unless the liver function is corrected and the kidneys recover, approximately half of these patients die within a few weeks.

Diagnosing Portal Hypertension

Unfortunately, there is no simple way or test to show if a person has portal hypertension. We cannot use a blood-pressure cuff like we can on an arm to measure "whole body" hypertension. Doctors become aware of portal hypertension when its signs and symptoms are first noticed. Imaging and laboratory tests suggest cirrhosis, which can be further diagnosed by a liver biopsy.

Some patients who undergo a biopsy will also have special pressure measurements taken in the liver at the same time to diagnose portal hypertension. Many of the imaging studies such as computed tomography (CT), magnetic resonance imaging (MRI), and ultrasound can also show signs of portal hypertension such as varices and enlargement of the spleen.

447

Treatment Options

Medical treatment of portal hypertension includes beta-blockers, which are known to many as drugs to improve blood pressure and heart function. This class of drugs helps to decrease blood flow into the portal vein system and to decrease the pressure. Beta-blockers also reduce the risk of bleeding from varices.

Minimally invasive procedures such as endoscopic variceal sclerotherapy (EVS), which involves the injection of a solution to seal the bleeding, and endoscopic variceal banding (EVB), which is the placement of a band from inside the esophagus to seal the bleeding, are used to stop bleeding from varices.

Another solution for portal hypertension is a procedure known as transjugular intrahepatic portosystemic shunt (TIPS) This procedure inserts a stent (a hollow wire tube) between a hepatic vein and a branch of the portal vein. The stent passes through the liver to connect these two vascular structures. With TIPS, blood moves through the stent and bypasses the liver. This procedure has both advantages and disadvantages. TIPS reduces portal vein pressure and bleeding from varices. However, because some blood bypasses the liver, some wastes are not cleared from the bloodstream. These nitrogen-containing compounds can cause confusion, which has to be treated with medications.

Some health professionals feel that there is no proof that someone lives longer after the TIPS procedure, that it is expensive and has a high failure rate within one year because the stent often becomes narrowed or blocked.

Other professionals believe that TIPS is the definitive lifesaving procedure for acute massive variceal hemorrhage at many institutions. While the TIPS procedure may be expensive, it is no more so than the other procedures described. TIPS did have a failure rate, but that is for the most part historical and misleading, Today TIPS is done with covered stents and patients are followed with ultrasound for restenosis. While many patients who have uncovered stents will have restenosis, this is caught on a surveillance program and easily remedied with balloon angioplasty.

Another treatment of portal hypertension is surgical shunting, a more invasive procedure than TIPS. However, some believe that surgical shunts, particularly in certain locations, improve long-term survival with portal hypertension. The only way to fully cure portal hypertension is with a liver transplant, which is expensive and afterward the patient needs lifelong medical attention. With liver transplantation continuing to be a difficult solution, a better understanding of portal hypertension is required, along with earlier diagnosis and management of the disease. Transplantation does not cure all forms of portal hypertension, and any mention of transplantation must include the proviso that not all patients are candidates for transplant and the waiting period can be very long. Then, patients with portal hypertension can have a better and longer life.

Section 41.3

Preeclampsia

"Preeclampsia or Toxemia: Pregnancy Induced Hypertension (PIH)," © 2006 American Pregnancy Association (www.americanpregnancy.org). Reprinted with permission.

Preeclampsia is a condition of high blood pressure during pregnancy. Your blood pressure goes up, you retain water, and protein is found in your urine. It is also called toxemia or pregnancy induced hypertension (PIH). The exact cause of preeclampsia is unknown.

Who is at risk for preeclampsia?

The following may increase the risk of developing preeclampsia:

- A first-time mom
- Women whose sisters and mothers had preeclampsia
- Women carrying multiple babies; teenage mothers; and women older than age forty
- Women who had high blood pressure or kidney disease prior to pregnancy

What are the symptoms of preeclampsia?

Mild preeclampsia: high blood pressure, water retention, and protein in the urine.

Severe preeclampsia: headaches, blurred vision, inability to tolerate bright light, fatigue, nausea/vomiting, urinating small amounts, pain in the upper right abdomen, shortness of breath, and tendency to bruise easily. Contact your doctor immediately if you experience blurred vision, severe headaches, abdominal pain, and/or urinating very infrequently.

How do I know if I have preeclampsia?

At each prenatal checkup your healthcare provider will check your blood pressure, urine levels, and may order blood tests which may show if you have preeclampsia.

Your physician may also perform other tests that include: checking kidney and blood-clotting functions; ultrasound scan to check your baby's growth; and Doppler scan to measure the efficiency of blood flow to the placenta.

How is preeclampsia treated?

Treatment depends on how close you are to your due date. If you are close to your due date, and the baby is developed enough, your health care provider will probably want to deliver your baby as soon as possible.

If you have mild preeclampsia and your baby has not reached full development, your doctor will probably recommend you do the following:

- rest, lying on your left side to take the weight of the baby off your major blood vessels;

- increase prenatal checkups;

- consume less salt;

- drink eight glasses of water a day.

If you have severe preeclampsia, your doctor may try to treat you with blood pressure medication until you are far enough along to deliver safely.

How does preeclampsia affect my baby?

Preeclampsia can prevent the placenta from getting enough blood. If the placenta doesn't get enough blood, your baby gets less oxygen and food. This can result in low birth weight.

Most women still can deliver a healthy baby if preeclampsia is detected early and treated with regular prenatal care.

450

How can I prevent preeclampsia?

Currently, there is no sure way to prevent preeclampsia. Some contributing factors to high blood pressure can be controlled and some can't. Follow your doctor's instruction about diet and exercise:

- Use little or no added salt in your meals.

- Drink six to eight glasses of water a day.

- Don't eat a lot of fried foods and junk food.

- Get enough rest.

- Exercise regularly.

- Elevate your feet several times during the day.

- Avoid drinking alcohol.

- Avoid beverages containing caffeine.

- Your doctor may suggest you take prescribed medicine and additional supplements.

Section 41.4

Renovascular Hypertension

Description

Renovascular hypertension is high blood pressure (greater than 140/80 mmHg) caused by renal artery disease. Normally, the kidneys regulate body fluid and blood pressure, as well as regulate blood chemistry and remove organic waste. Proper kidney function is disrupted, however, when the arteries that provide blood to the kidneys become narrowed, a condition called renal artery stenosis. When stenosis results in reduced blood flow, the kidney compensates by producing hormones that increase blood pressure. This response is a healthy one under normal circumstances. But when the reduction in blood flow is due to stenosis, blood pressure is increased unnecessarily. High blood pressure caused by renal artery disease may be difficult to control with medication. The good news is that renovascular hypertension is one of the few identifiable and treatable causes of high blood pressure—a condition that, if left untreated, can lead to heart attack, stroke, or kidney failure.

Primary hypertension is high blood pressure that has no apparent cause. Renovascular hypertension is the most common cause of secondary hypertension, high blood pressure that can be attributed to a specific cause. It is responsible for about 1 percent to 2 percent of the fifty million estimated cases of hypertension in the United States.

Symptoms

Clues that high blood pressure is being caused by renal artery stenosis include:

- significant high blood pressure at a young age;

- stable hypertension that suddenly gets worse;

- high blood pressure that occurs with impaired renal function;

- high blood pressure in someone with an abdominal aortic aneurysm or disease of the coronary, carotid, or the lower extremity arteries.

Risk factors

Patients who have atherosclerosis in some other part of the body are 30 percent to 50 percent more likely to develop renal artery stenosis.

Diagnosis

Renovascular disease can usually be diagnosed via duplex ultrasound scanning and other noninvasive tests. These include computed tomography (CT) angiography and magnetic resonance (MR) angiography. However, the definitive test is contrast angiography, a test that involves the injection of dye. If a blocked renal artery is discovered during an angiogram, treatment to open the artery may be performed during the same procedure.

Treatment

The most common treatment for renovascular hypertension caused by renal artery stenosis is balloon angioplasty to open the artery followed by stent placement to keep it open. The procedures involve the placement of a catheter in an artery of the groin through a small puncture in the skin. A balloon is advanced to the affected renal artery, where it is inflated, dilating the artery wall. A tube-like stent is then inserted to keep the artery open and the blood flowing freely. Patients usually stay in the hospital overnight and quickly resume normal activities.

Some patients may need open surgical repair of the renal arteries due to recurrent narrowing. During this open abdominal surgery, the artery is repaired using a graft from the aorta or some other healthy vessel.

Section 41.5

Hypotension (Low Blood Pressure)

Excerpted from "Hypotension," National Heart Lung and Blood Institute, National Institutes of Health, September 2008.

What Is Hypotension?

Hypotension is low blood pressure. Blood pressure is the force of blood pushing against the walls of the arteries as the heart pumps out blood.

Blood pressure is measured as systolic and diastolic pressures. Systolic blood pressure is the pressure when the heart beats while pumping blood. Diastolic blood pressure is the pressure when the heart is at rest between beats.

You will most often see blood pressure numbers written with the systolic number above or before the diastolic, such as 120/80 mmHg. (The mmHg is millimeters of mercury—the units used to measure blood pressure.)

Normal blood pressure in adults is lower than 120/80 mmHg. Hypotension is blood pressure that's lower than 90/60 mmHg.

Overview

Blood pressure changes during the day. It lowers as you sleep and rises when you wake up. It also can rise when you're excited, nervous, or active.

Your body is very sensitive to changes in blood pressure. Special cells in the arteries can sense if your blood pressure begins to rise or fall. When this happens, the cells trigger your body to try to bring blood pressure back to normal.

For example, if you stand up quickly, your blood pressure may drop. The cells will sense the drop and will quickly take action to make sure that blood continues to flow to your brain, kidneys, and other important organs.

Most forms of hypotension happen because your body can't bring blood pressure back to normal or can't do it fast enough.

Some people have low blood pressure all of the time. They have no signs or symptoms, and their low blood pressure is normal for them.

In other people, certain conditions or factors cause blood pressure to drop below normal.

Hypotension is a medical concern only if it causes signs or symptoms, such as dizziness, fainting, or, in extreme cases, shock.

Outlook

In a healthy person, low blood pressure without signs or symptoms usually isn't a problem and needs no treatment. If low blood pressure causes signs or symptoms, your doctor will try to find and treat the underlying condition that's causing it.

Hypotension can be dangerous. It can make a person fall because of dizziness or fainting. Shock, a severe form of hypotension, is a condition that's often fatal if not treated right away. With prompt and proper treatment, shock can be successfully treated.

Types of Hypotension

There are several types of hypotension. People who always have low blood pressure have chronic asymptomatic hypotension. They have no signs or symptoms and need no treatment. Their low blood pressure is normal for them.

Other types of hypotension occur only sometimes, when blood pressure suddenly drops too low. The symptoms and effects on the body range from mild to severe.

The three main types of this kind of hypotension are orthostatic hypotension, neurally mediated hypotension (NMH), and severe hypotension linked to shock.

Orthostatic Hypotension

This type of low blood pressure occurs when standing up from a sitting or lying down position. It can make you feel dizzy or lightheaded, or even make you faint.

Orthostatic hypotension occurs if your body isn't able to adjust blood pressure and blood flow fast enough for the change in position. This type of low blood pressure usually lasts for only a few seconds or minutes after you stand up. You may need to sit or lie down for a short time while your blood pressure returns to normal.

Orthostatic hypotension can occur in all age groups. However, it's more common in older adults, especially those who are frail or in poor health. It can be a symptom of other medical conditions, and treatment often focuses on treating the underlying condition(s).

Some people have orthostatic hypotension, but also have high blood pressure when lying down.

A form of orthostatic hypotension called postprandial hypotension is a sudden drop in blood pressure after a meal. This type of low blood pressure mostly affects older adults. It's also more likely to affect people who have high blood pressure or a central nervous system disorder, such as Parkinson disease.

Neurally Mediated Hypotension

With NMH, blood pressure drops after you've been standing for a long time. You may feel dizzy, faint, or sick to the stomach as a result. This type of low blood pressure also can occur if you have an unpleasant, upsetting, or scary experience.

NMH affects children and young adults more often than people in other age groups. Children often outgrow NMH.

Severe Hypotension Linked to Shock

People may say a person has "gone into shock" as a result of an upsetting event. But to doctors, the word "shock" has a different meaning.

Shock is a life-threatening condition in which blood pressure drops so low that the brain, kidneys, and other vital organs can't get enough blood to work properly. Blood pressure drops much lower in shock than in other types of hypotension.

Many factors can cause shock, such as major blood loss, certain severe infections, severe burns and allergic reactions, and poisoning. Shock can be fatal if it's not treated right away.

What Causes Hypotension?

Factors or conditions that disrupt the body's ability to control blood pressure cause hypotension. The different types of hypotension have different causes.

Orthostatic Hypotension

Orthostatic hypotension has many causes. Sometimes two or more factors combine to cause this type of low blood pressure.

Dehydration is the most common cause of orthostatic hypotension. Dehydration occurs when the body loses more water than it takes in. You may become dehydrated if you don't drink enough fluids or if you sweat a lot during physical activity. Fever, vomiting, and severe diarrhea also can lead to dehydration.

Orthostatic hypotension may occur during pregnancy, but it generally goes away after the birth.

Because an older body doesn't manage changes in blood pressure as well as a younger body, getting older also can lead to this type of hypotension.

Postprandial hypotension (a type of orthostatic hypotension) mostly affects older adults. Postprandial hypotension is a sudden drop in blood pressure after a meal.

Certain medical conditions can raise your risk for orthostatic hypotension, including the following:

- Heart conditions, such as heart attack, heart valve disease, bradycardia (a very low heart rate), and heart failure. These conditions prevent the heart from pumping enough blood to the body.

- Anemia.

- Severe infections.

- Endocrine conditions, such as thyroid disorders, Addison disease, low blood sugar, and diabetes.

- Disorders of the central nervous system, such as Parkinson disease.

- Pulmonary embolism.

Some medicines used to treat high blood pressure and heart disease can raise your risk for orthostatic hypotension. These medicines include the following:

- Diuretics, or "water pills"

- Calcium channel blockers

- Angiotensin-converting enzyme (ACE) inhibitors

- Angiotensin II receptor blockers

- Nitrates

- Beta blockers

Medicines used to treat conditions such as anxiety, depression, erectile dysfunction, and central nervous system disorders (like Parkinson disease) also can increase your risk for orthostatic hypotension.

Other substances, when taken with high blood pressure medicines, also can lead to orthostatic hypotension. These substances include alcohol, barbiturates, and some prescription and over-the-counter medicines.

Finally, other factors or conditions that can trigger orthostatic hypotension include being out in the heat or being immobile (not being able to move around very much) for a long time.

Neurally Mediated Hypotension

Neurally mediated hypotension (NMH) occurs when the brain and heart don't communicate with each other properly.

For example, when you stand for a long time, blood begins to pool in your legs. This causes your blood pressure to drop. In NHM, the body mistakenly tells the brain that blood pressure is high. In response, the brain slows the heart rate. This makes blood pressure drop even more, causing dizziness and other symptoms.

Severe Hypotension Linked to Shock

Many factors and conditions can cause severe hypotension linked to shock. Some of these factors also can cause orthostatic hypotension. In shock, though, blood pressure drops very low and doesn't return to normal on its own.

Shock is an emergency and must be treated right away. If a person has signs or symptoms of shock, someone should call 9-1-1 right away.

Certain severe infections can cause shock. This is known as septic shock. It can occur when bacteria enter the bloodstream. The bacteria release a toxin (a poison) that leads to a dangerous drop in blood pressure.

A severe loss of blood or fluids from the body also can cause shock. This is known as hypovolemic shock. Hypovolemic shock can happen as a result of the following things:

- Major external bleeding (for example, from a severe cut or injury)

- Major internal bleeding (for example, from a ruptured blood vessel or injury that causes bleeding inside the body)

- Major loss of body fluids from severe burns

- Severe swelling of the pancreas (an organ that produces enzymes and hormones, such as insulin)

- Severe diarrhea

- Severe kidney disease

- Overuse of diuretics

A major decrease in the heart's ability to pump blood also can cause shock. This is known as cardiogenic shock. Heart attack, pulmonary embolism, or arrhythmia (an irregular heartbeat) can cause this type of shock.

A sudden and extreme widening of the arteries and drop in blood pressure also can cause shock. This is known as vasodilatory shock. It can occur due to the following causes:

- A severe head injury

- A reaction to certain medicines

- Liver failure

- Poisoning

- A severe allergic reaction (called anaphylactic shock)

Who Is at Risk for Hypotension?

Hypotension can affect people of all ages. However, people in certain age groups are more likely to have certain types of low blood pressure.

Older adults are more likely to have orthostatic and postprandial hypotension. Children and young adults are more likely to have neurally mediated hypotension.

People who take certain medicines, such as high blood pressure medicines, are at higher risk for low blood pressure. People who have central nervous system disorders (such as Parkinson disease) or some heart conditions also are at higher risk for low blood pressure.

Other risk factors for hypotension include being immobile (not being able to move around very much) for long periods and pregnancy. Hypotension during pregnancy is normal and goes away after birth.

What Are the Signs and Symptoms of Hypotension?

Orthostatic Hypotension

The signs and symptoms of orthostatic hypotension may happen within a few seconds or minutes of standing up after you've been sitting or lying down. You may feel that you're going to faint, or you may actually faint. Signs and symptoms include the following:

- Dizziness or feeling lightheaded

- Blurry vision

- Confusion

- Weakness

- Nausea (feeling sick to your stomach)

These signs and symptoms go away if you sit or lie down for a few minutes until your blood pressure adjusts to normal.

Neurally Mediated Hypotension

The signs and symptoms of neurally mediated hypotension (NMH) are similar to those of orthostatic hypotension. They occur after standing for a long time or in response to an unpleasant, upsetting, or scary experience.

The drop in blood pressure with NMH doesn't last long and often goes away after sitting down.

Severe Hypotension Linked to Shock

In shock, not enough blood flows to the major organs, including the brain.

The early signs and symptoms of reduced blood flow to the brain include lightheadedness, sleepiness, and confusion. In the earliest stages of shock, it may be hard to detect any signs or symptoms. In older people, the first symptom may only be confusion.

Over time, as shock worsens, a person won't be able to sit up without passing out. If the shock continues, the person will lose consciousness. Shock is often fatal if not treated right away.

Other signs and symptoms of shock vary, depending on what's causing the shock. When low blood volume (from major blood loss, for example) or poor pumping action in the heart (from heart failure, for example) causes shock the following things occur:

- The skin becomes cold and sweaty. It often looks blue or pale. If pressed, the color returns to normal more slowly than usual. A bluish network of lines appears under the skin.

- The pulse becomes weak and rapid.

- The person begins to breathe very quickly.

When extreme widening or stretching of blood vessels (such as in septic shock) causes shock, a person feels warm and flushed at first. Later, the skin becomes cold and clammy and the person feels very sleepy.

Shock is an emergency and must be treated right away. If a person has signs or symptoms of shock, someone should call 9-1-1 right away.

How Is Hypotension Diagnosed?

Hypotension is diagnosed based on your medical history, a physical exam, and results from tests. Your doctor will want to know the following things:

• The type of low blood pressure you have and how severe it is

• Whether an underlying condition is causing the low blood pressure

Diagnostic Tests

When a person is in shock, someone should call 9-1-1 right away because emergency treatment is needed.

For other types of hypotension, your doctor may order tests to find out how your blood pressure responds in certain situations. The results will help your doctor understand why you're fainting or having other symptoms.

Blood tests. During a blood test, a small amount of blood is taken from your body. It's usually drawn from a vein in your arm using a thin needle. The procedure is quick and easy, although it may cause some short-term discomfort.

Blood tests can show whether anemia or low blood sugar is causing your hypotension.

Electrocardiogram (EKG). An EKG is a simple test that detects and records the heart's electrical activity. It shows how fast the heart is beating and the heart's rhythm (steady or irregular). An EKG also shows the strength and timing of electrical signals as they pass through each part of the heart.

Holter and event monitors. Holter and event monitors are medical devices that record the heart's electrical activity. These monitors are similar to an EKG. However, a standard EKG only records the heartbeat for a few seconds. It won't detect heart rhythm problems that don't occur during the test.

Holter and event monitors are small, portable devices. You can wear one while you do your normal daily activities. This allows the monitor to record your heart longer than an EKG can.

Echocardiography. Echocardiography is a test that uses sound waves to create a moving picture of your heart. The picture shows how well your heart is working and its size and shape.

There are several different types of echocardiography, including a stress echocardiogram, or "stress echo." This test is done as part of a stress test. A stress echo usually is done to find out whether you have decreased blood flow to your heart, a sign of coronary artery disease.

Stress test. Some heart problems are easier to diagnose when your heart is working hard and beating fast. During stress testing, you exercise (or are given medicine if you're unable to exercise) to make your heart work hard and beat fast while heart tests are done.

These tests may include nuclear heart scanning, echocardiography, and magnetic resonance imaging (MRI) and positron emission tomography (PET) scanning of the heart.

Valsalva maneuver. This is a simple test of the part of your nervous system that controls functions such as your heartbeat and the narrowing and widening of your blood vessels. If something goes wrong with this part of the nervous system, blood pressure problems may occur.

During this test you take a deep breath and then force the air out through your lips. You will do this several times. Your heart rate and blood pressure will be checked during the test.

Tilt table test. This test is used if you have fainting spells for no known reason. For the test, you lie on a table that moves from a lying down to an upright position. Your doctor checks your reaction to the change in position.

Doctors use a tilt table test to diagnose orthostatic hypotension and neurally mediated hypotension (NMH). People who have NMH usually faint during this test. The test can help your doctor find any underlying brain or nerve condition.

How Is Hypotension Treated?

Treatment depends on the type of hypotension you have and how severe your signs and symptoms are. The goals of treatment are to relieve signs and symptoms and manage any underlying condition(s) causing the hypotension.

Your response to treatment depends on your age, overall health, and strength. It also depends on how easily you can stop, start, or change medicines.

In a healthy person, low blood pressure without signs or symptoms usually needs no treatment.

If you have signs or symptoms of low blood pressure, you should sit or lie down right away. Put your feet above the level of your heart. If your symptoms don't go away quickly, you should seek medical care right away.

Orthostatic Hypotension

There are a number of treatments for orthostatic hypotension. If you have this type of low blood pressure, your doctor may advise making lifestyle changes such as the following:

- Drinking plenty of fluids, like water

- Drinking little or no alcohol

- Standing up slowly

- Not crossing your legs while sitting

- Gradually sitting up for longer periods if you've been immobile (not able to move around much) for a long time due to a medical condition

- Eating small, low-carbohydrate meals if you have postprandial hypotension (a form of orthostatic hypotension)

Talk to your doctor about using compression stockings. These stockings apply pressure to your lower legs. They help move blood throughout your body.

If medicine is causing your low blood pressure, your doctor may change the medicine or adjust the dose you take.

Several medicines also are used to treat orthostatic hypotension. These medicines, which raise blood pressure, include fludrocortisone and midodrine.

Neurally Mediated Hypotension

If you have neurally mediated hypotension (NMH), you may need to make lifestyle changes. These may include the following:

- Avoiding situations that trigger symptoms. For example, don't stand for long periods. Try to avoid unpleasant, upsetting, or scary situations.

- Drinking plenty of fluids, like water.

- Increasing your salt intake (as your doctor advises).

- Learning to recognize symptoms that occur before fainting and taking action to raise blood pressure. For example, sitting down and putting your head between your knees can help raise blood pressure.

If medicine is causing your low blood pressure, your doctor may change the medicine or adjust the dose you take. He or she also may prescribe a medicine to treat NMH.

Children who have NHM often outgrow it.

Treating Severe Hypotension Linked to Shock

Shock is a life-threatening emergency. People who have shock usually need to be treated in a hospital or by emergency medical personnel. If a person has signs or symptoms of shock, someone should call 9-1-1 right away.

The goals of treating shock are as follows:

- To restore blood flow to the organs as quickly as possible to prevent organ damage

- To find and reverse the cause of shock

Special fluid or blood injected into the bloodstream is often used to restore blood flow to the organs. Medicines can be used to raise blood pressure or make the heartbeat stronger. Depending on the cause of the shock, other treatments, such as antibiotics or surgery, may be needed.

Section 41.6

Shock

Shock is a life-threatening condition that occurs when the body is not getting enough blood flow. This can damage multiple organs. Shock requires immediate medical treatment and can get worse very rapidly.

Considerations

Major classes of shock include:

- cardiogenic shock (associated with heart problems);

- hypovolemic shock (caused by inadequate blood volume);

- anaphylactic shock (caused by allergic reaction);

- septic shock (associated with infections);

- neurogenic shock (caused by damage to the nervous system).

Causes

Shock can be caused by any condition that reduces blood flow, including:

- heart problems (such as heart attack or heart failure);

- low blood volume (as with heavy bleeding or dehydration);

- changes in blood vessels (as with infection or severe allergic reactions).

Shock is often associated with heavy external or internal bleeding from a serious injury. Spinal injuries can also cause shock.

Toxic shock syndrome is an example of a type of shock from an infection.

Symptoms

A person in shock has extremely low blood pressure. Depending on the specific cause and type of shock, symptoms will include one or more of the following:

• Anxiety or agitation

• Confusion

• Pale, cool, clammy skin

• Low or no urine output

• Bluish lips and fingernails

• Dizziness, lightheadedness, or faintness

• Profuse sweating, moist skin

• Rapid but weak pulse

• Shallow breathing

• Chest pain

• Unconsciousness

First Aid

Call 911 for immediate medical help.

Check the person's airways, breathing, and circulation. If necessary, begin rescue breathing and cardiopulmonary resuscitation (CPR).

Even if the person is able to breathe on his or her own, continue to check rate of breathing at least every five minutes until help arrives.

If the person is conscious and does *not* have an injury to the head, leg, neck, or spine, place the person in the shock position. Lay the person on the back and elevate the legs about twelve inches. Do *not* elevate the head. If raising the legs will cause pain or potential harm, leave the person lying flat.

Give appropriate first aid for any wounds, injuries, or illnesses.

Keep the person warm and comfortable. Loosen tight clothing.

If the person vomits or drools:

• Turn the head to one side so he or she will not choke. Do this as long as there is no suspicion of spinal injury.

• If a spinal injury is suspected, "log roll" him or her instead. Keep the person's head, neck, and back in line, and roll him or her as a unit.

Do Not

- Do not give the person anything by mouth, including anything to eat or drink.

- Do not move the person with a known or suspected spinal injury.

- Do not wait for milder shock symptoms to worsen before calling for emergency medical help.

When to Contact a Medical Professional

Call 911 any time a person has symptoms of shock. Stay with the person and follow the first aid steps until medical help arrives.

Prevention

Learn ways to prevent heart disease, falls, injuries, dehydration, and other causes of shock. If you have a known allergy (for example, to insect bites or stings), carry an epinephrine pen. Your doctor will teach you how and when to use it.

Once someone is already in shock, the sooner shock is treated, the less damage there may be to the person's vital organs (like the kidneys, liver, and brain). Early first aid and emergency medical help can save a life.

References

Marx JA, Hockberger RS, Walls RM, eds. *Rosen's Emergency Medicine: Concepts and Clinical Practice.* 5th ed. St. Louis, Mo: Mosby; 2002.

Goldman L, Ausiello D, eds. *Cecil Medicine.* 23rd ed. Philadelphia, Pa: Saunders; 2004.

Section 41.7

Syncope (Fainting)

"Syncope," reprinted with permission. © 2009 American Heart
Association, Inc. (www.americanheart.org).

What Is syncope?

Syncope (SIN'ko-pe) is temporary loss of consciousness and posture,
described as "fainting" or "passing out." It's usually related to temporary insufficient blood flow to the brain.

It most often occurs when the blood pressure is too low (hypotension)
and the heart doesn't pump a normal supply of oxygen to the brain.

What Causes Syncope?

It may be caused by emotional stress, pain, pooling of blood in the
legs due to sudden changes in body position, overheating, dehydration, heavy sweating or exhaustion. Syncope may occur during violent
coughing spells (especially in men) because of rapid changes in blood
pressure. It also may result from several heart, neurologic, psychiatric, metabolic, and lung disorders. And it may be a side effect of some
medicines.

Some forms of syncope suggest a serious disorder:

• Those occurring with exercise

• Those associated with palpitations or irregularities of the heart

• Those associated with family history of recurrent syncope or
  sudden death

What Is Neurally Mediated Syncope?

Neurally mediated syncope (NMS) is called also neurocardiogenic,
vasovagal, vasodepressor, or reflex mediated syncope. It's a benign
(and the most frequent) cause of fainting. However, life-threatening
conditions may also manifest as syncope. NMS is more common in

children and young adults, although it can occur at any age. NMS happens because blood pressure drops, reducing circulation to the brain and causing loss of consciousness. Typical NMS occurs while standing and is often preceded by a sensation of warmth, nausea, lightheadedness, and visual "grayout." If the syncope is prolonged, it can trigger a seizure. Placing the person in a reclining position will restore blood flow and consciousness and end the seizure.

American Heart Association (AHA) Recommendation

The majority of children and young adults with syncope have no structural heart disease or significant arrhythmia (abnormal heart rhythm). So, extensive medical work-up is rarely needed. A careful physical examination by a physician, including blood pressure and heart rate measured lying and standing, is generally the only evaluation required.

In other cases an electrocardiogram (EKG or ECG) is used to test for abnormal heart rhythms such as long Q-T syndrome. This is a genetic heart condition that can cause sudden cardiac death. Other tests, such as exercise stress test, Holter monitor, echocardiogram, etc. may be needed to rule out other cardiac causes of syncope.

If EKG and cardiac tests are normal, the person will undergo a tilt test. The blood pressure and heart rate will be measured while lying down on a board and after the board is tilted up. Someone who has NMS will usually faint during the tilt, due to the rapid drop in blood pressure and heart rate. As soon as the person is placed on his or her back again, blood flow and consciousness are restored.

To help prevent syncope, people with NMS should be on a high-salt diet and drink plenty of fluids to avoid dehydration and maintain blood volume. They should watch for the warning signs of fainting—dizziness, nausea, and sweaty palms—and sit or lie down if they feel the warning signs. Some people also may need medication.

Chapter 42

Carotid Artery Disease

What Are the Carotid Arteries?

The carotid arteries are the blood vessels that carry oxygen-rich blood away from the heart to the head and brain. Located on each side of the neck, these arteries can easily be felt pulsating by placing your fingers gently either side of your windpipe. The carotid arteries are essential as they supply blood to the large front part of the brain. This is the brain tissue where thinking, speech, personality, and sensory (our ability to feel) and motor (our ability to move) functions reside.

Another smaller set of arteries, the vertebral arteries, are located along the back of the neck adjacent to the spine, and supply blood to the back of the brain.

What Is Carotid Artery Disease?

Carotid artery disease is defined by the narrowing or blockage of this artery due to plaque build-up. The process that blocks these arteries (atherosclerosis) is basically the same as that which causes both coronary artery disease and that causes peripheral arterial disease (PAD). The slow build-up of plaque (which is a deposit of cholesterol, calcium, and other cells in the artery wall) is caused by high blood pressure, diabetes, tobacco use, high blood cholesterol, and other modifiable risk factors.

"Carotid Artery Disease," © 2008 Vascular Disease Foundation (www.vdf .org). Reprinted with permission.

Over time, this narrowing may eventually become so severe that a blockage decreases blood flow to the brain and may tragically cause a stroke. A stroke can also occur if a piece of plaque or a blood clot breaks off from the wall of the carotid artery and travels to the smaller arteries of the brain.

The brain survives on a continuous supply of oxygen and glucose carried to it by blood. Cells deprived of fresh blood for more than a few minutes will be damaged, a condition known as "ischemia," or the brain cells may die, a condition known as "infarction." When blood flow to the brain is blocked, the result is sometimes called "an ischemic event." This could be a stroke, which is permanent loss of brain function, or a "transient ischemic attack" (or TIA), which implies a temporary alteration of brain function. Brain damage can be permanent if this lack of blood flow lasts for more than three to six hours.

Stroke can also occur from other causes than carotid artery disease, for example from heart disease (heart valve problems, heart failure, or atrial fibrillation) or if bleeding occurs in brain tissue. Nevertheless, carotid artery disease is one of the most common causes of stroke. According to the National Stroke Council, more than half of the strokes in the United States occur because of carotid artery disease.

What Are the Symptoms of Carotid Artery Disease?

As for all artery diseases, there are usually no advanced warning signs for early forms of carotid artery disease. For many individuals, the first obvious sign often is a TIA or mini-stroke. Symptoms for a stroke or TIA are similar and may include blurring, dimming, or loss of vision; tingling around the mouth; difficulty with speech; the inability to normally move an arm or leg; the inability to feel (numbness) in a part of the body; and rarely, a sudden severe headache. The difference between a stroke and a TIA is that the symptoms of a TIA are not permanent and can last from a few minutes to twenty-four hours. A TIA is a very powerful warning sign; although the symptoms may resolve completely, the occurrence of a TIA offers an individual who is at risk of a permanent stroke an extra opportunity to take action. However, a TIA should still be treated as a medical emergency. If you think you are experiencing a stroke or TIA, get medical attention immediately!

What Are the Risk Factors for Carotid Artery Disease?

Carotid artery disease is part of the arterial circulatory system and has similar risk factors as PAD and coronary heart disease:

- Family history of atherosclerosis (build-up of plaque in the peripheral, coronary, or carotid arteries)

- Age (men have a higher risk before age seventy-five; women have a higher risk after age seventy-five)

- Smoking

- Hypertension

- Diabetes

- High cholesterol, and especially high amounts of "low density lipoprotein" (or LDL, the bad form of cholesterol)—although this risk factor appears to be less strong for stroke than it is for coronary artery disease

Most importantly, if you have an atherosclerotic artery disease such as PAD or coronary heart disease, you are at high risk for carotid artery disease and stroke.

How Is Carotid Artery Disease Diagnosed?

The diagnosis of carotid artery disease is usually based on the performance of an ultrasound study of the neck arteries (a carotid artery duplex scan). Alternatively, the artery can be visualized by a magnetic resonance angiogram (MRA) or standard angiogram.

How Is Carotid Artery Disease Treated?

Treatment for carotid artery disease normally consists of normalization of those risk factors that cause artery blockages, specific medications (usually antiplatelet medications), and sometimes treatment to open the narrowed carotid artery with an angioplasty and stent, or by a surgical procedure. Anyone with any degree of narrowing of a carotid artery, or with any history of stroke or TIA, should quit the use of all tobacco products immediately, control their high blood pressure, normalize their blood cholesterol by diet and medications, and exercise regularly.

Doctors also will want to reduce your risk for developing blood clots in order to prevent stroke or heart attack. Your doctor may prescribe a daily antiplatelet medication, such as aspirin, Plavix® (clopidogrel), Aggrenox® (aspirin combined with dipyridamole), or warfarin. The choice of medication is one that is best made by your own physician. Individuals with severe blockages of the carotid artery (usually at least 60 to 70 percent blockage) may be recommended for a surgical treatment called carotid endarterectomy. During this procedure the plaque from inside the artery wall will be surgically removed and the blood flow is restored to normal. Carotid endarterectomy is successful because the plaque in the carotid artery is limited to a very small area in the mid-portion of the artery in the neck. This allows the procedure to be performed through a small incision, and in many cases under regional anesthesia. Most patients can go home the morning after surgery.

Recovery from surgery is usually rapid and people can quickly resume their normal activities without any restrictions.

A new "nonsurgical" endovascular treatment uses angioplasty and stents to open blocked carotid arteries. This procedure's safety and efficacy continues to be studied in several medical centers. This procedure involves the placement of a small flexible tube (catheter) into an artery from the groin. The catheter is then directed to the neck to reach the carotid artery blockage. A balloon pushes open the artery wall and a stent (a small metallic coil) is often left to keep the artery open.

Prevention

Take care of your health through exercise and proper nutrition and take all medications as your doctor prescribes. If you have risk factors for carotid artery disease you should talk with your health care professional. If you have any symptoms, never hesitate or delay to seek help. Minutes are critical. It's up to you to do all you can to reduce your risk. No surprise—prevention is the best medicine!

Chapter 43

Coronary Artery and Heart Disease

Chapter Contents

Section 43.1

Coronary Artery Disease

Excerpted from "Coronary Artery Disease," National Heart Lung and
Blood Institute, National Institutes of Health, February 2009.

What Is Coronary Artery Disease?

Coronary artery disease (CAD), also called coronary heart disease, is a condition in which plaque builds up inside the coronary arteries. These arteries supply your heart muscle with oxygen-rich blood.

Plaque is made up of fat, cholesterol, calcium, and other substances found in the blood. When plaque builds up in the arteries, the condition is called atherosclerosis.

Plaque narrows the arteries and reduces blood flow to your heart muscle. It also makes it more likely that blood clots will form in your arteries. Blood clots can partially or completely block blood flow.

Overview

When your coronary arteries are narrowed or blocked, oxygen-rich blood can't reach your heart muscle. This can cause angina or a heart attack.

Angina is chest pain or discomfort that occurs when not enough oxygen-rich blood is flowing to an area of your heart muscle. Angina may feel like pressure or squeezing in your chest. The pain also may occur in your shoulders, arms, neck, jaw, or back.

A heart attack occurs when blood flow to an area of your heart muscle is completely blocked. This prevents oxygen-rich blood from reaching that area of heart muscle and causes it to die. Without quick treatment, a heart attack can lead to serious problems and even death.

Over time, CAD can weaken the heart muscle and lead to heart failure and arrhythmias. Heart failure is a condition in which your heart can't pump enough blood throughout your body. Arrhythmias are problems with the speed or rhythm of your heartbeat.

Outlook

CAD is the most common type of heart disease. It's the leading cause of death in the United States for both men and women. Lifestyle changes, medicines, and/or medical procedures can effectively prevent or treat CAD in most people.

What Causes Coronary Artery Disease?

Research suggests that coronary artery disease (CAD) starts when certain factors damage the inner layers of the coronary arteries. These factors include the following:

* Smoking

* High amounts of certain fats and cholesterol in the blood

* High blood pressure

* High amounts of sugar in the blood due to insulin resistance or diabetes

When damage occurs, your body starts a healing process. Excess fatty tissues release compounds that promote this process. This healing causes plaque to build up where the arteries are damaged.

The buildup of plaque in the coronary arteries may start in childhood. Over time, plaque can narrow or completely block some of your coronary arteries. This reduces the flow of oxygen-rich blood to your heart muscle.

Plaque also can crack, which causes blood cells called platelets to clump together and form blood clots at the site of the cracks. This narrows the arteries more and worsens angina or causes a heart attack.

Who Is at Risk for Coronary Artery Disease?

Coronary artery disease (CAD) is the leading cause of death in the United States for both men and women. Each year, more than half a million Americans die from CAD.

Certain traits, conditions, or habits may raise your chance of developing CAD. These conditions are known as risk factors.

You can control most risk factors and help prevent or delay CAD. Other risk factors can't be controlled.

Major Risk Factors

Many factors raise the risk of developing CAD. The more risk factors you have, the greater chance you have of developing CAD:

- **Unhealthy blood cholesterol levels.** This includes high amounts of low-density lipoprotein (LDL) cholesterol (sometimes called bad cholesterol) and low amounts of high-density lipoprotein (HDL) cholesterol (sometimes called good cholesterol).

- **High blood pressure.** Blood pressure is considered high if it stays at or above 140/90 mmHg over a period of time.

- **Smoking.** This can damage and tighten blood vessels, raise cholesterol levels, and raise blood pressure. Smoking also doesn't allow enough oxygen to reach the body's tissues.

- **Insulin resistance.** This condition occurs when the body can't use its own insulin properly. Insulin is a hormone that helps move blood sugar into cells where it's used.

- **Diabetes.** This is a disease in which the body's blood sugar level is high because the body doesn't make enough insulin or doesn't use its insulin properly.

- **Overweight or obesity.** Overweight is having extra body weight from muscle, bone, fat, and/or water. Obesity is having a high amount of extra body fat.

- **Metabolic syndrome.** Metabolic syndrome is the name for a group of risk factors linked to overweight and obesity that raise your chance for heart disease and other health problems, such as diabetes and stroke.

- **Lack of physical activity.** Lack of activity can worsen other risk factors for CAD.

- **Age.** As you get older, your risk for CAD increases. Genetic or lifestyle factors cause plaque to build in your arteries as you age. By the time you're middle-aged or older, enough plaque has built up to cause signs or symptoms. In men, the risk for CAD increases after age forty-five. In women, the risk for CAD risk increases after age fifty-five.

- **Family history of early heart disease.** Your risk increases if your father or a brother was diagnosed with CAD before fifty-five years of age, or if your mother or a sister was diagnosed with CAD before sixty-five years of age.

Although age and a family history of early heart disease are risk factors, it doesn't mean that you will develop CAD if you have one or both.

Making lifestyle changes and/or taking medicines to treat other risk factors can often lessen genetic influences and prevent CAD from developing, even in older adults.

Emerging Risk Factors

Scientists continue to study other possible risk factors for CAD.

High levels of a protein called C-reactive protein (CRP) in the blood may raise the risk for CAD and heart attack. High levels of CRP are proof of inflammation in the body. Inflammation is the body's response to injury or infection. Damage to the arteries' inner walls seems to trigger inflammation and help plaque grow.

Research is under way to find out whether reducing inflammation and lowering CRP levels also can reduce the risk of developing CAD and having a heart attack.

High levels of fats called triglycerides in the blood also may raise the risk of CAD, particularly in women.

Other Factors That Affect Coronary Artery Disease

Other factors also may contribute to CAD. These include the following:

- **Sleep apnea.** Sleep apnea is a disorder in which your breathing stops or gets very shallow while you're sleeping. Untreated sleep apnea can raise your chances of having high blood pressure, diabetes, and even a heart attack or stroke.

- **Stress.** Research shows that the most commonly reported "trigger" for a heart attack is an emotionally upsetting event—particularly one involving anger.

- **Alcohol.** Heavy drinking can damage the heart muscle and worsen other risk factors for heart disease. Men should have no more than two drinks containing alcohol a day. Women should have no more than one drink containing alcohol a day.

What Are the Signs and Symptoms of Coronary Artery Disease?

A common symptom of coronary artery disease (CAD) is angina. Angina is chest pain or discomfort that occurs when your heart muscle doesn't get enough oxygen-rich blood.

Angina may feel like pressure or a squeezing pain in your chest. You also may feel it in your shoulders, arms, neck, jaw, or back. This pain tends to get worse with activity and go away when you rest. Emotional stress also can trigger the pain.

Another common symptom of CAD is shortness of breath. This symptom happens if CAD causes heart failure. When you have heart failure, your heart can't pump enough blood throughout your body. Fluid builds up in your lungs, making it hard to breathe.

The severity of these symptoms varies. The symptoms may get more severe as the buildup of plaque continues to narrow the coronary arteries.

Signs and Symptoms of Heart Problems Linked to Coronary Artery Disease

Some people who have CAD have no signs or symptoms. This is called silent CAD. It may not be diagnosed until a person shows signs and symptoms of a heart attack, heart failure, or an arrhythmia (an irregular heartbeat).

Heart attack. A heart attack happens when an area of plaque in a coronary artery breaks apart, causing a blood clot to form.

The blood clot cuts off most or all blood to the part of the heart muscle that's fed by that artery. Cells in the heart muscle die because they don't receive enough oxygen-rich blood. This can cause lasting damage to your heart.

The most common symptom of heart attack is chest pain or discomfort. Most heart attacks involve discomfort in the center of the chest that lasts for more than a few minutes or goes away and comes back. The discomfort can feel like pressure, squeezing, fullness, or pain. It can be mild or severe. Heart attack pain can sometimes feel like indigestion or heartburn.

Heart attacks also can cause upper body discomfort in one or both arms, the back, neck, jaw, or stomach. Shortness of breath or fatigue (tiredness) often may occur with or before chest discomfort. Other symptoms of heart attack are nausea (feeling sick to your stomach), vomiting, lightheadedness or fainting, and breaking out in a cold sweat.

Heart failure. Heart failure is a condition in which your heart can't pump enough blood to your body. Heart failure doesn't mean that your heart has stopped or is about to stop working. It means that your heart can't fill with enough blood or pump with enough force, or both.

This causes you to have shortness of breath and fatigue that tends to increase with activity. Heart failure also can cause swelling in your feet, ankles, legs, and abdomen.

Arrhythmia. An arrhythmia is a problem with the speed or rhythm of the heartbeat. When you have an arrhythmia, you may notice that your heart is skipping beats or beating too fast. Some people describe arrhythmias as a fluttering feeling in their chests. These feelings are called palpitations.

Some arrhythmias can cause your heart to suddenly stop beating. This condition is called sudden cardiac arrest (SCA). SCA can make you faint and it can cause death if it's not treated right away.

How Is Coronary Artery Disease Diagnosed?

Your doctor will diagnose coronary artery disease (CAD) based on the following things:

- Your medical and family histories

- Your risk factors

- The results of a physical exam and diagnostic tests and procedures

Diagnostic Tests and Procedures

No single test can diagnose CAD. If your doctor thinks you have CAD, he or she will probably do one or more of the following tests.

Electrocardiogram (EKG). An EKG is a simple test that detects and records the electrical activity of your heart. An EKG shows how fast your heart is beating and whether it has a regular rhythm. It also shows the strength and timing of electrical signals as they pass through each part of your heart.

Certain electrical patterns that the EKG detects can suggest whether CAD is likely. An EKG also can show signs of a previous or current heart attack.

Stress testing. During stress testing, you exercise to make your heart work hard and beat fast while heart tests are performed. If you can't exercise, you're given medicine to speed up your heart rate.

When your heart is beating fast and working hard, it needs more blood and oxygen. Arteries narrowed by plaque can't supply enough oxygen-rich blood to meet your heart's needs. A stress test can show possible signs of CAD, such as the following:

- Abnormal changes in your heart rate or blood pressure

- Symptoms such as shortness of breath or chest pain

- Abnormal changes in your heart rhythm or your heart's electrical activity

During the stress test, if you can't exercise for as long as what's considered normal for someone your age, it may be a sign that not enough blood is flowing to your heart. But other factors besides CAD can prevent you from exercising long enough (for example, lung diseases, anemia, or poor general fitness).

Some stress tests use a radioactive dye, sound waves, positron emission tomography (PET), or cardiac magnetic resonance imaging (MRI) to take pictures of your heart when it's working hard and when it's at rest.

These imaging stress tests can show how well blood is flowing in the different parts of your heart. They also can show how well your heart pumps blood when it beats.

Echocardiography. This test uses sound waves to create a moving picture of your heart. Echocardiography provides information about the size and shape of your heart and how well your heart chambers and valves are working.

The test also can identify areas of poor blood flow to the heart, areas of heart muscle that aren't contracting normally, and previous injury to the heart muscle caused by poor blood flow.

Chest x-ray. A chest x-ray takes a picture of the organs and structures inside the chest, including your heart, lungs, and blood vessels.

A chest x-ray can reveal signs of heart failure, as well as lung disorders and other causes of symptoms that aren't due to CAD.

Blood tests. Blood tests check the levels of certain fats, cholesterol, sugar, and proteins in your blood. Abnormal levels may show that you have risk factors for CAD.

Electron-beam computed tomography. Your doctor may recommend electron-beam computed tomography (EBCT). This test finds and measures calcium deposits (called calcifications) in and around the coronary arteries. The more calcium detected, the more likely you are to have CAD. EBCT isn't used routinely to diagnose CAD, because its accuracy isn't yet known.

Coronary angiography and cardiac catheterization. Your doctor may ask you to have coronary angiography if other tests or factors show that you're likely to have CAD. This test uses dye and special x-rays to show the insides of your coronary arteries.

To get the dye into your coronary arteries, your doctor will use a procedure called cardiac catheterization. A long, thin, flexible tube called a catheter is put into a blood vessel in your arm, groin (upper thigh), or neck. The tube is then threaded into your coronary arteries, and the dye is released into your bloodstream. Special x-rays are taken while the dye is flowing through your coronary arteries.

Cardiac catheterization is usually done in a hospital. You're awake during the procedure. It usually causes little to no pain, although you may feel some soreness in the blood vessel where your doctor put the catheter.

How Is Coronary Artery Disease Treated?

Treatment for coronary artery disease (CAD) may include lifestyle changes, medicines, and medical procedures.

Lifestyle Changes

Making lifestyle changes can often help prevent or treat CAD. For some people, these changes may be the only treatment needed:

- Follow a heart healthy eating plan to prevent or reduce high blood pressure and high blood cholesterol and to maintain a healthy weight.

- Increase your physical activity. Check with your doctor first to find out how much and what kinds of activity are safe for you.

- Lose weight, if you're overweight or obese.

- Quit smoking, if you smoke. Avoid exposure to secondhand smoke.

- Learn to cope with and reduce stress.

Medicines

You may need medicines to treat CAD if lifestyle changes aren't enough. Medicines can do the following things:

- Decrease the workload on your heart and relieve CAD symptoms

- Decrease your chance of having a heart attack or dying suddenly

- Lower your cholesterol and blood pressure

- Prevent blood clots

- Prevent or delay the need for a special procedure (for example, angioplasty or coronary artery bypass grafting [CABG])

Medicines used to treat CAD include anticoagulants, aspirin and other antiplatelet medicines, angiotensin-converting enzyme (ACE) inhibitors, beta blockers, calcium channel blockers, nitroglycerin, glycoprotein IIb-IIIa, statins, and fish oil and other supplements high in omega-3 fatty acids.

Medical Procedures

You may need a medical procedure to treat CAD. Both angioplasty and CABG are used as treatments.

Angioplasty opens blocked or narrowed coronary arteries. During angioplasty, a thin tube with a balloon or other device on the end is threaded through a blood vessel to the narrowed or blocked coronary artery. Once in place, the balloon is inflated to push the plaque outward against the wall of the artery. This widens the artery and restores the flow of blood.

Angioplasty can improve blood flow to your heart, relieve chest pain, and possibly prevent a heart attack. Sometimes a small mesh tube called a stent is placed in the artery to keep it open after the procedure.

In CABG, arteries or veins from other areas in your body are used to bypass (that is, go around) your narrowed coronary arteries. CABG can improve blood flow to your heart, relieve chest pain, and possibly prevent a heart attack.

You and your doctor can discuss which treatment is right for you.

How Can Coronary Artery Disease Be Prevented or Delayed?

Taking action to control your risk factors can help prevent or delay coronary artery disease (CAD). Your chance of developing CAD goes up with the number of risk factors you have.

Making lifestyle changes and taking prescribed medicines are important steps.

Know your family history of health problems related to CAD. If you or someone in your family has CAD, be sure to tell your doctor. Also, let your doctor know if you smoke.

Section 43.2

Angina

Angina is chest pain or a sensation of pressure that occurs when
the heart muscle is not getting enough oxygen. It tends to develop in
women at a later age than in men.

A form of angina—angina decubitus—occurs when a person is lying down (not necessarily during sleep). It occurs because the fluids
in the body are redistributed in this position due to gravity, and the
heart has to work harder.

Another form—variant angina—occurs from a spasm in the arteries
on the surface of the heart. It produces pain during rest rather than
physical activity. It also produces changes that are detectable with
electrocardiography (ECG) while it is happening.

Unstable angina is when the pattern of symptoms changes. Usually, the condition in each individual usually remains constant, so any
change—increased pain, more frequent attacks, or occurrence at lesser
levels of activity or at rest—is a serious matter. It could mean that
the coronary artery disease is getting worse rapidly and the risk of a
heart attack is high. Unstable angina should be considered a medical
emergency.

There is a form of angina called cardiac syndrome X. In this form,
there is neither a spasm nor any detectable block in the coronary
arteries. In some people, the pain and pressure in the chest may be a
result of a temporary narrowing of the smaller arteries of the heart.
No one knows what causes this, but it may be the result of a chemical
imbalance in the heart or abnormalities in the arteries.

Symptoms of Angina

Angina symptoms usually first appear during physical activity or
emotional distress, both of which make the heart work harder and need
more oxygen. But if the reduced blood flow is severe enough, angina
can occur when a person is at rest.

When angina occurs it usually lasts only a few moments and goes away with rest. Sometimes it is worse when a person is active after having eaten. It is usually worse in cold weather or when moving from a warm room to a cold one. Sometimes experiencing a strong emotion while resting (or having a bad dream) can trigger it.

Typically, a person will feel pain or an ache or a sensation of pressure just beneath the breastbone. Many people describe the feel as discomfort or heaviness rather than pain. The ache or pressure might also be felt in either shoulder or down the inside of the arms, the back, or in the throat, jaw, or teeth.

The symptoms of angina that are felt by older people or by women may be different and easily misdiagnosed. Pain may be felt in the stomach area, especially after a meal. It may resemble indigestion.

Causes of Angina and Risk Factors

Fatty deposits in the arteries that feed the heart or sometimes because of other abnormalities that interfere with the flow of blood to the heart muscle are the main causes. Not everyone with coronary artery disease has angina.

Angina can also be caused by severe anemia—a condition in which the body has fewer red blood cells or less hemoglobin, which carries oxygen. Rarer causes of angina are severe high blood pressure, a narrowing of the aortic valve (aortic valve stenosis), leakage from the aortic valve, thickening of the walls of the ventricles. All of these factors make the heart work and increase its need for oxygen. Abnormalities of the aortic valve may also reduce the blood flow through the arteries of the heart. The openings for these arteries are just beyond the aorta.

Diagnosis of Angina

Angina is usually diagnosed on the basis of the symptoms that an individual describes. If the symptoms are typical, it's usually easy for a doctor to diagnose the condition. The kind of pain, its location, and its association with exertion, meals, weather, and other factors are also helpful.

This is especially so if there are other risk factors for coronary artery disease present. These tests may be done to determine if the person has coronary artery disease and how severe it is:

- Exercise stress testing

- Radionuclide imaging

- Echocardiography

- Coronary angiography

- Continuous electrocardiogram monitoring with a Holter monitor

Treatment of Angina

Angina is a symptom of coronary artery disease. How the angina is treated depends on the stability and severity of the symptoms. Treatment may include:

- Eliminating or minimizing risk factors of coronary artery disease by treating high blood pressure, lowering high cholesterol levels, quitting smoking, exercise, and weight loss if needed.

- Lowering low-density lipoprotein (LDL) cholesterol levels as much as possible using drugs.

- Drug therapy, including beta-blockers, nitrates (such as nitroglycerin), calcium channel blockers, angiotensin-converting enzyme (ACE) inhibitors, and anti-clotting drugs.

- Hospitalization if the symptoms get worse quickly.

- Angiography may be performed if symptoms do not improve to help determine if coronary artery bypass surgery or angioplasty is needed.

- Transmyocardial laser revascularization (TMR) is a new technique for relieving severe angina or coronary artery disease in patients unable to have bypass surgery or angioplasty.

Ultimately treatment of the coronary artery disease is required.

Section 43.3

Heart Attack

"Heart Attack (Myocardial Infarction)," © 2008 Cedars-Sinai Heart Institute (www.csmc.edu/2266.html). Reprinted with permission.

A heart attack or myocardial infarction is a medical emergency in which the supply of blood to the heart is suddenly and severely reduced or cut off, causing the muscle to die from lack of oxygen. More than 1.1 million people experience a heart attack (myocardial infarction) each year, and for many of them, the heart attack is their first symptom of coronary artery disease. A heart attack may be severe enough to cause death or it may be silent. As many as one out of every five people have only mild symptoms or none at all, and the heart attack may only be discovered by routine electrocardiography done some time later.

Heart Attack Symptoms

Not everyone has the same heart attack symptoms when having a myocardial infarction. Common ones include:

- About two out of every three people who have heart attacks have chest pain, shortness of breath, or feel tired a few days or weeks before the attack.

- A person who has angina (temporary chest pain) may find that it happens more often after less and less physical activity. A change in the pattern of angina should be taken seriously.

- During a heart attack, a person may feel pain in the middle of the chest that can spread to the back, jaw, or arms. The pain may also be felt in all of these places and not the chest. Sometimes the pain is felt in the stomach area, where it may be taken for indigestion. The pain is like that of angina but usually more severe, longer lasting, and does not get better by resting or taking a nitroglycerin pill.

- About one out of every three people who have heart attacks do not feel any chest pain. These people are more likely to be women, non-Caucasian, older than seventy-five, someone with heart failure or diabetes, and someone who has had a stroke.

- Faintness.

- Sudden sweating.

- Nausea.

- Shortness of breath, especially in older people.

- Heavy pounding of the heart.

- Abnormal heart rhythms (arrhythmias), which occur in more than 90 percent of the people who have had a heart attack.

- Loss of consciousness, which sometimes is the first symptom of a heart attack.

- Feelings of restlessness, sweatiness, anxiety, and a sense of impending doom.

- Bluishness of the lips, hands, or feet.

- Older people may have symptoms that resemble a stroke and may become disoriented.

- Older people, especially women, often take longer than younger people to admit they are ill or to seek medical help.

During the early hours of a heart attack, heart murmurs and other abnormal heart sounds may be heard through a stethoscope.

Causes of Heart Attacks and Risk Factors

A heart attack (myocardial infarction) is usually caused by a blood clot that blocks an artery of the heart. The artery has often already been narrowed by fatty deposits on its walls. These deposits can tear or break open, reducing the flow of blood and releasing substances that make the platelets of the blood sticky and more likely to form clots. Sometimes a clot forms inside the heart itself, then breaks away and gets stuck in an artery that feeds the heart. A spasm in one of these arteries can cause the blood flow to stop.

Diagnosis of Heart Attacks

Because a heart attack (myocardial infarction) can be life threatening, men older than thirty-five or women older than fifty who have chest pain should be examined to see if they area having a heart attack. However, similar pain can be caused by pneumonia, a blood clot in the lung (pulmonary embolism), pericarditis, a rib fracture, spasm of the esophagus, indigestion, or chest muscle tenderness after injury or exertion. A heart attack can be confirmed within a few hours of its occurrence by:

- Electrocardiography (ECG).

- Blood tests to measure levels of serum markers. The presence of these markers shows that there has been damage to or death of the heart muscle. These markers are normally found in the heart muscle, but they are released into the blood when the heart muscle is damaged.

- Echocardiography can be performed if the above tests do not give enough information.

- Radionuclide imaging can also be done.

Treatment of Heart Attacks (Myocardial Infarction)

Half the deaths from a heart attack occur in the first three or four hours after symptoms begin. It is crucial that symptoms of a heart attack be treated as a medical emergency. A person with these symptoms should be taken to the emergency department of a hospital in an ambulance with trained personnel.

The sooner that treatment of a heart attack begins, the better. Chewing an aspirin tablet after an ambulance has been called can help reduce the size of the blood clot. A beta-blocker may be given to slow the heart rate so the heart is not working as hard and to reduce the damage to the heart muscle. Often a person who is having a heart attack is given oxygen, which also helps heart tissue damage to be less.

People who may be having a heart attack are usually admitted to a hospital that has a cardiac care unit. Heart rhythm, blood pressure, and the amount of oxygen in the blood are closely monitored so that heart damage can be assessed. Nurses in these units are specially trained to care for people with heart problems and to handle cardiac emergencies.

Drugs may be used to dissolve blood clots in the artery so that heart tissue can be saved. To be effective, these drugs must be given intravenously within six hours of the start of the symptoms of a heart attack. After six hours, most damage is permanent. (People who have bleeding conditions or severe high blood pressure and those who have had recent surgery or a stroke cannot be given these drugs.)

Instead of drug therapy, angioplasty or coronary artery bypass surgery may be performed immediately after a heart attack to clear the arteries. This approach is preferred for people who cannot take thrombolytic drugs and for those who are very ill after having a massive heart attack.

Because most people who have had a heart attack (myocardial infarction) are anxious and uncomfortable, morphine is often given to calm them and reduce the work load on the heart. Nitroglycerin, which opens up the arteries of the heart and relieves pain, may also be given. Angiotensin-converting enzyme (ACE) inhibitors can reduce heart enlargement and increase the chance of survival for many people. Therefore, these drugs are usually given in the first few days after a heart attack and prescribed indefinitely.

A person who has just had a heart attack needs rest and as little emotional distress or excitement as possible. If there are no complications, most people can safely leave the hospital within five to seven days. If abnormal heart rhythms develop, the heart can no longer pump adequately, or there are complications, a person recovering from a heart attack will need to stay longer in the hospital.

Most people who survive for a few days after a heart attack (myocardial infarction) can expect a full recovery. One out of every ten people who have heart attacks, however, die within a year—usually within the first three or four months. Typically, these people continue to have chest pain, abnormal heart rhythms, or heart failure. Older people and smaller people tend to not do as well after a heart attack as younger people and larger people. This may be one reason why women tend to fare less well than men after a heart attack—they tend to be both older and smaller, as well as have other disorders. They also tend to wait longer after a heart attack before going to the hospital.

After a heart attack (myocardial infarction), a doctor may require additional tests or treatment, including:

- wearing a Holter monitor for continuous monitoring of the heart's electrical activity;

- an exercise stress test;

- drug therapy, including taking a daily aspirin, beta-blockers, or ACE inhibitors;

- coronary angiography;

- angioplasty;

- bypass surgery;

- lowering cholesterol levels;

- rehabilitation.

Chapter 44

Fibromuscular Dysplasia

What is fibromuscular dysplasia?

Fibromuscular dysplasia (FMD) is an uncommon disorder characterized by abnormal cellular growth in the walls of medium and large arteries. This abnormal cellular growth may lead to a beaded appearance of the affected artery and narrowing (stenosis) in some cases. Most cases—60 to 75 percent—occur in the renal artery, the artery leading from the abdominal aorta to the kidneys. Approximately 30 percent of cases involve the carotid arteries, the arteries in the neck that connect the heart and the brain. FMD also can affect the arteries to the legs or, less frequently, arteries in other parts of the body. In many cases, there is FMD found in multiple arteries of the body.

Who is affected by FMD?

FMD is most common in women between ages thirty and fifty, but may also occur in children and the elderly in some cases. FMD occurs two to ten times more frequently in women than in men.

What causes FMD?

The causes of FMD are still unknown and are the focus of considerable research. The disease most likely has multiple underlying causes. Some of the factors that may play a role include:

- **Hormonal influences:** The disease occurs most commonly in women of childbearing age.

- **Genetics:** About 10 percent of cases are familial, and there also seems to be an overlap of FMD with other genetic abnormalities that affect the blood vessels.

- **Internal mechanical stress:** This includes trauma or stress to the artery walls.

- **Loss of oxygen supply to the blood vessel wall:** This occurs when the tiny blood vessels in the artery walls that supply them with oxygenated blood get blocked by fibrous lesions.

Are there different types of fibromuscular dysplasia?

Artery walls have three layers: the tunica intima (the inside layer), the tunica media (the middle layer), and the adventitia (the outside layer). Fibromuscular dysplasia is described in terms of the affected layer and the composition of the lesions. Depending on the type of FMD, the narrowing (stenosis) of the artery is caused by an excess of either the fibrous or muscular components of the arterial wall. While the type of FMD can only be determined with 100 percent accuracy by analyzing the artery wall under the microscope, such as after a biopsy or surgical procedure, this is rarely done in modern times. In most cases, it is possible to distinguish the type of FMD on the basis of the appearance of the arteries affected with a dye angiogram test.

The five types of dysplasia, from most common to least common, are:

- Medial fibroplasia (75 to 80 percent of FMD lesions are this type):

  - Affects the tunica media

  - Characterized by areas of fibrous lesions alternating with bulging areas (aneurysms)

  - Has a classic "beads on a string" appearance on a dye angiogram

- Intimal fibroplasia (less than 10 percent of FMD lesions are this type):

  - Caused by collagen (fibrous tissue) deposits around the inside layer of the artery wall, the tunica intima

- Concentric, smooth narrowing (without beads) on a dye angiogram

- Perimedial fibroplasia (less than 10 percent of FMD lesions are this type):

  - Extensive collagen deposits in the outer portion of the tunica media

  - Irregular thickening of the artery walls

  - Has a different "beads on a string" appearance than medial fibroplasia, with beads that have a small diameter compared to the normal artery

  - Risk for total blockage of affected arteries

- Medial hyperplasia (1 to 2 percent of lesions are this type):

  - Caused by excessive formation of smooth muscle cells

  - Fibrous deposits are absent

  - Appearance on angiogram similar to intimal fibroplasias

- Periarterial hyperplasia (Rare, fewer than 1 percent of FMD cases are this type):

  - Caused by expansion of the adventitia

  - Collagen extends into the surrounding fat layers

  - Characterized by inflammation of the artery and surrounding area

What are the symptoms of FMD and how is it diagnosed?

Many people with FMD do not have any symptoms, but symptoms can occur if the stenosis is severe enough to restrict the blood flow through the affected artery:

- Symptoms of moderate FMD in the carotid artery may include headaches, ringing or a "swishing" noise in the ears, or light-headedness. More advanced FMD can cause stroke or transient ischemic attacks (TIAs, mini-strokes).

- FMD of the carotid or vertebral arteries (which supply blood to the back of the brain) may also present with a tear in the artery, known as carotid dissection. The symptoms of carotid dissection include headache, sudden neck pain, along with symptoms of stroke or mini-stroke in severe cases.

- FMD of the renal artery(ies) frequently causes high blood pressure in these arteries (renovascular hypertension) and/or diminished kidney function (renal insufficiency). FMD usually does not progress to the point where it causes kidney failure.

FMD is often diagnosed incidentally when the person is having an x-ray or scan for another problem that identifies the beaded appearance in the arteries. In other cases, a patient may be diagnosed with FMD after her or his physician hears a bruit (swishing noise indicating abnormal flow) in the neck or abdomen during a routine physical examination.

When a patient is diagnosed with FMD in one part of the body, additional imaging studies may be obtained to evaluate the other blood vessels. For example, if a patient is found to have carotid FMD and has high blood pressure, a test to evaluate the renal arteries may be requested by her physician. Noninvasive imaging studies such as duplex ultrasound, magnetic resonance angiography (MRA), and computed tomography angiography (CTA) can be used to confirm the diagnosis of FMD and determine the extent of the lesions. In some cases, it is recommended that the patient undergo a dye angiogram, which is considered the gold standard for diagnosing FMD. In general, dye angiogram studies are reserved for cases in which the diagnosis of FMD is not clear when a patient may require a therapeutic procedure during the same procedure, such as a balloon angioplasty.

It is generally recommended that patients diagnosed with carotid or vertebral artery FMD undergo an imaging study of the blood vessels within the brain to exclude the presence of an intracranial aneurysm that may require additional treatment.

What treatments are available for FMD?

When FMD is present without any symptoms, it usually is benign and does not require intervention. For these patients, the physician may prescribe an antiplatelet medication to prevent blood clots. This may be a prescription or simply aspirin taken on a regular schedule. All other risk factors for vascular disease, such as blood pressure, blood sugar, and blood cholesterol should be assessed and appropriately treated. These patients should have an imaging study (duplex ultrasound, MRA, or CTA) performed at regular intervals, generally annually, to monitor disease progression. This is particularly important when an aneurysm is present in the internal carotid arteries or the patient has had a carotid or vertebral artery dissection.

Patients with renovascular hypertension due to FMD may be treated with blood pressure medications, particularly with the angiotensin converting enzyme inhibitors (Ace inhibitors). In certain cases, percutaneous angioplasty of the renal arteries is considered the state-of-the-art treatment. Similar to the procedure used to treat blockages in the heart arteries, it involves using a catheter to place a tiny balloon inside the artery at the site of the stenosis. The balloon is inflated to re-open the blood vessel; then the balloon and the catheter are withdrawn. Using a stent (a tiny metal coil) to hold open the artery has not been proven to make the treatment of renal FMD more effective or longer-lasting. In general, renal artery stents should only be placed when absolutely necessary when the results of angioplasty alone are not adequate to improve blood flow to the kidney.

Angioplasty also is recommended for patients with FMD of the internal carotid artery who experience TIAs or stroke related to severe narrowings. In unusual cases of patients with FMD who have had carotid or vertebral artery dissection or who have a carotid aneurysm, stenting may be necessary.

Reconstructive surgery may be used in patients with complex FMD of the renal arteries or with an aneurysm of the internal carotid or vertebral arteries. The surgery depends upon the location and the extent of disease, but generally involves removing or bypassing the affected portion of the artery to restore normal blood flow.

FMD is a very different disorder than atherosclerosis, which is the plaque formation that is the most common cause of blocked arteries. Both percutaneous angioplasty and reconstructive surgery are technically demanding procedures and should be performed only by a physician experienced in these procedures and in the care of patients with FMD.

This information is not intended to replace the medical advice of your doctor or health care provider. Please consult your health care provider for advice about a specific medical condition.

Chapter 45

Klippel-Trénaunay Syndrome

What is Klippel-Trénaunay syndrome (KTS)?

Although Klippel-Trénaunay syndrome is a rare congenital (present at birth) disorder, it is the most common condition involving combined vascular malformations. The syndrome is characterized by a localized or diffuse capillary malformation (port-wine stain) that overlies a venous malformation and/or lymphatic malformation with associated soft tissue and bone hypertrophy (excessive growth). The port-wine stain is typically substantial, varicose veins are often quite numerous, and bone and soft tissue hypertrophy is variable. The affected limb is either larger or smaller than the unaffected limb. Hypertrophy occurs most commonly in the lower limbs, but may affect the arms, the face, the head, or internal organs. Additionally, a wide range of other skeletal and skin abnormalities sometimes coexists.

Bony enlargement is usually not present at birth, but may appear within the first few months or years of life and may become particularly problematic during puberty. The affected area grows longer and thicker due to increased blood supply. Sometime after puberty and before age thirty, the port-wine stain develops small vesicles (blood-filled bubble-like lesions) that can bleed spontaneously.

In some patients, small lymphatic vesicles may appear. These vesicles may leak clear or blood-tinged fluid.

In young adults, the port-wine stain may thicken and become more prominent.

What symptoms are associated with Klippel-Trénaunay syndrome?

Symptoms vary according to the severity of the dominant vascular component and its location. If lymphatic malformations are dominant, soft tissue swelling and enlargement will occur. If venous malformations are dominant, episodes of painful thrombosis (clotting) will occur. This group of patients often experiences muscle cramping or joint pain when walking. When the lower gastrointestinal tract (intestines) is involved, rectal bleeding often occurs. When there is bladder involvement, blood is often seen in the urine.

How is Klippel-Trénaunay syndrome diagnosed?

In many patients, a thorough medical history and physical examination are sufficient to make the diagnosis. When there are complications, however, a number of imaging studies are useful. Evaluation of the deep venous system can be done by Doppler ultrasonography (type of ultrasonography in which blood vessels are seen) and magnetic resonance imaging (MRI) studies. MRI is also helpful in imaging the soft tissue hypertrophy.

Careful clinical and radiologic assessment of the affected limb should be done at regular intervals to assess limb length discrepancy and to formulate an approach for prevention and treatment of overgrowth. For lower-limb overgrowth beyond a two-centimeter (bit less than one inch) differential, orthopedic intervention may be necessary.

What are the possible complications of Klippel-Trénaunay syndrome?

Patients with Klippel-Trénaunay syndrome can have numerous complications. Skin changes can cause bleeding, infection (cellulitis), or chronic ulceration (skin breakdown). Patients can have internal lesions that bleed or become infected. Chronic pain is a serious issue secondary to the above issues. Venous varicosities may lead to phlebitis (inflammation of the lining of the vein) and the development of small clots and phleboliths (calcium deposits in the veins). Because of the venous and lymphatic involvement, patients can have clotting abnormalities. Blood clots in the legs and lungs can be life threatening.

Hypertrophy (overgrowth) of a limb can lead to curvature of the spine (vertebral scoliosis) and can affect how patients walk. Also, it can compromise function.

How is Klippel-Trénaunay syndrome managed?

Management of Klippel-Trénaunay syndrome is dependent upon individual symptoms. Although both nonoperative and surgical approaches are used, treatment is primarily nonoperative and supportive.

Supportive care:

- **Compression therapy:** Compression garments are often advised for chronic venous insufficiency, lymphedema, recurrent cellulitis, and recurrent bleeding. They also protect the limb from trauma. Intermittent pneumatic compression pumps also may be beneficial.

- **Pain medication, antibiotics, and limb elevation:** These treatments are all used to manage cellulitis.

- **Anticoagulant therapy (the use of substances that prevent blood clotting):** This approach is indicated in cases of acute thrombosis (clotting) and is also used as a preventive measure prior to surgical procedures.

- **Heel inserts:** These are sometimes used to manage limb length discrepancies that are less than one inch. For greater discrepancies, orthopedic surgery may be considered.

Surgical interventions:

- **Laser therapy:** The flashlamp pulsed-dye laser is not as effective in lightening the color of the port-wine stain as it is in a patient with a port-wine stain only. Many treatments are typically required to achieve a desirable result. Laser treatment is also indicated when there is ulceration, since it tends to effect quicker healing.

- **Surgery:** Depending on individual circumstances and anatomical involvement, removal of a problematic area of abnormal tissue (debulking surgery) is sometimes advised.

Other treatment:

- **Sclerotherapy:** This treatment consists of the injection of a chemical into the vein causing inflammation. As the inner wall of the vein becomes inflamed, blood cannot flow through it. The vein then collapses and forms scar tissue.

Chapter 46

Peripheral Vascular Disease

Chapter Contents

503

Section 46.1

Buerger Disease (Thromboangiitis Obliterans)

What Is Buerger Disease?

Also known as thromboangiitis obliterans (TAO), it is a rare disorder characterized by inflammation of the small and medium arteries and veins. It affects about 8 to 11 persons per 100,000 in North America. The inflammation in TAO frequently leads to blockages of arteries of the lower segments of the arms and legs, and may cause claudication or rest pain and nonhealing sores or ulcers, a condition known as critical limb ischemia (CLI).

TAO is different from peripheral arterial disease or PAD, because it is not caused by atherosclerosis (plaque) buildup that causes a narrowing of the artery. Instead TAO is caused by inflammation of the artery wall, along with the development of clots in the small and medium-sized arteries of the arms or legs causing the arteries to become blocked. Without blood flow below the inflamed artery or clots, the fingers, toes, and skin tissue do not receive adequate blood. This usually leads to enormous pain at rest or with exercise, plus sores may develop and may be slow to heal.

Symptoms of Buerger Disease

Symptoms of TAO are generally rest pain and skin ulcerations in the feet or hands. This is often referred to as critical limb ischemia (CLI). The pain may also be felt in the leg or foot when exercising. Pain may become steadily worse and eventually become more constant, occurring at night while lying in bed. Foot sores may be present.

Individuals may also feel a coldness, numbness, or tingling in their feet and hands.

504

Risk Factors for Buerger Disease

TAO occurs:

- exclusively in individuals with a history of tobacco exposure of any kind, including smoking, chewing, or snuff;
- mostly in individuals between twenty and forty years old;
- more commonly in men;
- in those with a history of high cholesterol, high blood pressure, or diabetes.

Diagnosis of Buerger Disease

There are four key factors physicians use to diagnose TAO:

- Rest pain or ulceration before fifty years of age.
- Tobacco use.
- Tests indicating the arteries are blocked. Typical tests include artery blood flow measurements (such as the ankle-brachial index [ABI], or other vascular laboratory tests, such as ultrasound), arteriography (pictures of the affected blood vessel obtained by injecting a dye via catheter), and/or biopsy of the affected artery.
- No other causes for artery blockage or clot development. A physician would want to be sure that a clot did not develop from the heart or a large blood vessel and travel to the arm or leg (an embolus). The doctor would also want to be certain there had been no blood vessel injury or trauma, no local lesions such as a blood vessel cyst, no autoimmune diseases such as scleroderma, and no blood clotting diseases.

What Are the Treatment Options?

The treatment for TAO is immediate and complete tobacco cessation. It is absolutely essential. Mayo Clinic physicians have found that TAO patients who continue to smoke have a high rate of amputation that persists up to seventeen years after first diagnosis. The risk of amputation in TAO patients who stop smoking is much lower.

What Else Should I Know about TAO?

Unfortunately, knowledge about TAO is limited, and the long-term (greater than fifteen year) risk of amputation and death is not well known. One widely cited study of 112 patients was gathered from the Cleveland Clinic Foundation from 1970 to 1987. The study revealed that skin ulcerations occurred among 76 percent of TAO patients. Additionally, 27 percent of TAO patients underwent one or more amputations (15 percent finger, 33 percent toe, 10 percent forefoot, 36 percent below the knee, 5 percent above the knee). Clots in the superficial veins of the arms and legs and Raynaud phenomenon (fingers turning white and painful upon cold exposure) are also common. Despite these statistics, there is also good news. Long-term survival in TAO patients is slightly lower than for the U.S. population as a whole. The cause of this is not known but may be related to ongoing tobacco use.

Section 46.2

Claudication

Reprinted from "Intermittent Claudication," Walter Reed Army Medical Center. The text of this document is available online at http://www.wramc .army.mil/Patients/healthcare/surgery/vascular/Pages/claudication.aspx; accessed December 2, 2009.

What Is Claudication?

Claudication refers to pain or fatigue in the muscles of the lower extremities, such as in the calf region, aggravated by walking and relieved with rest. Claudication develops in a muscle below a complete or partial obstruction of a main artery or arteries to the lower extremities. Because of the obstruction(s) in a main arterial vessel(s), not enough blood reaches an exercising muscle to meet its energy needs. Pain occurs with exercise since the flow of blood is not adequate enough to remove waste materials that collect after activity.

What Causes Claudication?

This condition is due to buildup of atherosclerotic plaque on the inner lining of the arteries. The end result is a partial or complete blockage of blood flow through the arteries to the lower extremities. Diabetes mellitus, high blood pressure, high blood lipids/fats, and the use of tobacco are among the factors that can lead to the development of atherosclerosis. In addition to claudication, some individuals may also show signs of disease in the heart, kidneys, and major vessels supplying the brain due to the process of atherosclerosis.

Signs and Symptoms

- Cramping pain commonly occurs in the calf region.
- Fatigue, a feeling of tiredness, or pain may also occur in the buttock or thigh areas.
- Foot pain usually is associated with advanced peripheral vascular disease.

The symptoms of claudication recur after a similar level of activity is reached on a consistent basis. When pain occurs at rest, it usually is located in the foot. Elevation of the leg worsens this type of pain and standing or dangling the leg relieves it. With advanced peripheral vascular disease, the feet may feel cold and/or numb.

Prognosis

Intermittent claudication is considered a "benign process" in the majority of individuals with peripheral vascular disease. This means that the chance of losing a limb due to poor circulation is small when you carefully follow your prescribed medical regimen. As demonstrated by several studies, the majority of people with claudication do not require surgery, but can be managed conservatively with medical therapy.

Medical Treatment

The goals of medical therapy focus primarily on the reduction of risk factors, exercise program, and avoidance of foot trauma or injury.

Reduction of Risk Factors

- Stop smoking. Use of cigarettes is a primary risk factor for the development of atherosclerosis.
- Achieve and maintain a well-controlled blood pressure.
- If you have diabetes mellitus, keep your blood sugar under tight control.
- Maintain ideal body weight.
- Maintain a healthy diet. Reduce your intake of fatty foods. Keep your cholesterol level down.

Follow an Exercise Program

Several studies have shown that progressive exercise programs improve exercise performance, relieve the pain or discomfort of claudication, and allow you to perform your activities of daily living.

Walking stimulates the development of collateral circulation. Collateral circulation refers to the development of blood vessels that branch off large and medium-sized arteries. These vessels help to increase blood flow around the area of a blocked artery or arteries. Exercise also decreases levels of low-density lipoproteins (bad fat) and increases high-density lipoproteins (good fat).

Exercise at least thirty minutes daily to the onset of your symptom(s) of claudication, rest until the pain goes away, and then continue your exercise regimen. Follow the exercise regimen prescribed for you by your physician.

Avoid Foot Trauma or Injury

- Inspect your feet daily for cuts, ulcerations, or infection.
- Use moisturizing cream on areas of dry skin.
- Avoid wearing ill-fitting or worn-out shoes.
- Seek professional assistance with trimming toenails or calluses.
- Do not apply a heating pad or hot pack to your feet.
- Avoid walking barefoot.

Surgical Treatment

If indicated, your surgeon will determine the type of procedure to treat your poor circulation and discuss this with you. Several options include a bypass procedure or angioplasty.

Bypass Surgery

This procedure can treat a blockage in the abdomen or leg. A leg vein or man-made graft can create a path around the blockage. Blood then flows through this new path, "bypassing" the obstruction and improving the circulation to the affected area (s).

Angioplasty

This procedure requires the use of a catheter (hollow tube) placed in a major artery, such as the femoral artery. A small balloon, located at the end of the catheter, is inflated at the level of the blockage in order to widen the passageway for blood flow. Sometimes a stent (small hollow tube) can be placed inside the artery to prevent it from closing after the angioplasty.

When to Seek Medical Attention

Notify your doctor if the following problems occur:

- Nonhealing ulcers
- Black discoloration or "gangrene" of any tissue located in your lower extremities
- Rest pain
- Lifestyle-limiting claudication (inability to perform your activities of daily living despite following a prescribed medical regimen)

Section 46.3

Critical Limb Ischemia

"Critical Limb Ischemia," © 2009 University of California-Davis Vascular Center (www.ucdmc.ucdavis.edu/vascular). Reprinted with permission.

Critical limb ischemia (CLI) is a severe blockage in the arteries of the lower extremities, which markedly reduces blood flow. It is a serious form of peripheral arterial disease, or PAD, but less common than claudication. PAD is caused by atherosclerosis, the hardening and narrowing of the arteries over time due to the buildup of fatty deposits called plaque.

CLI is a chronic condition that results in severe pain in the feet or toes, even while resting. Complications of poor circulation can include sores and wounds that won't heal in the legs and feet. Left untreated, the complications of CLI will result in amputation of the affected limb.

Symptoms

The most prominent features of critical limb ischemia (CLI) are called ischemic rest pain—severe pain in the legs and feet while a person is not moving, or nonhealing sores on the feet or legs:

509

- Pain or numbness in the feet
- Shiny, smooth, dry skin of the legs or feet
- Thickening of the toenails
- Absent or diminished pulse in the legs or feet
- Open sores, skin infections, or ulcers that will not heal
- Dry gangrene (dry, black skin) of the legs or feet

Risk Factors

Risk factors for chronic limb ischemia are the same as those for atherosclerosis, hardening and narrowing of the arteries due to the buildup of fatty deposits, called plaque:

- Age
- Smoking
- Diabetes
- Overweight or obesity
- Sedentary lifestyle
- High cholesterol
- High blood pressure
- Family history of atherosclerosis or claudication

Diagnosis

Your doctor may identify and locate the cause of blockages associated with critical limb ischemia (CLI) using one or more of the following methods:

- **Auscultation:** The presence of a bruit, or "whooshing" sound, in the arteries of the legs is confirmed using a stethoscope.
- **Ankle-brachial index (ABI):** The systolic blood pressure in the arm is divided by the systolic pressure at the ankle.
- **Doppler ultrasound:** This form of ultrasound can measure the direction and velocity of blood flow through the vessels.
- **Computed tomography (CT) angiography:** An advanced x-ray procedure that uses a computer to generate three-dimensional images.

- **Magnetic resonance angiography (MR angiography):** The patient is exposed to radiofrequency waves in a strong magnetic field. The energy that is released is measured by a computer and used to construct two- and three-dimensional images of the blood vessels.

- **Angiogram:** An x-ray study of the blood vessels is taken using contrast dyes.

Treatment

Critical limb ischemia is a serious condition that requires immediate treatment to re-establish blood flow to the affected area. The number one priority is to preserve the limb.

Endovascular Treatments

Minimally invasive endovascular therapy is often an option in the care of CLI. The treatment recommended depends on the location and severity of the blockages. Most patients with CLI have multiple arterial blockages, including blockages of the arteries below the knee. In general, puncture of the groin, under local anesthesia, with insertion of a catheter into the artery in the groin will allow access to the diseased portion of the artery. Some of the endovascular procedures used to treat CLI include:

- **Angioplasty:** A tiny balloon is inserted through a puncture in the groin. The balloon is inflated one or more times, using a saline solution, to open the artery:

  - *Cutting balloon:* A balloon imbedded with micro-blades is used to dilate the diseased area. The blades cut the surface of the plaque, reducing the force necessary to dilate the vessel.

  - *Cold balloon (cryoplasty):* Instead of using saline, the balloon is inflated using nitrous oxide. The gas freezes the plaque. The procedure is easier on the artery; the growth of the plaque is halted; and little scar tissue is generated.

- **Stents:** Metal mesh tubes that provide scaffolding are left in place after an artery has been opened using a balloon angioplasty:

  - *Balloon-expanded:* A balloon is use to expand the stent. These stents are stronger but less flexible.

  - *Self-expanding:* Compressed stents are delivered to the diseased site. They expand upon release. These stents are more flexible.

- **Laser atherectomy:** Small bits of plaque are vaporized by the tip of a laser probe.

- **Directional atherectomy:** A catheter with a rotating cutting blade is used to physically remove plaque from the artery, opening the flow channel.

Recovery from these procedures usually takes one or two days, and most of these procedures are done on an outpatient basis. Treatment includes management of the risk factors of atherosclerosis.

Surgical Treatments

Treatment of wounds or ulcers may require additional surgical procedures or other follow-up care. If the arterial blockages are not favorable for endovascular therapy, surgical treatment is often recommended. This typically involves bypass around the diseased segment with either a vein from the patient or a synthetic graft. Hospitalization after a bypass operation varies from a few days to more than a week. Recovery from surgery may take several weeks.

Section 46.4

Erythromelalgia

This information is reprinted with permission from DermNet, the website of the New Zealand Dermatological Society. Visit www.dermnetnz.org for patient information on numerous skin conditions and their treatment. © 2008 New Zealand Dermatological Society.

What is erythromelalgia?

Erythromelalgia is a condition characterized by intense burning pain, erythema (marked redness), and increased skin temperature, primarily of the feet and hands. The condition is classified into primary and secondary erythromelalgia. It has also been classified into early-onset and late-onset forms. Symptoms of the disease vary markedly between individuals; in some patients there is a continual burning pain while others experience "flare-ups" or bouts of the condition lasting from minutes to days.

Erythromelalgia is also known as "erythermalgia." It may be considered a type of neuropathic pain syndrome (pain related to conditions affecting the nerves themselves), where there is dilation of the small blood vessels that become congested with blood.

What causes erythromelalgia and who gets it?

The actual cause of erythromelalgia is unknown in most cases. Primary erythromelalgia develops spontaneously without any associated underlying disease associated, and is sometimes called "idiopathic erythromelalgia." Secondary erythromelalgia develops secondarily to medical conditions such as neurological diseases (e.g., multiple sclerosis, peripheral neuropathy), autoimmune diseases (e.g., lupus, diabetes mellitus), or more commonly the myeloproliferative disorders. In these disorders the bone marrow produces excessive numbers of cells, e.g., polycythemia vera (increased red cells), and essential thrombocythemia (increased platelets). Erythromelalgia presents before the appearance of the myeloproliferative disorder in 85 percent of cases.

People with early-onset erythromelalgia develop it before they are twenty-five. Although the disease is of unknown origin in most cases, sometimes it can be traced back through generations of a family (Weir-Mitchell disease). This has recently been shown to be due to mutations in a gene called Na(v)1.7., which encodes a sodium channel within certain cells.

Late-onset erythromelalgia occurs most often around forty to sixty years of age and is primary in about 60 percent of cases.

What are the signs and symptoms?

Lower extremities such as the soles of feet and toes are most commonly involved. Rarely does the pain extend up to include the knees. Upper extremity involvement includes the fingers and hands. Often both feet and hands are involved and both sides of the body (bilateral) are affected. It may affect one side of the body (unilateral), particularly in secondary cases. Less frequently, symptoms may also appear in the face, ears, and other parts of the body.

The classic description of erythromelalgia is red, painful, warm hands or feet, brought on by warming or hanging the limb downward, and relieved with cooling and elevation:

- Some patients notice a continual burning while others are troubled with "flare-ups."

- Flare-ups may last minutes to days and typically occur late in the day and continue through the night.

- Usually attacks begin with an itching sensation, progressing to a more severe pain with a burning sensation.

- During an attack the affected extremity becomes warm, tender, swollen, and appears dusky red and sometimes mottled.

- Pain may be so intense that the patient cannot walk.

- Cooling (with fan or immersion in cold water) and elevating the extremity can relieve symptoms.

Symptoms often become so bad that normal functioning and quality of life are greatly affected. Patients avoid warm weather and may even relocate to cooler climates. Many cannot wear socks or closed shoes even in winter. Some patients become virtually housebound by continuous flare-ups and pain.

How is the diagnosis made?

Investigation for underlying causes is essential in all new cases of the disease. Erythromelalgia may be an early sign of polycythemia or thrombocythemia, where symptoms may precede diagnosis of the myeloproliferative disorder by 2.5 years. Dramatic relief with aspirin is typical of this type and can be used as an aid to diagnosis.

Diagnosis is based fairly much on the clinical picture, hence is often difficult because of the intermittent nature of the disease. Provided the patient gives a good description of their symptoms, a tentative diagnosis may be made. If in doubt, immersing an affected area in hot water for ten to thirty minutes may sometimes provoke an attack.

When no known underlying cause has been found, the erythromelalgia is considered primary.

What treatment is available?

The underlying cause must be treated where possible in secondary erythromelalgia. The treatment of symptoms of both primary and secondary erythromelalgia is through general nonmedical measures, drug therapy, and surgical intervention:

- General nonmedical measures such as cooling or elevating the extremity may relieve symptoms. Care is needed around cold water immersions; although it will provide temporary relief, it can cause many other serious problems. Frequent immersion into cold water can create a vicious cycle as the changes in temperature may cause reactive flaring. This can also lead to maceration of the skin, nonhealing ulcers, infection, gangrene, and amputation.

- Topical treatment with capsaicin cream has been reported with varying results.

- A variety of oral medications have been used to relieve symptoms, including:

  - **Aspirin:** Promptly relieves symptoms of erythromelalgia involving myeloproliferative disorders;

  - **Serotonin re-uptake inhibitors:** Venlafaxine, sertraline, fluoxetine, paroxetine;

  - **Tricyclic antidepressants:** Amitriptyline, imipramine;

  - **Anticonvulsants:** Gabapentin;

  - **Calcium antagonists:** Nifedipine, diltiazem;

  - **Prostaglandins:** Misoprostol.

- Intravenous infusions of nitroprusside, lignocaine (lidocaine) and prostaglandin.

- Surgical sympathectomy (a procedure in which the sympathetic nerve fibers are selectively cut).

Patients respond quite variably to drug therapy and no single therapy has proved consistently effective. Spontaneous remissions have also been known to occur.

Section 46.5

Peripheral Artery Disease

Excerpted from "Peripheral Arterial Disease," National Heart Lung and
Blood Institute, National Institutes of Health, September 2008.

What Is Peripheral Arterial Disease?

Peripheral arterial disease (PAD) occurs when plaque builds up in
the arteries that carry blood to your head, organs, and limbs. Plaque
is made up of fat, cholesterol, calcium, fibrous tissue, and other substances in the blood.

When plaque builds up in arteries, the condition is called atherosclerosis. Over time, plaque can harden and narrow the arteries. This
limits the flow of oxygen-rich blood to your organs and other parts of
your body.

What Causes Peripheral Arterial Disease?

The most common cause of peripheral arterial disease (PAD) is
atherosclerosis. The exact cause of atherosclerosis isn't known.

The disease may start when certain factors damage the inner layers
of the arteries. These factors include the following:

- Smoking

- High amounts of certain fats and cholesterol in the blood

- High blood pressure

- High amounts of sugar in the blood due to insulin resistance or
  diabetes

When damage occurs, your body starts a healing process. The healing may cause plaque to build up where the arteries are damaged.

Over time, the plaque may crack. Blood cell fragments called platelets stick to the injured lining of the artery and may clump together
to form blood clots.

The buildup of plaque or blood clots can severely narrow or block
the arteries and limit the flow of oxygen-rich blood to your body.

Who Is at Risk for Peripheral Arterial Disease?

The major risk factors for PAD are smoking, age, and having certain diseases or conditions, including diabetes, high blood pressure, high blood cholesterol, heart disease, or stroke.

What Are the Signs and Symptoms of Peripheral Arterial Disease?

At least half of the people who have peripheral arterial disease (PAD) don't have any signs or symptoms of it. Others may have a number of signs and symptoms.

Even if you don't have signs or symptoms, discuss with your doctor whether you should get checked for PAD if you're:

- aged seventy or older;

- aged fifty or older and have a history of smoking or diabetes;

- younger than fifty and have diabetes and one or more risk factors for atherosclerosis.

Intermittent Claudication

People who have PAD may have symptoms when walking or climbing stairs. These may include pain, numbness, aching, or heaviness in the leg muscles. Symptoms also may include cramping in the affected leg(s) and in the buttocks, thighs, calves, and feet. Symptoms may ease after resting.

These symptoms are called intermittent claudication. During physical activity, your muscles need increased blood flow. If your blood vessels are narrowed or blocked, your muscles won't get enough blood. When resting, the muscles need less blood flow, so the pain goes away.

Other Signs and Symptoms

Other signs and symptoms of PAD include the following:

- Weak or absent pulses in the legs or feet

- Sores or wounds on the toes, feet, or legs that heal slowly, poorly, or not at all

- A pale or bluish color to the skin

- A lower temperature in one leg compared to the other leg

- Poor nail growth on the toes and decreased hair growth on the legs

- Erectile dysfunction, especially among men who have diabetes

How Is Peripheral Arterial Disease Diagnosed?

Peripheral arterial disease (PAD) is diagnosed based on your medical and family histories, a physical exam, and results from tests.

PAD often is diagnosed after symptoms are reported. An accurate diagnosis is important, because people who have PAD are at increased risk for coronary artery disease (CAD), heart attack, stroke, and transient ischemic attack ("mini-stroke"). If you have PAD, your doctor also may want to look for signs of these conditions.

Diagnostic Tests

Ankle-brachial index. A simple test called an ankle-brachial index (ABI) is often used to diagnose PAD The ABI compares blood pressure in your ankle to blood pressure in your arm. This test shows how well blood is flowing in your limbs. ABI can show whether PAD is affecting your limbs, but it won't show which blood vessels are narrowed or blocked.

A normal ABI result is 1.0 or greater (with a range of 0.90 to 1.30). The test takes about ten to fifteen minutes to measure both arms and both ankles. This test may be done yearly to see whether PAD is getting worse.

Doppler ultrasound. A Doppler ultrasound is a test that uses sound waves to show whether a blood vessel is blocked. This test uses a blood pressure cuff and special device to measure blood flow in the veins and arteries of the limbs. A Doppler ultrasound can help find out how severe PAD is.

Treadmill test. A treadmill test can show how severe your symptoms are and what level of exercise brings them on. For this test, you walk on a treadmill. This shows whether you have any problems during normal walking.

You may have an ABI test done before and after the treadmill test. This will help compare blood flow in your arms and legs before and after exercise.

Magnetic resonance angiogram. A magnetic resonance angiogram (MRA) uses magnetic and radio wave energy to take pictures of blood vessels inside your body. An MRA is a type of magnetic resonance imaging (MRI).

An MRA can find the location of a blocked blood vessel and show how severe the blockage is.

If you have a pacemaker, man-made joint, stent, surgical clips, mechanical heart valve, or other metallic devices in your body, you might not be able to have an MRA. Ask your doctor whether an MRA is an option for you.

Arteriogram. An arteriogram provides a "road map" of the arteries. It's used to find the exact location of a blocked artery.

For this test, dye is injected through a needle or catheter (tube) into an artery. This may make you feel mildly flushed. After the dye is injected, an x-ray is taken. The pictures from the x-ray can show the location, type, and extent of the blockage in the artery.

Some hospitals use a newer method of arteriogram that uses tiny ultrasound cameras that take pictures of the insides of the blood vessels. This method is called intravascular ultrasound.

Blood tests. Your doctor may recommend blood tests to check for PAD risk factors. For example, you may get a blood test to check for diabetes. You may also get a blood test to check your cholesterol levels.

How Is Peripheral Arterial Disease Treated?

Treatments for peripheral arterial disease (PAD) include lifestyle changes, medicines, and surgery or procedures.

The overall goals of treating PAD are to reduce symptoms, improve quality of life, and prevent complications. Treatment is based on your signs and symptoms, risk factors, and results from a physical exam and tests.

Lifestyle Changes

Treatment often includes making long-lasting lifestyle changes, such as the following:

• Quitting smoking

• Lowering blood pressure

• Lowering high blood cholesterol levels

• Lowering blood glucose levels if you have diabetes

• Getting regular physical activity

Follow a healthy eating plan that's low in total fat, saturated fat, trans fat, cholesterol, and sodium (salt). Eat more fruits, vegetables, and low-fat dairy products. If you're overweight or obese, work with your doctor to create a reasonable weight-loss plan.

Medicines

Your doctor may prescribe medicines to do the following things:

• Lower high blood cholesterol levels and high blood pressure

• Thin the blood to prevent clots from forming due to low blood flow

• Help ease leg pain that occurs when you walk or climb stairs

Surgery or Procedures

Bypass grafting. Your doctor may recommend bypass grafting surgery if blood flow in your limb is blocked or nearly blocked. For this surgery, your doctor uses a blood vessel from another part of your body or a man-made tube to make a graft.

This graft bypasses (goes around) the blocked part of the artery, which allows blood to flow around the blockage. This surgery doesn't cure PAD, but it may increase blood flow to the affected limb.

Angioplasty. Your doctor may recommend angioplasty to restore blood flow through a narrowed or blocked artery.

During this procedure, a catheter with a balloon or other device on the end is inserted into a blocked artery. The balloon is then inflated, which pushes the plaque outward against the wall of the artery. This widens the artery and restores blood flow.

A stent (a small mesh tube) may be placed in the artery during angioplasty. A stent helps keep the artery open after angioplasty is done. Some stents are coated with medicine to help prevent blockages in the artery.

Other Types of Treatment

Researchers are studying cell and gene therapies to treat PAD. However, these treatments aren't yet available outside of clinical trials.

Section 46.6

Raynaud Phenomenon

Excerpted from "Fast Facts about Raynaud's Phenomenon," National
Institute of Arthritis and Musculoskeletal and Skin Diseases, National
Institutes of Health, April 2009.

What is Raynaud phenomenon?

Raynaud phenomenon is a disorder that affects blood vessels, mostly in
the fingers and toes. It causes the blood vessels to narrow when you are:

• cold;

• feeling stress.

Primary Raynaud phenomenon happens on its own. Secondary Raynaud phenomenon happens along with some other health problem.

Who gets Raynaud phenomenon?

People of all ages can have Raynaud phenomenon. Raynaud phenomenon may run in families, but more research is needed.

The primary form is the most common. It most often starts between age fifteen and twenty-five. It is most common in the following
populations:

• Women

• People living in cold places

The secondary form tends to start after age thirty-five to forty. It is
most common in people with connective tissue diseases, such as scleroderma, Sjögren syndrome, and lupus. Other possible causes include
the following:

• Carpal tunnel syndrome, which affects nerves in the wrists

• Blood vessel disease

• Some medicines used to treat high blood pressure, migraines, or
cancer

- Some over-the-counter cold medicines
- Some narcotics

People with certain jobs may be more likely to get the secondary form:

- Workers who are around certain chemicals
- People who use tools that vibrate, such as a jackhammer

What are the symptoms of Raynaud phenomenon?

The body saves heat when it is cold by slowing the supply of blood to the skin. It does this by making blood vessels more narrow.

With Raynaud phenomenon, the body's reaction to cold or stress is stronger than normal. It makes blood vessels narrow faster and tighter than normal. When this happens, it is called an "attack."

During an attack, the fingers and toes can change colors. They may go from white to blue to red. They may also feel cold and numb from lack of blood flow. As the attack ends and blood flow returns, fingers or toes can throb and tingle. After the cold parts of the body warm up, normal blood flow returns in about fifteen minutes.

What is the difference between primary and secondary Raynaud phenomenon?

Primary Raynaud phenomenon is often so mild a person never seeks treatment.

Secondary Raynaud phenomenon is more serious and complex. It is caused when diseases reduce blood flow to fingers and toes.

How does a doctor diagnose Raynaud phenomenon?

It is fairly easy to diagnose Raynaud phenomenon. But it is harder to find out whether a person has the primary or the secondary form of the disorder.

Doctors will diagnose which form it is using a complete history, an exam, and tests. Tests may include the following:

- Blood tests
- Looking at fingernail tissue with a microscope

What is the treatment for Raynaud phenomenon?

Treatment aims to do the following:

- Reduce how many attacks you have

- Make attacks less severe

- Prevent tissue damage

- Prevent loss of finger and toe tissue

Primary Raynaud phenomenon does not lead to tissue damage, so nondrug treatment is used first. Treatment with medicine is more common with secondary Raynaud.

Severe cases of Raynaud can lead to sores or gangrene (tissue death) in the fingers and toes. These cases can be painful and hard to treat. In severe cases that cause skin ulcers and serious tissue damage, surgery may be used.

Nondrug treatments and self-help measures. To reduce how long and severe attacks are, do the following things: keep your hands and feet warm and dry; warm your hands and feet with warm water; avoid air conditioning; wear gloves to touch frozen or cold foods; wear many layers of loose clothing and a hat when it's cold; use chemical warmers, such as small heating pouches that can be placed in pockets, mittens, boots, or shoes; talk to your doctor before exercising outside in cold weather; don't smoke; avoid medicines that make symptoms worse; control stress; and exercise regularly.

Treatment with medications. People with secondary Raynaud phenomenon are often treated with blood pressure medicines or medicines that relax blood vessels. One kind can be put on the fingers to heal ulcers. If blood flow doesn't return and finger loss is a risk, you will need other medicines.

Pregnant woman should not take these medicines. Sometimes Raynaud phenomenon gets better or goes away when a woman is pregnant.

Chapter 47

Renovascular Artery Stenosis and Thrombosis

Renal Artery Stenosis

Renal artery stenosis (RAS) is the narrowing of one or both arteries that carry blood to the two kidneys. "Renal" means "kidney" and "stenosis" means "narrowing." RAS can cause high blood pressure and reduce kidney function. RAS is often overlooked as a cause of high blood pressure.

You are at greater risk of developing RAS if you smoke or are overweight. RAS is most common in men between the ages of fifty and seventy, but women and younger adults can also have it. High cholesterol, diabetes, and a family history of cardiovascular disease are also risk factors for RAS. High blood pressure is both a cause and result of RAS.

What Are the Kidneys?

Your two kidneys are bean-shaped organs, each about the size of a fist. They are located just below the ribcage, one on each side of the spine. The arteries that carry blood to the kidneys—called the renal arteries—branch off directly from the abdominal aorta, the main vessel from the heart that supplies blood to most of the body's organs.

"Renal Artery Stenosis" is reprinted from "Renal Artery Stenosis," National Institute of Diabetes and Digestive and Kidney Diseases, National Institutes of Health, NIH Publication No. 07-6020, May 2007. "Renal Vein Thrombosis" is reprinted from "Renal Vein Thrombosis," © 2009 A.D.A.M., Inc. Reprinted with permission.

525

Healthy kidneys filter out wastes and extra fluid from the blood that passes through them. Those wastes and extra fluid become urine, which flows from the kidneys to the bladder through tubes called ureters. Urine is stored in the bladder until released through urination.

What Causes RAS?

In an overwhelming majority of cases, RAS is caused by atherosclerosis, hardening of the kidney arteries. Thus, RAS develops when a material called plaque builds up on the inner wall of one or both of the renal arteries. The plaque makes the artery wall hard and narrow. This narrowing reduces or cuts off the blood supply, possibly damaging the kidney. The damaged kidney is less efficient at removing wastes and extra fluid from the blood. This plaque is similar to plaques blocking the arteries supplying the heart, which cause heart attacks, and those blocking arteries supplying the brain, which cause strokes.

In renal artery stenosis, plaque builds up on the inner wall of the artery that supplies blood to the kidney.

When the kidneys fail, wastes and extra fluid build up in the blood. This condition, called uremia, causes nausea, headaches, fatigue, and swelling in the legs and abdomen. With total kidney failure, you will need dialysis or a kidney transplant to stay alive.

What Are the Symptoms of RAS?

RAS can be silent, meaning you will not feel any symptoms, until it becomes severe.

The first sign of RAS may be high blood pressure that stays high even when you take blood pressure medicine. High blood pressure caused by RAS is called renovascular hypertension. Your doctor cannot diagnose RAS based on blood pressure alone because many conditions can cause your blood pressure to rise. If you develop high blood pressure suddenly and have no family history of high blood pressure, or if your blood pressure is difficult to control, your doctor might suspect RAS.

How Is RAS Diagnosed?

When blood flows through a narrow vessel, it makes a whooshing sound, called a bruit. Your doctor may place a stethoscope on the front or the side of your abdomen to listen for this sound. The absence of this sound, however, by no means excludes the possibility of RAS.

For a more accurate diagnosis, your doctor may order an ultrasound or an angiogram to get a picture of the artery. An ultrasound uses harmless sound waves to create images of internal organs; it does not require intravenous injection or oral administration of any substances. An angiogram is a special kind of x-ray in which a thin, flexible tube called a catheter is threaded through the large arteries, often from the groin, to the artery of interest—in this case, the renal artery. A special dye is injected through the catheter so the renal artery will show up more clearly on the x-ray. The advantage of angiograms is that they give a better picture and therefore more accurate diagnosis of RAS; the disadvantage is that this procedure is more invasive.

More recently, doctors have been using computerized tomography (CT) scans and magnetic resonance angiograms (MRA) to evaluate RAS. CT scans use multiple x-ray images combined by a computer to create a three-dimensional image of your internal organs. MRAs use moving magnets to create similar three-dimensional images. CT scans and MRAs are less invasive than conventional angiograms, but the results may not be as clear or accurate. Researchers are exploring ways to improve these imaging techniques and make them more reliable for evaluating RAS.

How Is RAS Treated?

Approaches to RAS are threefold:

- Preventing RAS from getting worse

- Treating high blood pressure that results from RAS

- Relieving the blockage of the renal arteries

Lifestyle changes. The first step in treating RAS is making lifestyle changes that promote healthy blood vessels in general. Exercising, controlling your weight, and choosing healthy foods will help keep your arteries clean and flexible. If you smoke, quitting is one of the best things you can do to save your kidneys and other organs.

Blood pressure medicines. RAS causes high blood pressure, which can damage the kidneys. Damaged kidneys, in turn, can make your blood pressure even higher. If left uncontrolled, this vicious cycle can lead to kidney failure and damage the heart and blood vessels throughout the body.

Controlling renovascular hypertension is often difficult but usually achievable. It may require two or more different kinds of blood pressure medicine. Blood pressure medicines work in different ways.

Sometimes, by combining two or more blood pressure medicines that work in different ways, you may be able to control your blood pressure and stop the progression of kidney failure. Each type of blood pressure medicine has its own potential side effects; therefore, the choice of medicine is best determined by you and your doctor.

In addition to blood pressure medicines, your doctor may prescribe a cholesterol-lowering drug to prevent the plaques from forming in the arteries, and a blood thinner, such as aspirin, to help the blood flow more easily through the arteries.

Surgery. If RAS advances until the artery is nearly or completely blocked, you may need surgery to open up the flow of blood to the kidney. Different types of surgery for RAS include the following:

- *Angioplasty and stenting:* Angioplasty is a procedure in which a catheter is put into the renal artery, usually through the groin, just as in a conventional angiogram. In addition, for angioplasty, a tiny balloon at the end of the catheter can be inflated to flatten the plaque against the wall of the artery. Then your doctor may position a small mesh tube, called a stent, to keep plaque flattened and the artery open.

- *Endarterectomy:* In an endarterectomy, a vascular surgeon cleans out the plaque, leaving the inside lining of the artery smooth and clear.

- *Bypass surgery:* To create a bypass, a vascular surgeon uses a vein or synthetic tube to connect the kidney to the aorta. This new path serves as an alternate route for blood to flow around the blocked artery into the kidney.

Hope through Research

The National Institute of Diabetes and Digestive and Kidney Diseases (NIDDK) conducts and supports research into many kinds of kidney disease, including RAS. Researchers supported by the NIDDK are exploring ways to improve the diagnosis of this disease using new MRA techniques that provide more information about blood flow to the kidney and how well the kidney is functioning. These studies will point the way to more effective treatments for RAS and healthy kidneys.

Renal Vein Thrombosis

Renal vein thrombosis is a blood clot that develops in the vein that drains blood from the kidney.

Causes

Renal vein thrombosis is a fairly uncommon situation that may happen after trauma to the abdomen or back, or it may occur due to:

- scar formation;

- stricture;

- tumor.

It may be associated with nephrotic syndrome.

In some children, it occurs after severe dehydration and is a more serious condition than in adults. Dehydration is the most common cause of renal vein thrombosis in infants.

Symptoms

- Bloody urine

- Decreased urine output

- Flank pain or low back pain

Exams and Tests

An examination may not reveal the specific problem, but may indicate nephrotic syndrome or other causes of renal vein thrombosis:

- Abdominal computed tomography (CT) scan, abdominal magnetic resonance imaging (MRI), or abdominal ultrasound may show obstruction of the renal vein.

- Urinalysis may show large quantities of protein in the urine, or red blood cells in the urine.

- X-ray of the kidney veins (venography) may show renal vein thrombosis.

Treatment

The treatment is focused on preventing new clot formations and reducing the risk of the clot traveling to other locations in the body (embolization).

You may get medications that prevent blood clotting (anticoagulants) to stop new clots from forming. Your doctor may recommend bed rest or limited activity for a brief period.

Outlook (Prognosis)

Renal vein thrombosis usually gets better over time without permanently injuring the kidneys.

Possible Complications

- Acute renal failure (if thrombosis occurs in a dehydrated child)
- Embolization of the blood clot to the lungs (pulmonary embolism)
- Formation of new blood clots

When to Contact a Medical Professional

Call your health care provider if you have symptoms of renal vein thrombosis.

If you have experienced renal vein thrombosis, call your health care provider if you develop decreased urine output, difficulty breathing, or other new symptoms.

Prevention

There is no specific prevention for renal vein thrombosis. Maintaining fluids in the body to avoid dehydration may help to reduce its risk.

Alternative Names

Clot in the renal vein; occlusion—renal vein

References

Kanso AA, Hassan NMA, Badr KF. Microvascular and macrovascular diseases of the kidney. In: Brenner BM, ed. *Brenner and Rector's The Kidney*. 8th ed. Philadelphia, Pa; Saunders Elsevier; 2007: chap 32.

Chapter 48

Sepsis

Alternative Names

Systemic inflammatory response syndrome (SIRS)

Definition

Sepsis is a severe illness in which the bloodstream is overwhelmed by bacteria.

Causes

Sepsis is caused by a bacterial infection that can begin anywhere in the body. Common places where an infection might start include:

- the bowel (usually seen with peritonitis);
- the kidneys (upper urinary tract infection);
- the liver or the gall bladder;
- the lungs (bacterial pneumonia);
- the skin (cellulitis).

Sepsis may also accompany meningitis. In children, sepsis may accompany infection of the bone (osteomyelitis). In hospitalized patients, common sites of infection include intravenous lines, surgical wounds, surgical drains, and sites of skin breakdown known as bedsores (decubitus ulcers).

The infection is often confirmed by a blood test. But, a blood test may not reveal infection in people who have been receiving antibiotics.

In sepsis, blood pressure drops, resulting in shock. Major organs and systems, including the kidneys, liver, lungs, and central nervous system, stop functioning normally.

A change in mental status and hyperventilation may be the earliest signs of sepsis coming on.

Sepsis is often life threatening, especially in people with a weakened immune system or with other illness.

Symptoms

- Chills
- Confusion or delirium
- Decreased urine output
- Fever or low body temperature (hypothermia)
- Hyperventilation

- Lightheadedness
- Rapid heart beat
- Shaking
- Skin rash
- Warm skin

Exams and Tests

The following may indicate sepsis:

- Blood culture that reveals bacteria
- Blood gases that reveal acidosis
- Kidney function tests that are abnormal (early in the course of disease)
- Platelet count that is lower than normal
- White blood cell count that is lower or higher than normal

This disease may also change the normal results of the following tests:

- Blood differential: Showing immature white blood cells
- Fibrin degradation products: Often higher than normal, a condition that may be associated with a tendency to bleed
- Peripheral smear: May show a low platelet count and destruction of red blood cells

Treatment

People with sepsis usually need to be in an intensive care unit (ICU). As soon as sepsis is suspected, "broad spectrum" (able to destroy a wide array of bacteria) intravenous (directly in the vein) antibiotic therapy is begun.

The number of antibiotics may be decreased when blood tests reveal which particular bacteria are causing the infection. The source of the infection should be discovered, if possible. This could mean more testing. Infected intravenous lines or surgical drains should be removed, and any abscesses should be surgically drained.

Oxygen, intravenous fluids, and medications that increase blood pressure may be needed. Dialysis may be necessary if there is kidney failure, and a breathing machine (mechanical ventilation) if there is respiratory failure.

Outlook (Prognosis)

The death rate can be as high as 60 percent for people with underlying medical problems. The death rate is somewhat lower in those without other medical problems.

Possible Complications

- Death
- Disseminated intravascular coagulation
- Impaired blood flow to vital organs (brain, heart, kidneys)
- Septic shock

Prevention

The risk of sepsis can be reduced, especially in children, by following the recommended immunization schedule.

References

Enrione MA, Powell KR. Sepsis, septic shock, and systemic inflammatory response syndrome. In: Kliegman RM, Behrman RE, Jenson HB, Stanton BF, eds. Nelson Textbook of Pediatrics. 18th Ed. Philadelphia, Pa: Saunders Elsevier; 2007: chap 176.

Shapiro NI, Zimmer GD, Barkin AZ. Sepsis syndrome. In: Marx, JA, ed. Rosen's Emergency Medicine: Concepts and Clinical Practice. 6th ed. Philadelphia, Pa: Mosby Elsevier; 2006: chap 136.

Chapter 49

Stroke

What is stroke?

A stroke is serious, just like a heart attack. A stroke is sometimes called a "brain attack." Most often, stroke occurs when blood flow to the brain stops because it is blocked by a clot. When this happens, the brain cells in the immediate area begin to die.

Some brain cells die because they stop getting the oxygen and nutrients they need to function. Other brain cells die because they are damaged by sudden bleeding into or around the brain.

The brain cells that don't die immediately remain at risk for death. These cells can linger in a compromised or weakened state for several hours. With timely treatment these cells can be saved. Knowing stroke symptoms, calling 911 immediately, and getting to a hospital as quickly as possible are critical.

Who gets stroke?

Stroke occurs in all age groups, in both sexes, and in all races in every country. It can even occur before birth, when the fetus is still in the womb. Nearly three-quarters of all strokes occur in people over the age of sixty-five. And the risk of having a stroke more than doubles each decade after the age of fifty-five.

Excerpted from "Stroke," NIH Senior Health, National Institutes of Health, November 13, 2007.

535

What are the different kinds of stroke?

There are two kinds of stroke. The most common kind of stroke is called ischemic stroke. It accounts for approximately 80 percent of all strokes. An ischemic stroke is caused by a blood clot that blocks or plugs a blood vessel in the brain.

The other kind of stroke is called hemorrhagic stroke. A hemorrhagic stroke is caused by a blood vessel that breaks and bleeds into the brain.

What disabilities can result from stroke?

Stroke damage in the brain can affect the entire body—resulting in mild to severe disabilities. These include paralysis, problems with thinking, problems with speaking, emotional problems, and pain.

What are the warning signs of stroke?

Warning signs are clues your body sends to tell you that your brain is not receiving enough oxygen. These are warning signs of a stroke, or brain attack:

- Sudden numbness or weakness of the face, arm, or leg, especially on one side of the body

- Sudden confusion, trouble speaking or understanding

- Sudden trouble seeing in one or both eyes

- Sudden trouble walking, dizziness, loss of balance or coordination

- Sudden severe headache with no known cause

If you observe one or more of these signs, don't wait. Call a doctor or 911 right away!

What is a transient ischemic attack, or TIA?

Transient ischemic attacks, or TIAs, occur when the warning signs of stroke last only a few moments and then disappear. These brief episodes are also sometimes called "mini-strokes." Although brief, they identify an underlying serious condition that isn't going away without medical help. Unfortunately, since they clear up, many people ignore them. Don't ignore them. Heeding them can save your life.

What are the risk factors for stroke?

A risk factor is a condition or behavior that increases your chances of getting a disease. Having a risk factor for stroke doesn't mean you'll have a stroke. On the other hand, not having a risk factor doesn't mean you'll avoid a stroke. But your risk of stroke grows as the number and severity of risk factors increases.

The risk factors for stroke include high blood pressure, diabetes, cigarette smoking, and heart disease. Experiencing warning signs and having a history of stroke are also risk factors for stroke.

What is atherosclerosis?

Atherosclerosis, also known as hardening of the arteries, is the most common blood vessel disease. It is caused by the buildup of fatty deposits in the arteries, and is a risk factor for stroke.

Is stroke preventable?

Yes. Stroke is preventable. A better understanding of the causes of stroke has helped people make lifestyle changes that have cut the stroke death rate nearly in half in the last two decades.

While family history of stroke plays a role in your risk, there are many risk factors you can control:

- If you have high blood pressure, work with your doctor to get it under control. Managing your high blood pressure is the most important thing you can do to avoid stroke.

- If you smoke, quit.

- If you have diabetes, learn how to manage it. Many people do not realize they have diabetes, which is a major risk factor for heart disease and stroke.

- If you are overweight, start maintaining a healthy diet and exercising regularly.

- If you have high cholesterol, work with your doctor to lower it. A high level of total cholesterol in the blood is a major risk factor for heart disease, which raises your risk of stroke.

How is stroke diagnosed?

Doctors have several techniques and imaging tools to help diagnose stroke quickly and accurately. The first step in diagnosis is a short neurological examination, or an evaluation of the nervous system.

When a possible stroke patient arrives at a hospital, a health care professional, usually a doctor or nurse, will ask the patient or a companion what happened and when the symptoms began. Blood tests, an electrocardiogram, and a brain scan such as computed tomography or CT, or magnetic resonance imaging or MRI, will often be done.

What are the treatments for stroke?

With stroke, treatment depends on the stage of the disease. There are three treatment stages for stroke: prevention, therapy immediately after stroke, and rehabilitation after stroke. Stroke treatments include medications, surgery, and rehabilitation.

In treating a stroke that has just occurred, every minute counts. Ischemic strokes—the most common kind—can be treated with thrombolytic drugs. These drugs halt the stroke by dissolving the blood clot that is blocking blood flow to the brain. But a person needs to be at the hospital as soon as possible after symptoms start to be evaluated and receive treatment.

A thrombolytic drug known as t-PA can be effective if a person receives it intravenously within three hours after his or her stroke symptoms have started. Since thrombolytic drugs can increase bleeding, t-PA should be used only after the doctor is certain that the patient has suffered an ischemic and not a hemorrhagic stroke.

What other medications are used to treat stroke?

Medication or drug therapy is the most common treatment for stroke. The most popular kinds of drugs to prevent or treat stroke are antithrombotics—which include antiplatelet agents and anticoagulants—and thrombolytics.

Antithrombotics prevent the formation of blood clots that can become stuck in an artery of the brain and cause strokes. In the case of stroke, doctors prescribe antiplatelet drugs mainly for prevention. The most widely known and used antiplatelet drug is aspirin. Other antiplatelet drugs include clopidogrel, ticlopidine, and dipyridamole.

Anticoagulants reduce the risk of stroke by reducing the clotting property of the blood. The most commonly used anticoagulants include warfarin, also known as Coumadin®, heparin, and enoxaparin, also known as Lovenox®.

Neuroprotectants are medications that protect the brain from secondary injury caused by stroke. Although the Food and Drug Administration has not approved any neuroprotectants for use in stroke at this time, many are being tested in clinical trials.

Which surgeries are used to treat stroke?

Surgery can be used to prevent stroke, treat stroke, repair damage to the blood vessels, or correct malformations in and around the brain. The two most common types of surgery for stroke are carotid endarterectomy and extracranial/intracranial bypass, or EC/IC bypass. Extracranial refers to the area outside the cranium, or skull, and intracranial refers to the area inside the skull.

Carotid endarterectomy is a surgical procedure in which a doctor removes fatty deposits, or plaque, from the inside of one of the carotid arteries. The procedure is performed to prevent stroke. The carotid arteries are located in the neck and are the main suppliers of blood to the brain.

EC/IC bypass surgery is a procedure that restores blood flow to a blood-deprived area of brain tissue. The surgeon reroutes a healthy artery in the scalp to the area of brain tissue affected by a blocked artery.

What kinds of therapies are available to help rehabilitate patients after stroke?

For most stroke patients, rehabilitation mainly involves physical therapy. The aim of physical therapy is to have the stroke patient relearn simple motor activities such as walking, sitting, standing, lying down, and the process of switching from one type of movement to another.

Another type of therapy to help patients relearn daily activities is occupational therapy. This type of therapy also involves exercise and training. Its goal is to help the stroke patient relearn everyday activities such as eating, drinking and swallowing, dressing, bathing, cooking, reading and writing, and toileting.

Speech therapy helps stroke patients relearn language and speaking skills, or learn other forms of communication. It is appropriate for patients who have no deficits in cognition or thinking, but have problems understanding speech or written words, or problems forming speech.

Talk therapy, along with the right medication, can help ease some of the mental and emotional problems that result from stroke.

What research is being done on stroke?

The National Institute of Neurological Disorders and Stroke sponsors a wide range of basic and clinical research aimed at finding better ways to prevent, diagnose, and treat stroke, and to restore functions lost as a result of stroke.

Currently, scientists are conducting stroke studies in animals. One promising area of animal research involves hibernation. If scientists can discover how animals hibernate without experiencing brain damage, they may discover ways to stop the brain damage associated with decreased blood flow in stroke patients.

Scientists are also working to develop new and better ways to help the brain repair itself to restore important functions to stroke patients. New advances in imaging and rehabilitation have shown that the brain can compensate for functions lost as a result of stroke.

Clinical trials—another avenue of stroke research—give scientists a way to test new treatments in humans. Clinical trials test surgical devices and procedures, medications, and rehabilitation therapies. They also test methods to improve lifestyles and mental and social skills. The goal of clinical trials is to find safe and effective treatments and to establish the right levels of treatment.

Scientists are using clinical trials to study ways of restoring blood flow to the brain. They hope to find methods that are safer, more effective, and available to more stroke victims. Some of these studies are testing new types of thrombolytic drugs—drugs that halt the stroke by dissolving the blood clot that is blocking blood flow to the brain.

Other studies are testing techniques such as combining thrombolytic drugs with other drugs or with ultrasound, delivering clot-dissolving drugs directly into the clot, and pulling the clot out with a device unaided by drugs.

Researchers are also testing the use of brain imaging to identify patients who may benefit from treatment even beyond three hours, since many have their strokes in their sleep or are brought to the hospital too late for standard therapy.

What is brain plasticity?

Brain plasticity is the brain's ability to learn and change, allowing it to adapt to deficits and injury and to take over the functions of damaged cells. When cells in an area of the brain responsible for a particular function die after a stroke, the patient becomes unable to perform that function. However, the brain's ability to rewire the connections between its nerve cells allows it to compensate for lost functions.

Chapter 50

Vascular Birthmarks: Hemangiomas and Vascular Malformations

What Is a Vascular Birthmark?

Every day, many children—as many as one in ten—are born with some type of birthmark (also called a vascular anomaly). Birthmarks vary in size and can range in color from brown to blue to shades of red or pink. Although in some children a birthmark is a minor flaw that they can live with, 50 to 60 percent of all children with a birthmark will require some treatment.

There are essentially two very different type of vascular birth marks:

- Hemangiomas
- Vascular malformations

Hemangiomas

Hemangiomas are benign (noncancerous) tumors that may not be apparent at birth, but usually become visible within one to four weeks after birth. Hemangiomas usually occur on the head or neck, but they can occur anywhere, including the internal organs. The hemangioma will grow rapidly and change for the first twelve months of life and then "involute" or regress. The involution can last from three to ten years. Typically, 70 percent of hemangiomas disappear by seven years of age. However, surgical or medical treatment may be required if the hemangioma blocks off any vision or hearing, or if it interferes with breathing.

Vascular Malformations

Vascular malformations are benign (noncancerous) lesions. These lesions are present at birth and grow with the child. Unlike hemangiomas, vascular malformations do not have a rapid growth cycle followed by regression—they continue to slowly grow throughout life. Types of vascular malformations include:

- **Port wine stains:** These birthmarks are present at birth; are flat; and appear pink, purple, or reddish in color. They vary in size and can appear anywhere on the body. They are thought to be associated with a deficiency in the nerve supply to the blood vessels. They are more superficial and can be treated with laser therapy.

- **Venous:** Often confused with a hemangioma, these malformations will always grow, are soft to the touch, and the color disappears when compressed. Most commonly found on the jaw, cheek, tongue, and lips. These lesions have low blood flow and can sometimes be injected or sclerosed.

- **Lymphatic:** Formed when excess fluid accumulates within the lymphatic vessels. Lymphatic malformations are very difficult to treat but newer injection therapies are available.

- **Arteriovenous:** Caused when an abnormal amount of blood goes into the capillary beds and engorges the vessels. These are high flow lesions.

Causes of Vascular Birthmarks

Currently, there are no known causes or risk factors for developing vascular birthmarks. Some initial research shows a potential genetic link, but this is inconclusive at this time.

Treatment of Vascular Birthmarks

Your child's pediatrician and treatment team will work with you and your child to determine your child's needs and determine the best course of treatment. Current treatment options include:

- **Steroid treatment:** This can be an oral medication or injected.

- **Laser surgery:** Especially useful for ulceration or in combination with other treatments.

- **Surgery:** Surgical removal of the lesion.

- **Radiology:** For embolization or sclerosis.

- **Combinations of the above.**

Chapter 51

Vasculitis

What Is Vasculitis?

Vasculitis is a condition that involves inflammation in the blood vessels. The condition occurs if your immune system attacks your blood vessels by mistake. This may happen as the result of an infection, a medicine, or another disease or condition.

The inflammation can lead to serious problems. Complications depend on which blood vessels, organs, or other body systems are affected.

Overview

Vasculitis can affect any of the body's blood vessels. These include arteries, veins, and capillaries. Arteries carry blood from your heart to your body's organs. Veins carry blood from your organs and limbs back to your heart. Capillaries connect the small arteries and veins.

When a blood vessel is inflamed, it can narrow or close off. This limits or prevents blood from getting through the vessel. Rarely, the blood vessel will stretch and weaken, causing it to bulge. This bulge is known as an aneurysm.

The disruption in blood flow from inflammation can damage the body's organs. Signs and symptoms depend on which organs have been damaged and the extent of the damage.

"Vasculitis," National Heart Lung and Blood Institute, National Institutes of Health, March 2009.

Typical symptoms of inflammation, such as fever and general aches and pains, are common among people who have vasculitis.

Outlook

There are many types of vasculitis, but overall the condition is rare. If you have vasculitis, the outlook depends on the following:

- The type of vasculitis you have
- Which organs are affected
- How quickly the condition worsens
- How severe the condition is

Treatment often works well if the condition is diagnosed and treated early. In some cases, vasculitis may go into remission. "Remission" means the condition isn't active, but it can come back, or "flare," at any time.

Some cases of vasculitis are chronic (ongoing) and never go into remission. Long-term treatment with medicines often can control the signs and symptoms of chronic vasculitis.

Rarely, vasculitis doesn't respond well to treatment. This can lead to disability and even death.

Much is still unknown about vasculitis. However, researchers continue to learn more about the condition and its various types, causes, and treatments.

Types of Vasculitis

There are many types of vasculitis. Each type involves inflamed blood vessels. However, most types differ in whom they affect and the organs that are involved.

The types of vasculitis often are grouped based on the size of the blood vessels they affect.

Mostly Large Vessel Vasculitis

These types of vasculitis usually, but not always, affect the larger blood vessels.

Behçet disease. Behçet disease can cause recurrent, painful ulcers in the mouth, ulcers on the genitals, acne-like skin lesions, and eye inflammation called uveitis.

The disease occurs most often in people aged twenty to forty. Men are more likely to get it, but it also can affect women. It's more common in people of Mediterranean, Middle Eastern, and Far Eastern descent, although it rarely affects blacks.

Researchers believe that a gene called the HLA-B51 gene may play a role in Behçet disease. However, not everyone who has the gene gets the disease.

Cogan syndrome. Cogan syndrome can occur in people who have a systemic vasculitis that affects the large vessels, especially the aorta and aortic valve. The aorta is the main artery that carries oxygen-rich blood from the heart to the body. A systemic vasculitis is a type of vasculitis that affects you in a general or overall way.

Cogan syndrome can lead to eye inflammation called interstitial keratitis. It also can cause hearing changes, including sudden deafness.

Giant cell arteritis. Giant cell arteritis usually affects the temporal artery, an artery on the side of your head. This condition also is called temporal arteritis. Symptoms of this condition can include headache, scalp tenderness, jaw pain, blurred vision, double vision, and acute (sudden) vision loss.

Giant cell arteritis is the most common form of vasculitis in adults older than fifty. It's more likely to occur in people of Scandinavian origin, but it can affect people of any race.

Polymyalgia rheumatica. Polymyalgia rheumatica, or PMR, commonly affects the large joints in the body, such as the shoulders and hips. PMR typically causes stiffness and pain in the muscles of the neck, shoulders, lower back, hips, and thighs.

Most often, PMR occurs by itself, but 10 to 20 percent of people who have PMR also develop giant cell arteritis. Also, about half of the people who have giant cell arteritis also can have PMR.

Takayasu arteritis. Takayasu arteritis affects medium- and large-sized arteries, particularly the aorta and its branches. The condition is sometimes called aortic arch syndrome.

Though rare, Takayasu arteritis occurs mostly in teenage girls and young women. The condition is more common in Asians, but it can affect people of all races and occur throughout the world.

Takayasu arteritis is a systemic disease. A systemic disease is one that affects you in a general or overall way. Symptoms of Takayasu arteritis may include tiredness and a sense of feeling unwell, fever, night sweats, sore joints, loss of appetite, and weight loss. These symptoms usually occur before other signs develop that point to arteritis.

Mostly Medium Vessel Vasculitis

These types of vasculitis usually, but not always, affect the medium-sized blood vessels.

Buerger disease. Buerger disease, also known as thromboangiitis obliterans, typically affects blood flow to the hands and feet. In this disease, the blood vessels in the hands and feet tighten or become blocked. This causes less blood to flow to the affected tissues, which can lead to pain and tissue damage.

Rarely, Buerger disease also can affect blood vessels in the brain, abdomen, and heart. The disease usually affects men aged twenty to forty of Asian or Eastern European descent. The disease is strongly linked to cigarette smoking.

Symptoms of Buerger disease include pain in the calves or feet when walking, or pain in the forearms and hands with activity. Other symptoms include blood clots in the surface veins of the limbs and Raynaud phenomenon.

In severe cases, ulcers may develop on the fingers and toes, leading to gangrene. The term "gangrene" refers to the death or decay of body tissues.

Surgical bypass of the blood vessels may help restore blood flow to some areas. Medicines generally aren't effective treatments. The best treatment is to stop using tobacco of any kind.

Central nervous system vasculitis. Central nervous system (CNS) vasculitis usually occurs as a result of a systemic vasculitis. A systemic vasculitis is one that affects you in a general or overall way.

Very rarely, vasculitis affects only the brain and/or spinal cord. When it does, the condition is called isolated vasculitis of the CNS or primary angiitis of the CNS.

Symptoms of CNS vasculitis are headache, problems thinking clearly or changes in mental function, or stroke-like symptoms, such as muscle weakness and paralysis (an inability to move).

Kawasaki disease. Kawasaki disease is a rare childhood disease in which the walls of the blood vessels throughout the body become inflamed. The disease can affect any blood vessel in the body, including arteries, veins, and capillaries. Kawasaki disease also is known as mucocutaneous lymph node syndrome.

Sometimes the disease affects the coronary arteries, which carry oxygen-rich blood to the heart. As a result, a small number of children who have Kawasaki disease may develop serious heart problems.

Polyarteritis nodosa. Polyarteritis nodosa can affect many parts of the body. It often affects the kidneys, the digestive tract, the nerves, and the skin.

Symptoms often include fever, a general feeling of being unwell, weight loss, and muscle and joint aches, including pain in the calf muscles that develops over weeks or months. Other signs and symptoms include anemia (a low red blood cell count), a lace- or web-like rash, bumps under the skin, and abdominal pain after eating.

Researchers believe that this type of vasculitis is very rare, although the symptoms can be similar to those of other types of vasculitis. Some cases of polyarteritis nodosa seem to be linked to hepatitis B or C infections.

Mostly Small Vessel Vasculitis

These types of vasculitis usually, but not always, affect the small blood vessels.

Churg-Strauss syndrome. Churg-Strauss syndrome is a very rare disorder that causes blood vessel inflammation. It's also known as allergic angiitis and granulomatosis.

This disorder can affect many organs, including the lungs, skin, kidneys, nervous system, and heart. Symptoms can vary widely. They may include asthma, higher than normal levels of white blood cells in the blood and tissues, and tissue formations known as granulomas.

Essential mixed cryoglobulinemia. Essential mixed cryoglobulinemia can occur alone, or it may be linked to a systemic vasculitis. A systemic vasculitis is one that affects the body in a general or overall way.

Symptoms often include joint aches; weakness; nerve changes, such as numbness, tingling, and pain in the limbs; kidney inflammation; and a raised, bumpy, reddish-purple skin rash known as palpable purpura.

While essential mixed cryoglobulinemia can occur with other conditions, it most often is linked to chronic hepatitis C infection.

Henoch-Schönlein purpura. Henoch-Schönlein purpura (HSP) is a type of vasculitis that affects the smallest blood vessels—the capillaries—in the skin, joints, intestines, and kidneys.

Symptoms often include abdominal pain, aching and swollen joints, and signs of kidney damage, such as blood in the urine. Another symptom is a bruise-like rash that mostly shows up as reddish-purple blotches on the lower legs and buttocks (although it can appear anywhere on the body).

HSP is more common in children, but it also can affect teens and adults. In children, about half of all cases follow a viral or bacterial upper respiratory infection. Most people get better in a few weeks and have no lasting problems.

Hypersensitivity vasculitis. Hypersensitivity vasculitis affects the skin. This condition also is known as allergic vasculitis, cutaneous vasculitis, or leukocytoclastic vasculitis.

A common symptom is red spots on the skin, usually on the lower legs. For people who are bedridden, the rash appears on the lower back.

An allergic reaction to a medicine or infection often causes this type of vasculitis. Stopping the medicine or treating the infection usually clears up the vasculitis. However, some people may need to take anti-inflammatory medicines, such as corticosteroids, for a short time. These medicines help reduce inflammation.

Microscopic polyangiitis. Microscopic polyangiitis affects small vessels, particularly those in the kidneys and the lungs. This disease mainly occurs in middle-aged people; it affects men slightly more often than women.

The symptoms often aren't specific, and they can begin gradually with fever, weight loss, and muscle aches. In some cases, the symptoms come on suddenly and progress quickly, leading to kidney failure.

If the lungs are involved, the first symptom may be coughing up blood. In some cases, the disease occurs along with a vasculitis that affects the intestinal tract, the skin, and the nervous system.

The signs and symptoms of microscopic polyangiitis are similar to those of the vasculitis condition called Wegener granulomatosis. However, microscopic polyangiitis usually doesn't affect the nose and sinuses or cause abnormal tissue formations in the lungs and kidneys.

The results of certain blood tests can suggest inflammation. These results include a higher than normal erythrocyte sedimentation rate (ESR); lower than normal hemoglobin and hematocrit levels (which suggest anemia); and higher than normal white blood cell and platelet counts.

Also, more than half of the people with microscopic polyangiitis have certain antibodies called antineutrophil cytoplasmic autoantibodies (ANCA) in their blood. These antibodies also are seen in people who have Wegener granulomatosis.

Testing for ANCA can't be used to diagnose either of these two types of vasculitis. However, testing can help evaluate people who have vasculitis-like symptoms.

Wegener granulomatosis. Wegener granulomatosis is a rare vasculitis. It affects men and women equally, but occurs more often in whites than in African Americans. This type of vasculitis can occur at any age, but it is more common in middle-aged people.

Wegener granulomatosis typically affects the sinuses, nose, and throat; the lungs; and the kidneys. Other organs also can be involved.

In addition to inflamed blood vessels, the affected tissues also develop abnormal formations called granulomas. If granulomas develop in the lungs, they can destroy the lung tissue. The damage can be mistaken for pneumonia or even lung cancer.

Symptoms of Wegener granulomatosis often are not specific and can begin gradually with fever, weight loss, and muscle aches. Sometimes, the symptoms come on suddenly and progress rapidly, leading to kidney failure. If the lungs are involved, the first symptom may be coughing up blood.

The results of certain blood tests can suggest inflammation. These results include a higher than normal ESR; lower than normal hemoglobin and hematocrit levels (which suggest anemia); and higher than normal white blood cell and platelet counts.

Another test looks for antiproteinase-3 (an antineutrophil cytoplasmic autoantibody) in the blood. Most people who have active Wegener granulomatosis will have this antibody. A small portion may have another ANCA known as antimyeloperoxidase-specific ANCA.

Having either ANCA antibody isn't enough on its own to make a diagnosis of Wegener granulomatosis. However, testing for the antibodies can help support the diagnosis in patients who have other signs and symptoms of the condition.

A biopsy of an affected organ is the best way for your doctor to make a firm diagnosis. A biopsy is a procedure in which your doctor takes a small sample of your body tissue to examine under a microscope.

What Causes Vasculitis?

Vasculitis occurs when your immune system attacks your own blood vessels by mistake. What causes this to happen isn't fully known.

A recent or chronic (ongoing) infection may prompt the attack. Your body also may attack its own blood vessels in reaction to a medicine.

Sometimes an autoimmune disorder triggers vasculitis. Autoimmune disorders occur when the immune system makes antibodies (proteins) that attack and damage the body's own tissues or cells. Examples of such autoimmune disorders include lupus, rheumatoid arthritis, and scleroderma. You can have these disorders for years before developing vasculitis.

Vasculitis also may be linked to certain blood cancers, such as leukemia and lymphoma.

What Are the Signs and Symptoms of Vasculitis?

The signs and symptoms of vasculitis vary. They depend on the type of vasculitis you have, the organs involved, and how severe the condition is. Some people may have few signs and symptoms. Other people may become very sick.

Sometimes, the signs and symptoms develop gradually over months. Other times, the signs and symptoms develop faster, over days or weeks.

Systemic Signs and Symptoms

Systemic signs and symptoms are those that affect you in a general, or overall, way. Common systemic signs and symptoms of vasculitis are as follows:

- Fever

- Loss of appetite

- Weight loss

- Fatigue (tiredness)

- General aches and pains

Organ- or Body System–Specific Signs and Symptoms

Vasculitis can affect specific organs and body systems, causing a range of signs and symptoms.

Skin. If the condition affects your skin, you may notice a number of skin changes. For example, you may notice purple or red spots or bumps, clusters of small dots, splotches, bruises, or hives. Your skin also may itch.

Joints. If the condition affects your joints, you may ache or develop arthritis in one or more joints.

Lungs. If the condition affects your lungs, you may feel short of breath. You may even cough up blood. The results from a chest x-ray may show signs of pneumonia, even though that isn't what you have.

Gastrointestinal tract. If the condition affects your gastrointestinal tract, you may get ulcers in your mouth or have abdominal pain.

In severe cases, blood flow to the intestines can be blocked. This can cause the wall of the intestines to weaken and possibly rupture. A rupture can lead to serious problems or even death.

Sinuses, nose, throat, and ears. If the condition affects your sinuses, nose, throat, and ears, you may have sinus or chronic (ongoing) middle ear infections. Other symptoms include ulcers in the nose and, in some cases, hearing loss.

Eyes. If vasculitis affects your eyes, you may develop red, itchy, burning eyes. Your eyes also may become sensitive to light, and your vision may become blurry. In rare cases, certain types of vasculitis may cause blindness.

Brain. If vasculitis affects your brain, symptoms may include headache, problems thinking clearly or changes in mental function, or stroke-like symptoms, such as muscle weakness and paralysis (an inability to move).

Nerves. If the condition affects your nerves, you may have numbness, tingling, and weakness in various parts of your body. You also may have a loss of feeling or strength in your hands and feet and shooting pains in your arms and legs.

How Is Vasculitis Diagnosed?

Your doctor will diagnose vasculitis based on your signs and symptoms, your medical history, a physical exam, and the results from tests.

Diagnostic Tests and Procedures

Blood tests. Blood tests can show whether you have abnormal levels of certain blood cells and antibodies in your blood.

These tests may look at the following things:

- *Hemoglobin and hematocrit:* A low hemoglobin or hematocrit level suggests anemia, which may be a complication of vasculitis. Vasculitis can interfere with the body's ability to make enough red blood cells.

- *Antineutrophil cytoplasmic antibodies (ANCA):* These antibodies can be seen in certain types of vasculitis.

- *Erythrocyte sedimentation rate (ESR):* If the ESR is high, it can be a nonspecific sign of inflammation in the body.

- *The amount of C-reactive protein (CRP) in your blood:* A higher than normal CRP level suggests inflammation.

Biopsy. A biopsy often is the best way for your doctor to make a firm diagnosis of vasculitis. During a biopsy, your doctor takes a small sample of your body tissue to examine under a microscope.

To diagnose vasculitis, he or she will take a tissue sample from a blood vessel or an affected organ.

A pathologist will examine the sample for signs of inflammation or tissue damage. A pathologist is a doctor who specializes in identifying diseases by studying cells and tissues under a microscope.

Blood pressure. Blood pressure should be closely monitored in all cases of vasculitis. Blood pressure can become elevated in vasculitis that damages the kidneys.

Urinalysis. For this test, you'll provide a sample of urine for analysis. This test identifies abnormal levels of protein or blood cells in the urine. Abnormal levels of these substances can be a sign of vasculitis affecting the kidneys.

Electrocardiogram (EKG). An EKG is a simple, painless test that records the heart's electrical activity. You might have this test to show whether vasculitis is affecting your heart.

Echocardiography. Echocardiography is a painless test that uses sound waves to create pictures of your heart. The test provides your doctor with information about the size and shape of your heart and how well your heart's chambers and valves are working.

Chest x-ray. A chest x-ray is a painless test that creates pictures of the structures inside your chest, such as your heart, lungs, and blood vessels. Abnormal chest x-ray results may show changes that suggest that vasculitis is affecting your lungs or your large arteries (such as the aorta or the pulmonary arteries).

Lung function tests. Lung function tests measure the size of your lungs, how much air you can breathe in and out, how fast you can breathe air out, and how well your lungs deliver oxygen to your blood.

Lung function tests can help your doctor find out whether airflow into and out of your lungs is restricted or blocked.

Abdominal ultrasound. An abdominal ultrasound uses sound waves to create a picture of the organs and structures in your abdomen. If vasculitis affects your abdominal organs, this test may show abnormalities.

Computed tomography scan. A computed tomography (CT) scan is a type of x-ray that creates more detailed pictures of your internal organs than standard x-rays. If you have a type of vasculitis that affects your abdominal organs or blood vessels, this test can show abnormalities that have developed.

Magnetic resonance imaging. A magnetic resonance imaging (MRI) test uses radio waves, magnets, and a computer to create detailed pictures of your internal organs.

Angiography. Angiography is a test that uses dye and special x-rays to show blood flow through your blood vessels. The dye is injected into your bloodstream.

Special x-ray pictures are taken while the dye flows through your blood vessels. The dye helps highlight the vessels on the x-ray pictures.

Angiography is used to help find out whether your blood vessels are narrowed, swollen, deformed, or blocked as a result of inflammation.

How Is Vasculitis Treated?

Treatment for vasculitis will depend on the type of vasculitis you have, which organs are affected, and how severe the condition is.

People who have severe vasculitis are treated with prescription medicines. Rarely, surgery may be done. People who have mild vasculitis may find relief with over-the-counter pain medicines, such as acetaminophen, aspirin, ibuprofen, or naproxen.

Goals of Treatment

The main goal of vasculitis treatment is to reduce inflammation in the affected blood vessels. This usually is done by reducing or stopping the immune response that caused the inflammation.

Types of Treatment

Common prescription medicines used to treat vasculitis include corticosteroid and cytotoxic medicines.

Corticosteroids help reduce inflammation in your blood vessels. Examples of corticosteroids are prednisone, prednisolone, and methylprednisolone.

Cytotoxic medicines may be prescribed if vasculitis is severe or if corticosteroids don't work well. Cytotoxic medicines kill the cells that are causing the inflammation. Examples of these medicines are azathioprine, methotrexate, and cyclophosphamide.

Your doctor may prescribe both corticosteroids and cytotoxic medicines.

Other treatments may be used for certain types of vasculitis. For example, the standard treatment for Kawasaki disease is high-dose aspirin and immune globulin. Immune globulin is a medicine given intravenously (injected into a vein).

Certain types of vasculitis may require surgery to remove aneurysms that have formed as a result of the condition. (An aneurysm is an abnormal bulge in the wall of a blood vessel.)

Chapter 52

Venous Disorders

Chapter Contents

555

Section 52.1

Arteriovenous Fistula

"Arteriovenous Fistula," from *The Merck Manual of Medical Information—Second Home Edition*, edited by Robert Porter. Copyright 2008 by
Merck & Co., Inc., Whitehouse Station, NJ.

An arteriovenous fistula is an abnormal channel between an artery
and a vein:

- Although doctors may be able to hear the distinctive sound of
  blood flow though a fistula by using a stethoscope, imaging tests
  are often needed.

- Fistulas can be cut out or eliminated with laser therapy, or sometimes substances are injected into the fistula to block the blood flow.

Normally, blood flows from arteries into capillaries and then into
veins. When an arteriovenous fistula is present, blood flows directly
from an artery into a vein, bypassing the capillaries. A person may be
born with an arteriovenous fistula (congenital fistula), or a fistula may
develop after birth (acquired fistula).

Congenital arteriovenous fistulas are uncommon. Acquired arteriovenous fistulas can be caused by any injury that damages an artery and
a vein that lie side by side. Typically, the injury is a piercing wound,
as from a knife or bullet. The fistula may appear immediately or may
develop after a few hours. The area can swell quickly if blood escapes
into the surrounding tissues.

Some medical treatments, such as kidney dialysis, require that a
vein be pierced for each treatment. With repeated piercing, the vein
becomes inflamed and clotting can develop. Eventually, scar tissue may
develop and destroy the vein. To avoid this problem, doctors may delib-
erately create an arteriovenous fistula, usually between an adjoining
vein and artery in the arm. This procedure widens the vein, making
needle insertion easier and enabling the blood to flow faster. Faster
flowing blood is less likely to clot. Unlike some large arteriovenous
fistulas, these small, intentionally created fistulas do not lead to heart
problems, and they can be closed when no longer needed.

Symptoms and Diagnosis

When congenital arteriovenous fistulas are near the surface of the skin, they may appear swollen and reddish blue. In conspicuous places, such as the face, they appear purplish and may be unsightly.

If a large acquired arteriovenous fistula is not treated, a large volume of blood flows under high pressure from the artery into the vein network. Vein walls are not strong enough to withstand such high pressure, so the walls stretch and the veins enlarge and bulge (sometimes resembling varicose veins). In addition, blood flows more freely into the enlarged veins than it would if it continued its normal course through the arteries. As a result, blood pressure falls. To compensate for this fall in blood pressure, the heart pumps more forcefully and more rapidly, thus greatly increasing its output of blood. Eventually, the increased effort may strain the heart, causing heart failure. The larger the fistula, the more quickly heart failure can develop.

With a stethoscope placed over a large acquired arteriovenous fistula, doctors can hear a distinctive "to-and-fro" sound, like that of moving machinery. This sound is called a machinery murmur. Doppler ultrasonography is used to confirm the diagnosis and to determine the extent of the problem. For fistulas between deeper blood vessels (such as the aorta and vena cava), magnetic resonance imaging (MRI) is more useful.

Treatment

Small congenital arteriovenous fistulas can be cut out or eliminated with laser coagulation therapy. This procedure must be done by a skilled vascular surgeon, because the fistulas are sometimes more extensive than they appear to be on the surface. Arteriovenous fistulas near the eye, brain, or other major structures can be especially difficult to treat.

Acquired arteriovenous fistulas are corrected by a surgeon as soon as possible after diagnosis. Before the surgery, a radiopaque dye, which can be seen on x-rays, may be injected to outline the fistula more clearly in a procedure called angiography. If the surgeon cannot reach the fistula easily (for example, if it is in the brain), complex injection techniques that cause clots to form may be used to block blood flow through the fistula. For example, coils or plugs may be inserted into the fistula at the various points where the vein and the artery meet. This procedure is done using x-rays for guidance and does not require open surgery.

Section 52.2

Chronic Venous Insufficiency

What Is Chronic Venous Insufficiency?

When veins weaken and lose the ability to pump blood effectively, the condition is called chronic venous insufficiency, or CVI.

Symptoms of CVI include varicose veins; skin problems; leg and ankle swelling; tight calves; and legs that feel heavy, tired, restless, or achy.

What Are Risk Factors for Chronic Venous Insufficiency?

- High blood pressure can stretch and weaken vein walls causing CVI.
- A blockage of the blood flow through the veins.
- Family history of CVI.
- Obesity.
- Pregnancy.
- Sedentary lifestyle.
- Cigarette smoking.
- Jobs that require standing or sitting in one place for long periods of time.
- Women who are over fifty are most likely to develop serious cases.

Symptoms of Chronic Venous Insufficiency

Blood that is unable to flow back to the heart pools in the veins of the legs and may cause:

- swollen ankles;
- legs that feel heavy, tired, restless, or achy;

- pain during or after walking;

- varicose veins (blue, bulging, and twisted veins visible through the skin on the legs);

- skin irritation or sores;

- hardening and discoloration under the skin that looks like a rash on the calves or ankles;

- reddish or discolored skin;

- leg ulcers and sores;

- swelling of the leg.

Diagnosing Chronic Venous Insufficiency

After discussing symptoms and medical history, and performing a physical exam including measuring the blood pressure in the legs and examining any varicose veins, the following tests may be requested to confirm a diagnosis of CVI:

- Duplex ultrasound

- Plethysmography

- Venograms

Treatment Options

Chronic venous insufficiency does not usually pose a serious threat, and with proper treatment to minimize pain or disability, most people with this condition continue to lead active lives. Mild cases of chronic venous insufficiency can be treated on an outpatient basis with some of the following simple procedures:

- Elastic compression therapy (elastic stockings worn to squeeze the legs and veins—simply and effectively preventing blood from flowing backward and pooling in the legs).

- Elevate the legs (this allows gravity to drain swollen veins— beneficial even when done only periodically).

- Avoid sitting or standing for long periods.

- Flex or move the legs when sitting or standing for long periods is unavoidable.

More serious cases of chronic venous insufficiency may be treated with surgical or minimally invasive procedures including:

- sclerotherapy;

- vein stripping;

- deep vein bypass surgery (bypass surgery to treat CVI in the upper thigh);

- valve repair;

- in vein transplantation (a piece of a healthy vein from the person's own arm replaces a malfunctioning deep vein in the knee or thigh).

Section 52.3

Thrombophlebitis

"Thrombophlebitis," © 2009 A.D.A.M., Inc. Reprinted with permission.

Alternative Names

Phlebitis

Definition

Thrombophlebitis is swelling (inflammation) of a vein caused by a blood clot.

Causes

The following increase your chances for thrombophlebitis:

- Being hospitalized for a major surgery or with a major illness

- Disorders that make you more likely to develop blood clots

- Sitting for a long period of time (such as on a long airplane trip)
There are two main types of thrombophlebitis:

- Deep venous thrombosis (affects deeper, larger veins)

- Superficial thrombophlebitis (affects veins near the skin surface)

Symptoms

The following symptoms are often associated with thrombophlebitis:

- Inflammation (swelling) in the part of the body affected
- Pain in the part of the body affected
- Skin redness (not always present)
- Warmth and tenderness over the vein

Exams and Tests

The health care provider can usually diagnose the condition based on how the affected area looks. You may need to have your pulse, blood pressure, temperature, skin condition, and circulation frequently checked to make sure you don't have complications.

If the cause cannot be easily identified, one or more of the following tests may be done:

- Blood coagulation studies
- Doppler ultrasound
- Venography

Treatment

In general, treatment may include support stockings and wraps to reduce discomfort as well as medications such as:

- analgesics (pain killers);
- antibiotics (if infection is present);
- anticoagulants (blood thinners) to prevent new clots from forming;
- nonsteroidal anti-inflammatory drugs (NSAIDs) such as ibuprofen to reduce pain and inflammation;
- thrombolytics to dissolve an existing clot.

You may be told to do the following:

- Apply moist heat to reduce inflammation and pain.
- Keep pressure off of the area to reduce pain and decrease the risk of further damage.
- Raise the affected area to reduce swelling.

Surgical removal, stripping, or bypass of the vein is rarely needed but may be recommended in some situations.

Outlook (Prognosis)

Thrombophlebitis and other forms of phlebitis usually respond to prompt medical treatment.

Possible Complications

Superficial thrombophlebitis rarely causes complications.

Complications of deep vein thrombosis include blood clots in the lungs (pulmonary embolism) or chronic pain and swelling in the leg.

When to Contact a Medical Professional

Call your healthcare provider if you have symptoms of thrombophlebitis.

Call your healthcare provider promptly if thrombophlebitis symptoms do not improve with treatment, if symptoms get worse, or if new symptoms occur (such as an entire limb becoming pale, cold, or swollen).

Prevention

Routine changing of intravenous (IV) lines helps to prevent thrombophlebitis related to IVs.

If you are taking a long car or plane trip, walk or stretch your legs once in a while and drink plenty of liquids. Wearing support hose may help.

If you are hospitalized, your doctor may prescribe medicine to prevent deep venous thrombosis.

References

Ginsberg J. Peripheral venous disease. In: Goldman L, Ausiello D, eds. *Cecil Medicine*. 23rd ed. Philadelphia, Pa: Saunders Elsevier; 2007:chap 81.

Section 52.4

Varicose Veins and Spider Veins

"Frequently Asked Questions: Varicose Veins and Spider Veins," National Women's Health Information Center, December 1, 2005. Reviewed by David A. Cooke, M.D., November 2009.

What are varicose veins and spider veins?

Varicose veins are enlarged veins that can be flesh colored, dark purple, or blue. They often look like cords and appear twisted and bulging. They are swollen and raised above the surface of the skin. Varicose veins are commonly found on the backs of the calves or on the inside of the leg. During pregnancy, varicose veins called hemorrhoids can form in women in the vagina or around the anus.

Spider veins are similar to varicose veins, but they are smaller. They are often red or blue and are closer to the surface of the skin than varicose veins. They can look like tree branches or spider webs with their short jagged lines. Spider veins can be found on the legs and face. They can cover either a very small or very large area of skin.

What causes varicose veins and spider veins?

The heart pumps blood filled with oxygen and nutrients to the whole body. Arteries carry blood from the heart toward the body parts. Veins carry oxygen-poor blood from the body back to the heart.

The squeezing of the leg muscles pumps blood back to the heart from the lower body. Veins have valves that act as one-way flaps. These valves prevent the blood from flowing backward as it moves up the legs. If the one-way valves become weak, blood can leak back into the vein and collect there. This problem is called venous insufficiency. Pooled blood enlarges the vein and it becomes varicose. Spider veins can also be caused by the backup of blood. Hormone changes, inherited factors, and exposure to the sun can also cause spider veins.

How common are abnormal leg veins?

About 50 to 55 percent of American women and 40 to 45 percent of American men suffer from some form of vein problem. Varicose veins affect one out of two people age fifty and older.

Who usually has varicose veins and spider veins?

Many factors increase a person's chances of developing varicose or spider veins. These include the following:

- Increasing age.

- Having family members with vein problems or being born with weak vein valves.

- Hormonal changes. These occur during puberty, pregnancy, and menopause. Taking birth control pills and other medicines containing estrogen and progesterone also increases the risk of varicose or spider veins.

- Pregnancy. During pregnancy there is a huge increase in the amount of blood in the body. This can cause veins to enlarge. The expanding uterus also puts pressure on the veins. Varicose veins usually improve within three months after delivery. A growing number of abnormal veins usually appear with each additional pregnancy.

- Obesity, leg injury, prolonged standing, and other things that weaken vein valves.

- Sun exposure, which can cause spider veins on the cheeks or nose of a fair-skinned person.

Why do varicose veins and spider veins usually appear in the legs?

The force of gravity, the pressure of body weight, and the task of carrying blood from the bottom of the body up to the heart make legs the primary location for varicose and spider veins. Compared with other veins in the body, leg veins have the toughest job of carrying blood back to the heart. They endure the most pressure. This pressure can be stronger than the veins' one-way valves.

Are varicose veins and spider veins painful or dangerous?

Spider veins usually do not need medical treatment, but varicose veins usually enlarge and worsen over time. Severe varicose veins can cause health problems. These include the following:

- Severe venous insufficiency. This severe pooling of blood in the veins slows the return of blood to the heart. This condition can cause blood clots and severe infections. Blood clots can be very dangerous because they can move from leg veins and travel to the lungs. Blood clots in the lungs are life threatening because they can block the heart and lungs from functioning.

- Sores or skin ulcers on skin tissue around varicose veins.

- Ongoing irritation, swelling, and painful rashes of the legs.

What are the signs of varicose veins?

Some common symptoms of varicose veins include the following:

- Aching pain
- Easily tired legs
- Leg heaviness
- Swelling in the legs
- Darkening of the skin (in severe cases)
- Numbness in the legs
- Itching or irritated rash in the legs

How can I prevent varicose veins and spider veins?

Not all varicose and spider veins can be prevented. But some things can reduce your chances of getting new varicose and spider veins. These same things can help ease discomfort from the ones you already have:

- Wear sunscreen to protect your skin from the sun and to limit spider veins on the face.

- Exercise regularly to improve your leg strength, circulation, and vein strength. Focus on exercises that work your legs, such as walking or running.

- Control your weight to avoid placing too much pressure on your legs.

- Do not cross your legs when sitting.

- Elevate your legs when resting as much as possible.

- Do not stand or sit for long periods of time. If you must stand for a long time, shift your weight from one leg to the other every few minutes. If you must sit for long periods of time, stand up and move around or take a short walk every thirty minutes.

- Wear elastic support stockings and avoid tight clothing that constricts your waist, groin, or legs.

- Eat a low-salt diet rich in high-fiber foods. Eating fiber reduces the chances of constipation, which can contribute to varicose veins. High-fiber foods include fresh fruits and vegetables and whole grains, like bran. Eating too much salt can cause you to retain water or swell.

Should I see a doctor about varicose veins?

Has the varicose vein become swollen, red, or very tender or warm to the touch?

- If yes, see your doctor.

- If no, are there sores or a rash on the leg or near the ankle with the varicose vein, or do you think there may be circulation problems in your feet?

  - If yes, see your doctor.

  - If no, continue to follow the self-care tips above.

How are varicose and spider veins treated?

Besides a physical exam, your doctor can take x-rays or ultrasound pictures of the vein to find the cause and severity of the problem. You may want to speak with a doctor who specializes in vein diseases or phlebology. Talk to your doctor about what treatment options are best for your condition and lifestyle. Not all cases of varicose veins are the same.

Some available treatments include sclerotherapy, laser surgery, endovenous techniques (radiofrequency and laser), and surgery.

Sclerotherapy: This is the most common treatment for both spider veins and varicose veins. The doctor injects a solution into the vein that causes the vein walls to swell, stick together, and seal shut. This stops the flow of blood and the vein turns into scar tissue. In a few weeks, the vein should fade. The same vein may need to be treated more than once.

This treatment is very effective if done the right way. Most patients can expect a 50 to 90 percent improvement. Microsclerotherapy uses special solutions and injection techniques that increase the success rate for removal of spider veins. Sclerotherapy does not require anesthesia, and can be done in the doctor's office.

Possible side effects include the following:

- Temporary stinging or painful cramps where the injection was made

- Temporary red raised patches of skin where the injection was made
- Temporary small skin sores where the injection was made
- Temporary bruises where the injection was made
- Spots around the treated vein that usually disappear
- Brown lines around the treated vein that usually disappear
- Groups of fine red blood vessels around the treated vein that usually disappear

The treated vein can also become inflamed or develop lumps of clotted blood. This is not dangerous. Applying heat and taking aspirin or antibiotics can relieve inflammation. Lumps of coagulated blood can be drained.

Laser surgery: New technology in laser treatments can effectively treat spider veins in the legs. Laser surgery sends very strong bursts of light onto the vein. This makes the vein slowly fade and disappear. Lasers are very direct and accurate. So the proper laser controlled by a skilled doctor will usually damage only the area being treated. Most skin types and colors can be safely treated with lasers.

Laser surgery is more appealing to some patients because it does not use needles or incisions. Still, when the laser hits the skin, the patient feels a heat sensation that can be quite painful. Cooling helps reduce the pain. Laser treatments last for fifteen to twenty minutes. Depending on the severity of the veins, two to five treatments are generally needed to remove spider veins in the legs. Patients can return to normal activity right after treatment, just as with sclerotherapy. For spider veins larger than 3 mm, laser therapy is not very practical.

Possible side effects of laser surgery include the following:

- Redness or swelling of the skin right after the treatment that disappears within a few days.
- Discolored skin that will disappear within one to two months.
- Rarely burns and scars result from poorly performed laser surgery.

Endovenous techniques (radiofrequency and laser): These methods for treating the deeper varicose veins of the legs (the saphenous veins) have been a huge breakthrough. They have replaced surgery for the vast majority of patients with severe varicose veins. This technique is not very invasive and can be done in a doctor's office.

The doctor puts a very small tube called a catheter into the vein. Once inside, the catheter sends out radiofrequency or laser energy that shrinks and seals the vein wall. Healthy veins around the closed vein restore the normal flow of blood. As this happens, symptoms from the varicose vein improve. Veins on the surface of the skin that are connected to the treated varicose vein will also usually shrink after treatment. When needed, these connected varicose veins can be treated with sclerotherapy or other techniques.

Possible side effects include slight bruising.

Surgery: Surgery is used mostly to treat very large varicose veins. Types of surgery for varicose veins include surgical ligation and stripping, ambulatory phlebectomy, and endoscopic vein surgery.

Surgical ligation and stripping: With this treatment, problematic veins are tied shut and completely removed from the leg. Removing the veins does not affect the circulation of blood in the leg. Veins deeper in the leg take care of the larger volumes of blood. Most varicose veins removed by surgery are surface veins and collect blood only from the skin. This surgery requires either local or general anesthesia and must be done in an operating room on an outpatient basis.

Serious side effects or problems from this surgery are uncommon. Possible side effects include the following:

- With general anesthesia, a risk of heart and breathing problems.
- Bleeding and congestion of blood can be a problem. But the collected blood usually settles on its own and does not require any further treatment.
- Wound infection, inflammation, swelling, and redness.
- Permanent scars.
- Damage of nerve tissue around the treated vein. It is hard to avoid harming small nerve branches when veins are removed. This damage can cause numbness, burning, or a change in sensation around the surgical scar.
- A deep vein blood clot. These clots can travel to the lungs and heart. Injections of heparin, a medicine that reduces blood clotting, reduce the chance of these dangerous blood clots, but heparin also can increase the normal amount of bleeding and bruising after surgery.
- Significant pain in the leg and recovery time of one to four weeks depending on the extent of surgery is typical after surgery.

Ambulatory phlebectomy: With this surgery, a special light source marks the location of the vein. Tiny cuts are made in the skin, and surgical hooks pull the vein out of the leg. This surgery requires local or regional anesthesia. The vein usually is removed in one treatment. Very large varicose veins can be removed with this treatment while leaving only very small scars. Patients can return to normal activity the day after treatment.

Possible side effects include the following:

- Slight bruising

- Temporary numbness

Endoscopic vein surgery: With this surgery, a small video camera is used to see inside the veins. Then varicose veins are removed through small cuts. People who have this surgery must have some kind of anesthesia including epidural, spinal, or general anesthesia. Patients can return to normal activity within a few weeks.

Can varicose and spider veins return even after treatment?

Current treatments for varicose veins and spider veins have very high success rates compared to traditional surgical treatments. Over a period of years, however, more abnormal veins can develop. The major reason for this is that there is no cure for weak vein valves. So with time, pressure gradually builds up in the leg veins. Ultrasound can be used to keep track of how badly the valves are leaking (venous insufficiency). Ongoing treatment can help keep this problem under control.

The single most important thing a person can do to slow down the development of new varicose veins is to wear graduated compression support stockings as much as possible during the day.

Part Six

Additional Help and Information

Chapter 53

Glossary of Terms Related to Blood and Circulatory Disorders

acute: Sudden onset of symptoms or disease.

agnogenic myeloid metaplasia (AMM): Another name for idiopathic myelofibrosis.

anemia: A condition of the blood caused by a deficiency of red blood cells.

androgen: A male hormone that may be used to treat cancer.

antibody: A protein substance made by the body to help defend it against disease. If too many abnormal antibodies are made it can cause disease.

antigen: A protein that tells the body to produce antibodies.

anti-inflammatory: A medicine that helps to reduce inflammation of tissue in the body.

autoimmune disorder: Diseases caused by the immune system making antibodies against the tissue of its own body.

basophils: A type of white blood cell that plays a special role in allergic reactions.

B-lymphocytes: A type of lymphocyte, or white blood cell, used by the immune system. B-cells secrete antibodies into the body fluid to fight foreign substances that cause infections, disease, or poisoning.

biological therapy: A treatment that stimulates the body's own immune system to fight cancer or blood disorders.

bisphosphonates: Medicines that strengthen the bones and reduce bone pain and improve blood cell counts.

blood count: A blood test that counts the number of the various types of blood cells.

blood transfusions: Giving blood or blood parts directly into the bloodstream to treat blood loss or to treat anemia.

blood-clotting factors: The parts of plasma that are involved in the clotting of blood.

bone marrow: The spongy substance inside our vertebrae, pelvis, and the large bones that makes red blood cells, white blood cells, and platelets.

bone marrow biopsy: A test where a needle is inserted into the bone of the hip or sternum (breastbone) to obtain a marrow sample for study and examination.

chemotherapy: A treatment using medicines.

deciliter: One-tenth of a liter.

eosinophils: A type of white blood cell that plays a role in allergic reactions to foreign substances.

erythrocytes (red blood cells): The cells that carry oxygen.

essential thrombocythemia: A disorder that causes an overproduction of platelets.

external beam radiation therapy: Treating cancer and other disorders with radiation. Sometimes it is called radiation therapy.

extramedullary hematopoiesis: Making blood cells outside of the bone marrow, such as in the spleen.

femtoliters: 1/1,000,000,000,000,000 of a liter (this is very small!).

genetic disorder: A disorder passed down on genes through generations of a family.

gout: A painful inflammation in the joints, usually caused by too much uric acid in the body.

gram: A unit of mass, about the weight of a paperclip.

hematologist: A doctor who studies and treats diseases of blood and bone marrow.

hormonal therapy: A treatment that uses the body's hormones to treat cancer. This can be done by medicines, surgery to remove the hormone-producing glands, or radiation therapy.

idiopathic myelofibrosis (MF): A disorder that causes the bone marrow to slowly be replaced with fibrous scar tissue and the spleen or liver to become enlarged.

idiopathic thrombocytopenic purpura (ITP): A disorder that causes the immune system to make antibodies that destroy platelets, a type of blood cell. When the platelets are destroyed, a person is more likely to bruise and bleed.

immune system: A complex group of cells and substances that protect the body from infection and disease.

immunotherapy: A treatment that stimulates the body's immune system to fight cancer.

intravenous: Into a vein.

leukocytes: White blood cells.

liter: About a quart.

lymphocytes: A type of white blood cell. Three important kinds of lymphocytes are T-cells, B-cells, and natural killer cells. T-cells attack and destroy virus-infected cells, foreign tissue, and cancer cells; B-cells produce antibodies that help destroy foreign substances; natural killer cells destroy cancer cells and virus-infected cells.

microangiopathy: The clotting of blood in the small blood vessels of organs.

microliter: 1/1,000,000 of a liter. In a blood test, a microliter is a single drop of blood.

monoclonal antibody: Monoclonal antibodies are a type of biological therapy. In ITP and macroglobulinemia, monoclonal antibodies are used to decrease the number of cells making inappropriate antibodies.

monocytes: A type of white blood cell.

monitoring (or observation): Usually consists of regularly scheduled blood counts and appointments.

myelofibrosis: Where the bone marrow is replaced with fibrosis (scar) tissue.

neutrophils: A mature white blood cell that fights bacterial infections. Neutrophils are also called segmented neutrophils or segs.

petechiae: Small areas of pinpoint bleeding on the skin. This can be due to low platelet counts.

phlebotomy: The removal of blood from a vein.

picograms: 1/100,000,000,000 of a gram (this is very small!).

plasma: The fluid part of blood.

plasma exchange: In plasma exchange, blood is filtered through a machine that removes plasma and replaces it with plasma from healthy blood donors.

plasmapheresis: During this procedure, blood is filtered through a machine that removes the antibody-containing plasma and replaces it with a substitute. Plasmapheresis can be used to reduce the amount of antibodies in the blood for a short time.

plateletpheresis: A procedure that removes platelets from the blood.

platelets (thrombocytes): A blood cell that helps blood clot. Patients are at risk to bleed if the platelet count is less than 50,000.

polycythemia vera (PV): A type of blood disorder that causes an excess of red blood cells. Some patients may also have too many white blood cells and platelets.

radioactive: Giving off high-dose energy in the form of particles. Radioactive substances can be used to treat some blood disorders.

red blood cells (erythrocytes): The blood cells that carry oxygen and make the blood red.

splenectomy: Surgery to remove the spleen.

surgery: An operation.

thrombocytes (platelets): Cells used to make the blood clot.

thrombotic thrombocytopenic purpura (TTP): A disorder of multiple clots in small blood vessels of many organs of the body.

ultraviolet light: Light that is beyond the visible spectrum.

Waldenström macroglobulinemia: A rare disease that starts in the bone marrow and causes a rapid growth of B-lymphocytes, a type of white blood cell.

white blood cells: Blood cells used by the immune system to fight bacteria and viruses.

Chapter 54

Directory of Resources Related to Blood and Circulatory Disorders

General

American Society of Hematology
1900 M Street, NW, Suite 200
Washington, DC 20036
Phone: 202-776-0544
Fax: 202-776-0545
Website:
http://www.hematology.org
E-mail: ash@hematology.org

Iron Disorders Institute
P.O. Box 675
Taylors, SC 29687
Toll-Free: 888-565-IRON (4766)
Phone: 864-292-1175
Fax: 864-292-1878
Website: http://www.
irondisorders.org
E-mail: publications@
irondisorders.org

National Heart Lung and Blood Institute
NHLBI Health Information Center
P.O. Box 30105
Bethesda, MD 20824-0105
Phone: 301-592-8573
Fax: 240-629-3246
TTY: 240-629-3255
Website: http://www.nhlbi.nih.gov

National Institute of Arthritis and Musculoskeletal and Skin Diseases (NIAMS)
Information Clearinghouse
1 AMS Circle
Bethesda, MD 20892-3675
Toll-Free: 877-22-NIAMS (226-4267)
Phone: 301-495-4484
Fax: 301-718-6366
TTY: 301-565-2966
Website: http://www.niams.nih.gov
E-mail: NIAMSinfo@mail.nih.gov

The information in this chapter was compiled from various sources deemed accurate. All contact information was verified and updated in November 2009. Inclusion does not imply endorsement. This list is intended to serve as a starting point for information gathering; it is not comprehensive.

National Organization for Rare Disorders, Inc.
55 Kenosia Avenue
P.O. Box 1968
Danbury, CT 06813–1968
Toll-Free: 800-999-6673
Phone: 203-744-0100
Fax: 203-798-2291
Website: http://www.raherediseases.org
E-mail: orphan@rarediseases.org

Nemours Foundation
Website: http://kidshealth.org

Anemia

American Society of Hematology
1900 M Street NW
Suite 200
Washington, DC 20036
Phone: 202-776-0544
Fax: 202-776-0545
Website: http://www.hematology.org
E-mail: ash@hematology.org

Aplastic Anemia and MDS International Foundation, Inc.
100 Park Avenue
Suite 108
Rockville, MD 20850
Toll-Free: 800-747-2820
Phone: 301-279-7202
Fax: 301-279-7205
Website: http://www.aamds.org
E-mail: help@aamds.org

Fanconi Anemia Research Fund, Inc.
1801 Willamette Street
Suite 200
Eugene, OR 97401
Toll-Free: 888-FANCONI
(888-326-2664)
Phone: 541-687-4658
Fax: 541-687-0548
Website: http://www.fanconi.org
E-mail: info@fanconi.org

National Anemia Action Council
555 East Wells Street
Suite 1100
Milwaukee, WI 53202
Phone: 414-225-0138
Fax: 414-276-3349
Website: http://www.anemia.org
E-mail: info@anemia.org

National Center for Chronic Disease Prevention and Health Promotion
U.S. Centers for Disease Control and Prevention
4770 Buford Highway NE,
Mailstop K–40
Atlanta, GA 30341–3717
Toll-Free: 800-CDC-INFO
(800-232-4636)
Fax: 770-488-5966
TTY: 888-232-634
Website: http://www.cdc.gov/nccdphp
E-mail: ccdinfo@cdc.gov

Aneurysms

American Association of Neurological Surgeons
5550 Meadowbrook Drive
Rolling Meadows, IL 60008-3852
Toll-Free: 888-566-AANS (2267)
Phone: 847-378-0500
Fax: 847-378-0600
Website: http://www.aans.org
E-mail: info@aans.org

American Stroke Association
7272 Greenville Avenue
Dallas, TX 75231-4596
Toll-Free: 888-4STROKE
(478-7653)
Fax: 214-706-5231
Website:
http://www.strokeassociation.org
E-mail:
strokeassociation@heart.org

Brain Aneurysm Foundation
269 Hanover Street, Building 3
Hanover, MA 02339
Toll-Free:
888-BRAIN02 (272-4602)
Phone: 781-826-5556
Website: http://www.bafound.org
E-mail:office@bafound.org

Brain Resources and Information Network (BRAIN)
P.O. Box 5801
Bethesda, MD 20824
Phone: 301-496-5751
Toll-Free: 800-352-9424
Website: http://www.ninds.nih.gov

Antiphospholipid Antibody Syndrome

APS Foundation of America, Inc.
P.O. Box 801
LaCrosse, WI 54602-0801
Website: http://www.apsfa.org

Bleeding and Clotting Disorders

HHT Foundation International, Inc.
P.O. Box 329
Monkton, MD 21111
Toll-Free: 800-448-6389
Phone: 410-357-9932
Fax: 410-357-0655
Website: http://www.hht.org
E-mail: hhtinfo@hht.org

National Alliance for Thrombosis & Thrombophilia
120 White Plains Road, Suite 100
Tarrytown, NY 10591
Toll-Free: 877-4NO-CLOT
Phone: 914-220-5040
Website: http://stoptheclot.org
E-mail: info@stoptheclot.org

Blood Donation

AABB (formerly the American Association of Blood Banks)
8101 Glenbrook Road
Bethesda, MD 20814-2749
Phone: 301-907-6977
Fax: 301-907-6895
Website: http://www.aabb.org
E-mail: aabb@aabb.org

American Red Cross National Headquarters
2025 E Street, NW
Washington, DC 20006
Toll-Free: 800-REDCROSS
(800-733-2767)
Phone: 202-303-5000
Website: http://www.redcross.org

America's Blood Centers
725 15th Street NW
Suite 700
Washington, DC 20005
Phone: 202-393-5725
Fax: 202-393-1282
Website:
http://www.americasblood.org

Bone Marrow Donation

National Marrow Donor Program
3001 Broadway Street NE
Suite 100
Minneapolis, MN 55413-1753
Website:
http://www.marrow-donor.org

Circulatory Disorders

American Heart Association
National Center
7272 Greenville Avenue
Dallas, TX 75231
Toll-Free: 800-AHA-USA-1
(800-242-8721)
Website:
http://www.americanheart.org

The Erythromelalgia Association
200 Old Castle Lane
Wallingford, PA 19086
Website: http://www.
erythromelalgia.org

Fibromuscular Dysplasia Association of America (FMDSA)
20325 Center Ridge Road
Suite 620
Rocky River, OH 44116
Toll-Free: 888-709-7089
Phone: 216-834-2410
Website: http://www.fmdsa.org
E-mail: admin@fmdsa.org

UC Davis Vascular Center
Lawrence J. Ellison Ambulatory
Care Center
4860 Y Street, Suite 2100
Sacramento, CA 95817
Toll-Free: 800-2-UCDAVIS
(800-282-3284)
Phone: 916-734-3800
Fax: 916-734-8487
Website:
http://www.ucdmc.ucdavis.edu/
vascular/
E-mail: vascular.center
@ucdmc.ucdavis.edu

The Vascular Birthmarks Foundation
P.O. Box 106
Latham, NY 12110
Phone: 877-VBF-4646
(877-823-4646)
Website:
http://www.birthmark.org

Vascular Disease Foundation

1075 S. Yukon, Suite 320
Lakewood, CO 80226
Toll-Free: 888-VDF-4INFO
(888-833-4463)
Phone: 303-989-0500
Fax: 303-989-0200
Website: http://www.vdf.org

Vasculitis Foundation

P.O. Box 28660
Kansas City, MO 64188-8660
Toll-Free: 800-277-9474
Phone/Fax: 816-436-8211
Website:
http://www.vasculitisfounda
tion.org
E-mail:
vf@vasculitisfoundation.org

Hemochromatosis

American Hemochromatosis Society, Inc.

4044 West Lake Mary Boulevard
Unit #104 PMB 416
Lake Mary, FL 32746-2012
Toll-Free: 888-655-IRON (4766)
Phone: 407-829-4488
Fax: 407-333-1284
Website:
http://www.americanhs.org
E-mail: mail@americanhs.org

American Liver Foundation

75 Maiden Lane, Suite 603
New York, NY 10038-4810
Toll-Free: 800-GO-LIVER
(465-4837) or 888-443-7872
Phone: 212-668-1000
Fax: 212-483-8179
Website: http://www.
liverfoundation.org
E-mail: info@liverfoundation.org

Hemophilia

Hemophilia Federation of America

Toll-Free: 800-230-9797
Website: http://www.
hemophiliafed.org/site.php

National Hemophilia Foundation

116 West 32nd Street
11th Floor
New York, NY 10001
Toll-Free: 800-424-2634
Phone: 212-328-3700
Fax: 212-328-3777
Website:
http://www.hemophilia.org

World Federation of Hemophilia

1425 René Lévesque Blvd. W.
Suite 1010
Montreal, Quebec
H3G 1T7 Canada
Phone: 514-875-7944
Fax: 514-875-8916
Website: http://www.wfh.org
E-mail: wfh@wfh.org

Leukemia

American Cancer Society
Toll-Free: 800-ACS-2345
TTY: 866-228-4327
Website: http://www.cancer.org

Leukemia & Lymphoma Society
1311 Mamaroneck Ave.
White Plains, NY 10605
Toll-Free: 800-955-4572
Website: http://www
.leukemia-lymphoma.org

National Cancer Institute
NCI Public Inquiries Office
6116 Executive Boulevard
Room 3036A
Bethesda, MD 20892-8322
Toll-Free: 800-4-CANCER
(800-422-6237)
Website: http://www.cancer.gov

Myeloproliferative Disorders

Myelodysplastic Syndromes Foundation
P.O. BOX 353
Crosswicks, NJ 08515
Toll-Free: 800-MDS-0839
(800-637-0839)
Phone: 609-298-6746 (Outside U.S.)
Fax: 609-298-0590
Website:
http://www.mds-foundation.org

MPD Foundation
233 S. Wacker Drive, Suite 375
Chicago, IL 60606
Phone: 312-683-7243
Fax: 312-332-0840
Website:
http://www.mpdfoundation.org

Plasma Cell Disorders

Amyloid Treatment and Research Program
Boston University School of Medicine
72 East Concord Street., K503
Boston, MA 02118
Phone: 617-638-4317
Fax: 617-638-4493
Website: http://www.bu.edu/
amyloid/index.shtml
E-mail: amyloid@bu.edu

Amyloidosis Foundation, Inc.
7151 N. Main St. Suite 208
Clarkston, MI 48346
Toll-Free: 877-AMYLOID
(877-269-5643)
Phone: 248-922-9610
Fax: 248-922-9620
Website:
http://www.amyloidosis.org

International Waldenstrom's Macroglobulinemia Foundation (IWMF)
3932D Swift Road
Sarasota, FL 34231
Phone: 941-927-4963
Fax: 941-927-4467
Website: http://www.iwmf.com
E-mail: info@iwmf.com

Multiple Myeloma Research Foundation
383 Main Avenue, 5th floor
Norwalk, CT 06851
Phone: 203-229-0464
Fax: 203-229-0572
Website: http://www.
multiplemyeloma.org
E-mail: info@themmrf.org

Sickle Cell Disease

Sickle Cell Disease Association of America, Inc.
231 East Baltimore Street
Suite 800
Baltimore, Maryland 21202
Toll-Free: 800-421-8453
Phone: 410-528-1555
Fax: 410-528-1495
Website: http://www.
sicklecelldisease.org
E-mail: scdaa@sicklecelldisease.org

White Blood Cell Disorders

American Partnership For Eosinophilic Disorders
P.O. Box 29545
Atlanta, GA 30359
Phone: 713-493-7749
Website: http://apfed.org
E-mail: mail@apfed.org

Campaign Urging Research for Eosinophilic Disease (CURED)
P.O. Box 32
Lincolnshire, IL 60069
Website: http://www.
curedfoundation.org

Center for Pediatric Eosinophilic Disorders
Children's Hospital of Philadelphia
Website:
http://www.chop.edu/consumer/
jsp/division/generic.jsp?id=83824

Neutropenia Support Association Inc.
P.O. Box 243
905 Corydon
Winnipeg, Manitoba
Canada, R3M 3S7
Toll-Free: 800-6-NEUTRO
Phone: 204-489-8454
Website:
http://www.neutropenia.ca

Index

Index

Page numbers followed by 'n' indicate a footnote. Page numbers in *italics* indicate a table or illustration.

592

Health Reference Series
Complete Catalog
List price $93 per volume. School and library price $84 per volume.

Adolescent Health Sourcebook, 3rd Edition

Basic Consumer Health Information about Adolescent Growth and Development, Puberty, Sexuality, Reproductive Health, and Physical, Emotional, Social, and Mental Health Concerns of Teens and Their Parents, Including Facts about Nutrition, Physical Activity, Weight Management, Acne, Allergies, Cancer, Diabetes, Growth Disorders, Juvenile Arthritis, Infections, Substance Abuse, and More

Along with Information about Adolescent Safety Concerns, Youth Violence, a Glossary of Related Terms, and a Directory of Resources

Edited by Amy L. Sutton. 600 pages. 2010. 978-0-7808-1140-9.

Adult Health Concerns Sourcebook

Basic Consumer Health Information about Medical and Mental Concerns of Adults, Including Facts about Choosing Healthcare Providers, Navigating Insurance Options, Maintaining Wellness, Preventing Cancer, Heart Disease, Stroke, Diabetes, and Osteoporosis, and Understanding Aging-Related Health Concerns, Including Menopause, Cognitive Changes, and Changes in the Coronary and Vascular Systems

Along with Tips on Caring for Aging Parents and Dealing with Health-Related Work and Travel Issues, a Glossary, and a Directory of Resources for Additional Help and Information

Edited by Sandra J. Judd. 648 pages. 2008. 978-0-7808-0999-4.

"Provides a thorough list of topics that are important to adult health and for caregivers."
—CHOICE, Nov '08

"Written in easy-to-understand language... the content is well-organized and is intended to aid adults in making health care-related decisions."
—AORN Journal, Dec '08

AIDS Sourcebook, 4th Edition

Basic Consumer Health Information about Human Immunodeficiency Virus (HIV) and Acquired Immunodeficiency Syndrome (AIDS), Featuring Updated Statistics and Facts about Risks, Prevention, Screening, Diagnosis, Treatments, Side Effects, and Complications, and Including a Section about the Impact of HIV/AIDS on the Health of Women, Children, and Adolescents

Along with Tips on Managing Life with AIDS, Reports on Current Research Initiatives and Clinical Trials, a Glossary of Related Terms, and Resource Directories for Further Help and Information

Edited by Ivy L. Alexander. 680 pages. 2008. 978-0-7808-0997-0.

SEE ALSO Contagious Diseases Sourcebook, 2nd Edition

Alcoholism Sourcebook, 3rd Edition

Basic Consumer Health Information about Alcohol Use, Abuse, and Dependence, Featuring Facts about the Physical, Mental, and Social Health Effects of Alcohol Addiction, Including Alcoholic Liver Disease, Pancreatic Disease, Cardiovascular Disease, Neurological Disorders, and the Effects of Drinking during Pregnancy

Along with Information about Alcohol Treatment, Medications, and Recovery Programs, in Addition to Tips for Reducing the Prevalence of Underage Drinking, Statistics about Alcohol Use, a Glossary of Related Terms, and Directories of Resources for More Help and Information

Edited by Joyce Brennfleck Shannon. 600 pages. 2010. 978-0-7808-1141-6.

SEE ALSO Drug Abuse Sourcebook, 3rd Edition

Allergies Sourcebook, 3rd Edition

Basic Consumer Health Information about Allergic Disorders, Such as Anaphylaxis, Hives,

Eczema, Rhinitis, Sinusitis, and Conjunctivitis, and Their Triggers, Including Pollen, Mold, Dust Mites, Animal Dander, Insects, Chemicals, Food, Food Additives, and Medications

Along with Advice about the Diagnosis and Treatment of Allergy Symptoms, a Glossary of Related Terms, a Directory of Resources for Help and Information, and Suggestions for Additional Reading

Edited by Amy L. Sutton. 588 pages. 2007. 978-0-7808-0950-5.

SEE ALSO Asthma Sourcebook, 2nd Edition

Alzheimer Disease Sourcebook, 4th Edition

Basic Consumer Health Information about Alzheimer Disease, Other Dementias, and Related Disorders, Including Multi-Infarct Dementia, Dementia with Lewy Bodies, Frontotemporal Dementia (Pick Disease), Wernicke-Korsakoff Syndrome (Alcohol-Related Dementia), AIDS Dementia Complex, Huntington Disease, Creutzfeldt-Jacob Disease, and Delirium

Along with Information about Coping with Memory Loss and Forgetfulness, Maintaining Skills, and Long-Term Planning for People with Dementia, and Suggestions Addressing Common Caregiver Concerns, Updated Information about Current Research Efforts, a Glossary of Related Terms, and Directories of Sources for Additional Help and Information

Edited by Karen Bellenir. 603 pages. 2008. 978-0-7808-1001-3.

"An invaluable resource for persons who have received a diagnosis, for caregivers, and for family members dealing with this insidious disease. It is recommended for public, community college, and ready-reference sections in academic libraries."
—*American Reference Books Annual, 2009*

SEE ALSO Brain Disorders Sourcebook, 3rd Edition

Arthritis Sourcebook, 3rd Edition

Basic Consumer Health Information about the Risk Factors, Symptoms, Diagnosis, and Treatment of Osteoarthritis, Rheumatoid Arthritis, Juvenile Arthritis, Gout, Infectious Arthritis, and Autoimmune Disorders Associated with Arthritis

Along with Facts about Medications, Surgeries, and Self-Care Techniques to Manage Pain and Disability, Tips on Living with Arthritis, a Glossary of Related Terms, and Resources for Additional Help and Information

Edited by Amy L. Sutton. 600 pages. 2010. 978-0-7808-1077-8.

Asthma Sourcebook, 2nd Edition

Basic Consumer Health Information about the Causes, Symptoms, Diagnosis, and Treatment of Asthma in Infants, Children, Teenagers, and Adults, Including Facts about Different Types of Asthma, Common Co-Occurring Conditions, Asthma Management Plans, Triggers, Medications, and Medication Delivery Devices

Along with Asthma Statistics, Research Updates, a Glossary, a Directory of Asthma-Related Resources, and More

Edited by Karen Bellenir. 581 pages. 2006. 978-0-7808-0866-9.

SEE ALSO Lung Disorders Sourcebook; Respiratory Disorders Sourcebook, 2nd Edition

Attention Deficit Disorder Sourcebook

Basic Consumer Health Information about Attention Deficit/Hyperactivity Disorder in Children and Adults, Including Facts about Causes, Symptoms, Diagnostic Criteria, and Treatment Options Such as Medications, Behavior Therapy, Coaching, and Homeopathy

Along with Reports on Current Research Initiatives, Legal Issues, and Government Regulations, and Featuring a Glossary of Related Terms, Internet Resources, and a List of Additional Reading Material

Edited by Dawn D. Matthews. 447 pages. 2002. 978-0-7808-0624-5.

"Recommended reference source."
—*Booklist, Jan '03*

SEE ALSO Learning Disabilities Sourcebook, 3rd Edition

Autism and Pervasive Developmental Disorders Sourcebook

Basic Consumer Health Information about Autism Spectrum and Pervasive Developmental Disorders, Such as Classical Autism, Asperger Syndrome, Rett Syndrome, and Childhood Disintegrative Disorder, Including Information about Related Genetic Disorders and Medical Problems and Facts about Causes, Screening Methods, Diagnostic Criteria, Treatments and Interventions, and Family and Education Issues

Along with a Glossary of Related Terms, Tips for Evaluating the Validity of Health Claims, and a Directory of Resources for Additional Help and Information

Edited by Sandra J. Judd. 603 pages. 2007. 978-0-7808-0953-6.

"This book provides a current overview of disorders on the autism spectrum and information about various therapies, educational resources, and help for families with practical issues such as workplace adjustments, living arrangements, and estate planning. It is a useful resource for public and consumer health libraries."

—*American Reference Books Annual, 2009*

SEE ALSO *Learning Disabilities Sourcebook, 3rd Edition*

Back and Neck Disorders Sourcebook, 2nd Edition

Basic Consumer Health Information about Spinal Pain, Spinal Cord Injuries, and Related Disorders, Such as Degenerative Disk Disease, Osteoarthritis, Scoliosis, Sciatica, Spina Bifida, and Spinal Stenosis, and Featuring Facts about Maintaining Spinal Health, Self-Care, Pain Management, Rehabilitative Care, Chiropractic Care, Spinal Surgeries, and Complementary Therapies

Along with Suggestions for Preventing Back and Neck Pain, a Glossary of Related Terms, and a Directory of Resources

Edited by Amy L. Sutton. 607 pages. 2004. 978-0-7808-0738-9.

"Recommended... An easy to use, comprehensive medical reference book."

—*E-Streams, Sep '05*

"For anyone who has back or neck problems, this book is ideal. Its easy-to-understand language and variety of topics makes this sourcebook a worthwhile read. The price... is reasonable for the amount of information contained in the book"

—*Occupational Therapy in Health Care, 2007*

Blood & Circulatory Disorders Sourcebook, 3rd Edition

Basic Consumer Health Information about Blood and Circulatory System Disorders, Such as Anemia, Leukemia, Lymphoma, Rh Disease, Hemophilia, Thrombophilia, Other Bleeding and Clotting Deficiencies, and Artery, Vascular, and Venous Diseases, Including Facts about Blood Types, Blood Donation, Bone Marrow and Stem Cell Transplants, Tests and Medications, and Tips for Maintaining Circulatory Health

Along with a Glossary of Related Terms and a List of Resources for Additional Help and Information

Edited by Sandra J. Judd. 600 pages. 2010. 978-0-7808-1081-5.

SEE ALSO *Leukemia Sourcebook*

Brain Disorders Sourcebook, 3rd Edition

Basic Consumer Health Information about Acquired and Traumatic Brain Injuries, Brain Tumors, Cerebral Palsy and Other Genetic and Congenital Brain Disorders, Infections of the Brain, Epilepsy, and Degenerative Neurological Disorders Such as Dementia, Huntington Disease, and Amyotrophic Lateral Sclerosis (ALS)

Along with Information on Brain Structure and Function, Treatment and Rehabilitation Options, a Glossary of Terms Related to Brain Disorders, and a Directory of Resources for More Information

Edited by Joyce Brennfleck Shannon. 600 pages. 2010. 978-0-7808-1083-9.

SEE ALSO *Alzheimer Disease Sourcebook, 4th Edition*

Breast Cancer Sourcebook, 3rd Edition

Basic Consumer Health Information about Breast Health and Breast Cancer, Including Facts about Environmental, Genetic, and Other Risk Factors, Prevention Efforts, Screening and Diagnostic Methods, Surgical Treatment Options and Other Care Choices, Complementary and Alternative Therapies, and Post-Treatment Concerns

Along with Statistical Data, News about Research Advances, a Glossary of Related Terms, and Directories of Resources for Additional Information and Support

Edited by Karen Bellenir. 606 pages. 2009. 978-0-7808-1030-3.

"A very useful reference for people wanting to learn more about breast cancer and how to negotiate their care or the care of a loved one. The third edition is necessary as information/treatment options continue to evolve."

—*Doody's Review Service, 2009*

SEE ALSO *Cancer Sourcebook for Women, 3rd Edition, Women's Health Concerns Sourcebook, 3rd Edition*

Breastfeeding Sourcebook

Basic Consumer Health Information about the Benefits of Breastmilk, Preparing to Breastfeed, Breastfeeding as a Baby Grows, Nutrition, and More, Including Information on Special Situations and Concerns Such as Mastitis, Illness, Medications, Allergies, Multiple Births, Prematurity, Special Needs, and Adoption

Along with a Glossary and Resources for Additional Help and Information

Edited by Jenni Lynn Colson. 367 pages. 2002. 978-0-7808-0332-9.

SEE ALSO *Pregnancy and Birth Sourcebook, 3rd Edition*

Burns Sourcebook

Basic Consumer Health Information about Various Types of Burns and Scalds, Including Flame, Heat, Cold, Electrical, Chemical, and Sun Burns

Along with Information on Short-Term and Long-Term Treatments, Tissue Reconstruction, Plastic Surgery, Prevention Suggestions, and First Aid

Edited by Allan R. Cook. 604 pages. 1999. 978-0-7808-0204-9.

"This is an exceptional addition to the series and is highly recommended for all consumer health collections, hospital libraries, and academic medical centers."

—*E-Streams, Mar '00*

"This key reference guide is an invaluable addition to all health care and public libraries in confronting this ongoing health issue."

—*American Reference Books Annual, 2000*

SEE ALSO *Dermatological Disorders Sourcebook, 2nd Edition*

Cancer Sourcebook, 5th Edition

Basic Consumer Health Information about Major Forms and Stages of Cancer, Featuring Facts about Head and Neck Cancers, Lung Cancers, Gastrointestinal Cancers, Genitourinary Cancers, Lymphomas, Blood Cell Cancers, Endocrine Cancers, Skin Cancers, Bone Cancers, Metastatic Cancers, and More

Along with Facts about Cancer Treatments, Cancer Risks and Prevention, a Glossary of Related Terms, Statistical Data, and a Directory of Resources for Additional Information

Edited by Karen Bellenir. 1105 pages. 2007. 978-0-7808-0947-5.

"The 5th, updated edition of Cancer Sourcebook should be in every public and health lending library collection... An unparalleled discussion essential for any health collections considering an all-in-one basic general reference."

—*California Bookwatch, Aug '07*

SEE ALSO *Breast Cancer Sourcebook, 3rd Edition, Cancer Survivorship Sourcebook, Leukemia Sourcebook*

Cancer Sourcebook for Women, 4th Edition

Basic Consumer Health Information about Gynecologic Cancers and Other Cancers of Special Concern to Women, Including Cancers of the Breast, Cervix, Colon, Lung, Ovaries, Thyroid, and Uterus

Along with Facts about Benign Conditions of the Female Reproductive System, Cancer Risk

Factors, Diagnostic and Treatment Procedures, Side Effects of Cancer and Cancer Treatments, Women's Issues in Cancer Survivorship, a Glossary of Related Terms, and a Directory of Resources for Additional Help and Information

Edited by Karen Bellenir. 600 pages. 2010. 978-0-7808-1139-3.

SEE ALSO Breast Cancer Sourcebook, 3rd Edition, Women's Health Concerns Sourcebook, 3rd Edition

Cancer Survivorship Sourcebook

Basic Consumer Health Information about the Physical, Educational, Emotional, Social, and Financial Needs of Cancer Patients from Diagnosis, through Cancer Treatment, and Beyond, Including Facts about Researching Specific Types of Cancer and Learning about Clinical Trials and Treatment Options, and Featuring Tips for Coping with the Side Effects of Cancer Treatments and Adjusting to Life after Cancer Treatment Concludes

Along with Suggestions for Caregivers, Friends, and Family Members of Cancer Patients, a Glossary of Cancer Care Terms, and Directories of Related Resources

Edited by Karen Bellenir. 633 pages. 2007. 978-0-7808-0985-7.

"Well organized and comprehensive in coverage, the book speaks to issues encountered both during and after cancer treatment. Recommended for consumer health and public libraries."
—Library Journal, Aug 1 '07

"Cancer Survivorship Sourcebook will be useful to anyone who has a friend or loved one with a cancer diagnosis."
—American Reference Books Annual, 2008

SEE ALSO Cancer Sourcebook, 5th Edition, Disease Management Sourcebook

Cardiovascular Disorders Sourcebook, 4th Edition

Basic Consumer Health Information about Heart and Blood Vessel Diseases and Disorders, Such as Angina, Heart Attack, Heart Failure, Cardiomyopathy, Arrhythmias, Valve Disease, Atherosclerosis, Aneurysms, and

Congenital Heart Defects, Including Information about Cardiovascular Disease in Women, Men, Children, Adolescents, and Minorities

Along with Facts about Diagnosing, Managing, and Preventing Cardiovascular Disease, a Glossary of Related Medical Terms, and a Directory of Resources for Additional Information

Edited by Amy L. Sutton. 600 pages. 2010. 978-0-7808-1080-8.

Caregiving Sourcebook

Basic Consumer Health Information for Caregivers, Including a Profile of Caregivers, Caregiving Responsibilities and Concerns, Tips for Specific Conditions, Care Environments, and the Effects of Caregiving

Along with Facts about Legal Issues, Financial Information, and Future Planning, a Glossary, and a Listing of Additional Resources

Edited by Joyce Brennfleck Shannon. 583 pages. 2001. 978-0-7808-0331-2.

"Essential for most collections."
—Library Journal, Apr 1 '02

"An ideal addition to the reference collection of any public library. Health sciences information professionals may also want to acquire the Caregiving Sourcebook for their hospital or academic library for use as a ready reference tool by health care workers interested in aging and caregiving."
—E-Streams, Jan '02

Child Abuse Sourcebook, 2nd Edition

Basic Consumer Health Information about the Physical, Sexual, and Emotional Abuse of Children, Neglect, Münchhausen Syndrome by Proxy (MSBP), and Shaken Baby Syndrome, and Featuring Facts about Withholding Medical Care, Corporal Punishment, Child Maltreatment in Youth Sports, and Parental Substance Abuse

Along with Information about Child Protective Services, Foster Care, Adoption, Parenting Challenges, Abuse Prevention Programs, and Intervention, Treatment, and Recovery Guidelines, a Glossary of Related Terms, and Resources for Additional Help and Information

Edited by Joyce Brennfleck Shannon. 600 pages. 2009. 978-0-7808-1037-2.

SEE ALSO *Domestic Violence Sourcebook, 3rd Edition*

Childhood Diseases and Disorders Sourcebook, 2nd Edition

Basic Consumer Health Information about the Physical, Mental, and Developmental Health of Pre-Adolescent Children, Including Facts about Infectious Diseases, Asthma, Allergies, Diabetes, and Other Acute and Chronic Conditions Affecting the Gastrointestinal Tract, Ears, Nose, Throat, Liver, Kidneys, Heart, Blood, Brain, Muscles, Bones, and Skin

Along with Reports on Recommended Childhood Vaccinations, Wellness Guidelines, a Glossary of Related Medical Terms, and a List of Resources for Parents

Edited by Sandra J. Judd. 694 pages. 2009. 978-0-7808-1031-0.

"The strength of this source is the wide range of information given about childhood health issues... It is most appropriate for public libraries and academic libraries that field medical questions."
—*American Reference Books Annual, 2009*

SEE ALSO *Healthy Children Sourcebook*

Colds, Flu and Other Common Ailments Sourcebook

Basic Consumer Health Information about Common Ailments and Injuries, Including Colds, Coughs, the Flu, Sinus Problems, Headaches, Fever, Nausea and Vomiting, Menstrual Cramps, Diarrhea, Constipation, Hemorrhoids, Back Pain, Dandruff, Dry and Itchy Skin, Cuts, Scrapes, Sprains, Bruises, and More

Along with Information about Prevention, Self-Care, Choosing a Doctor, Over-the-Counter Medications, Folk Remedies, and Alternative Therapies, and Including a Glossary of Important Terms and a Directory of Resources for Further Help and Information

Edited by Chad T. Kimball. 622 pages. 2001. 978-0-7808-0435-7.

"A good starting point for research on common illnesses. It will be a useful addition to public and consumer health library collections."
—*American Reference Books Annual, 2002*

"Will prove valuable to any library seeking to maintain a current, comprehensive reference collection of health resources... Excellent reference."
—*The Bookwatch, Aug '01*

SEE ALSO *Contagious Diseases Sourcebook, 2nd Edition*

Communication Disorders Sourcebook

Basic Information about Deafness and Hearing Loss, Speech and Language Disorders, Voice Disorders, Balance and Vestibular Disorders, and Disorders of Smell, Taste, and Touch

Edited by Linda M. Ross. 533 pages. 1996. 978-0-7808-0077-9.

"This is skillfully edited and is a welcome resource for the layperson. It should be found in every public and medical library."
—*Booklist Health Sciences Supplement, Oct '97*

Complementary & Alternative Medicine Sourcebook, 4th Edition

Basic Consumer Health Information about Ayurveda, Acupuncture, Aromatherapy, Chiropractic Care, Diet-Based Therapies, Guided Imagery, Herbal and Vitamin Supplements, Homeopathy, Hypnosis, Massage, Meditation, Naturopathy, Pilates, Reflexology, Reiki, Shiatsu, Tai Chi, Traditional Chinese Medicine, Yoga, and Other Complementary and Alternative Medical Therapies

Along with Statistics, Tips for Selecting a Practitioner, Treatments for Specific Health Conditions, a Glossary of Related Terms, and a Directory of Resources for Additional Help and Information

Edited by Amy L. Sutton. 600 pages. 2010. 978-0-7808-1082-2.

Congenital Disorders Sourcebook, 2nd Edition

Basic Consumer Health Information about Nonhereditary Birth Defects and Disorders

Related to Prematurity, Gestational Injuries, Congenital Infections, and Birth Complications, Including Heart Defects, Hydrocephalus, Spina Bifida, Cleft Lip and Palate, Cerebral Palsy, and More

Along with Facts about the Prevention of Birth Defects, Fetal Surgery and Other Treatment Options, Research Initiatives, a Glossary of Related Terms, and Resources for Additional Information and Support

Edited by Sandra J. Judd. 619 pages. 2007. 978-0-7808-0945-1.

"Congenital Disorders Sourcebook provides an excellent, non-technical overview of many aspects of pregnancy with the focus on congenital disorders."
—American Reference Books Annual, 2008

"An excellent readable reference aimed at the lay public for difficult to understand medical problems. An excellent starting point for the interested parent or family member who may then be motivated to seek more information."
—Doody's Review Service, 2007

SEE ALSO Pregnancy and Birth Sourcebook, 3rd Edition

Contagious Diseases Sourcebook, 2nd Edition

Basic Consumer Health Information about Diseases Spread from Person to Person through Direct Physical Contact, Airborne Transmissions, Sexual Contact, or Contact with Blood or Other Body Fluids, Including Pneumococcal, Staphylococcal, and Streptococcal Diseases, Colds, Influenza, Lice, Measles, Mumps, Tuberculosis, and Others

Along with Facts about Self-Care and Over-the-Counter Medications, Antibiotics and Drug Resistance, Disease Prevention, Vaccines, and Bioterrorism, a Glossary, and a Directory of Resources for More Information

Edited by Joyce Brennfleck Shannon. 600 pages. 2010. 978-0-7808-1075-4.

SEE ALSO AIDS Sourcebook, 4th Edition, Hepatitis Sourcebook

Cosmetic and Reconstructive Surgery Sourcebook, 2nd Edition

Basic Consumer Information about Plastic Surgery and Non-Surgical Appearance-Enhancing Procedures, Including Facts about Botulinum Toxin, Collagen Replacement, Dermabrasion, Chemical Peels, Eyelid Surgery, Nose Reshaping, Lip Augmentation, Liposuction, Breast Enlargement and Reduction, Tummy Tucking, and Other Skin, Hair, Facial, and Body Shaping Procedures

Along with Information about Reconstructive Procedures for Congenital Disorders, Disfiguring Diseases, Burns, and Traumatic Injuries, a Glossary of Related Terms, and a Directory of Additional Resources

Edited by Karen Bellenir. 483 pages. 2007. 978-0-7808-0951-2.

"A comprehensive source for people considering cosmetic surgery... also recommended for medical students who will perform these procedures later in their careers; and public librarians and academic medical librarians who may assist patrons interested in this information."
—Medical Reference Services Quarterly, Fall '08

"A practical guide for health care consumers and health care workers... This easy-to-read reference guide would be useful for novice and veteran health care consumers, surgical technology students, nursing students, and perioperative nurses new to plastic and reconstructive surgery. It also may be helpful for medical-surgical nurses as a guide for patient teaching in their practices."
—AORN Journal, Aug '08

SEE ALSO Surgery Sourcebook, 2nd Edition

Death and Dying Sourcebook, 2nd Edition

Basic Consumer Health Information about End-of-Life Care and Related Perspectives and Ethical Issues, Including End-of-Life Symptoms and Treatments, Pain Management, Quality-of-Life Concerns, the Use of Life Support, Patients' Rights and Privacy Issues, Advance Directives, Physician-Assisted Suicide, Caregiving, Organ and Tissue Donation, Autopsies, Funeral Arrangements, and Grief

Along with Statistical Data, Information about the Leading Causes of Death, a Glossary, and Directories of Support Groups and Other Resources

Edited by Joyce Brennfleck Shannon. 626 pages. 2006. 978-0-7808-0871-3.

Dental Care and Oral Health Sourcebook, 3rd Edition

Basic Consumer Health Information about Dental Care and Oral Health Throughout the Lifespan, Including Facts about Cavities, Bad Breath, Cold and Canker Sores, Dry Mouth, Toothaches, Gum Disease, Malocclusion, Temporomandibular Joint and Muscle Disorders, Oral Cancers, and Dental Emergencies

Along with Information about Mouth Hygiene, Crowns, Bridges, Implants, and Fillings, Surgical, Orthodontic, and Cosmetic Dental Procedures, Pain Management, Health Conditions that Impact Oral Care, a Glossary of Related Terms, and a Directory of Additional Resources

Edited by Amy L. Sutton. 619 pages. 2008. 978-0-7808-1032-7.

"Could serve as turning point in the battle to educate consumers in issues concerning oral health. Tightly written in terms the average person can understand, yet comprehensive in scope and authoritative in tone, it is another excellent sourcebook in the Health Reference Series... Should be in the reference department of all public libraries, and in academic libraries that have a public constituency."
—American Reference Books Annual, 2009

Depression Sourcebook, 2nd Edition

Basic Consumer Health Information about Unipolar Depression, Bipolar Disorder, Dysthymia, Seasonal Affective Disorder, Postpartum Depression, and Other Depressive Disorders, Including Facts about Populations at Special Risk, Coexisting Medical Conditions, Symptoms, Treatment Options, and Suicide Prevention

Along with Statistical Data, a Glossary of Related Terms, and a Directory of Resources for Additional Help and Information

Edited by Sandra J. Judd. 646 pages. 2008. 978-0-7808-1003-7.

"Recommended for public libraries."
—American Reference Books Annual, 2009

SEE ALSO Mental Health Disorders Sourcebook, 4th Edition

Dermatological Disorders Sourcebook, 2nd Edition

Basic Consumer Health Information about Conditions and Disorders Affecting the Skin, Hair, and Nails, Such as Acne, Rosacea, Rashes, Dermatitis, Pigmentation Disorders, Birthmarks, Skin Cancer, Skin Injuries, Psoriasis, Scleroderma, and Hair Loss, Including Facts about Medications and Treatments for Dermatological Disorders and Tips for Maintaining Healthy Skin, Hair, and Nails

Along with Information about How Aging Affects the Skin, a Glossary of Related Terms, and a Directory of Resources for Additional Help and Information

Edited by Amy L. Sutton. 617 pages. 2006. 978-0-7808-0795-2.

"Well organized... presents a plethora of information in a manner that is appropriate in style and readability for the intended audience."
—Physical Therapy, Nov '06

"Helpfully brings together... sources in one convenient place, saving the user hours of research time."
—American Reference Books Annual, 2006

SEE ALSO Burns Sourcebook

Diabetes Sourcebook, 4th Edition

Basic Consumer Health Information about Type 1 and Type 2 Diabetes Mellitus, Gestational Diabetes, Monogenic Forms of Diabetes, and Insulin Resistance, with Guidelines for Lifestyle Modifications and the Medical Management of Diabetes, Including Facts about Insulin, Insulin Delivery Devices, Oral Diabetes Medications, Self-Monitoring of Blood Glucose, Meal Planning, Physical Activity Recommendations, Foot Care, and Treatment Options for People with Kidney Failure

Along with a Section about Diabetes Complications and Co-Occurring Conditions, a Glossary of Related Terms, and Directories of Resources for Additional Help and Information

Edited by Karen Bellenir. 627 pages. 2008. 978-0-7808-1005-1.

"Completely and comprehensively covering almost everything a student or physician would need to know... well worth the investment."

—Internet Bookwatch, Dec '08

SEE ALSO *Endocrine and Metabolic Disorders Sourcebook, 2nd Edition*

Diet and Nutrition Sourcebook, 3rd Edition

Basic Consumer Health Information about Dietary Guidelines and the Food Guidance System, Recommended Daily Nutrient Intakes, Serving Proportions, Weight Control, Vitamins and Supplements, Nutrition Issues for Different Life Stages and Lifestyles, and the Needs of People with Specific Medical Concerns, Including Cancer, Celiac Disease, Diabetes, Eating Disorders, Food Allergies, and Cardiovascular Disease

Along with Facts about Federal Nutrition Support Programs, a Glossary of Nutrition and Dietary Terms, and Directories of Additional Resources for More Information about Nutrition

Edited by Joyce Brennfleck Shannon. 605 pages. 2006. 978-0-7808-0800-3.

"A valuable resource tool for any individual."
—Journal of Dental Hygiene, Apr '07

"From different recommended eating habits to reduce disease and common ailments to nutrition advice for those with specific conditions, Diet and Nutrition Sourcebook is especially important because so much is changing in this area, and so rapidly."
—California Bookwatch, Jun '06

SEE ALSO *Eating Disorders Sourcebook, 2nd Edition, Vegetarian Sourcebook*

Digestive Diseases and Disorders Sourcebook

Basic Consumer Health Information about Diseases and Disorders that Impact the Upper and Lower Digestive System, Including Celiac Disease, Constipation, Crohn's Disease, Cyclic Vomiting Syndrome, Diarrhea, Diverticulosis and Diverticulitis, Gallstones, Heartburn, Hemorrhoids, Hernias, Indigestion (Dyspepsia), Irritable Bowel Syndrome, Lactose Intolerance, Ulcers, and More

Along with Information about Medications and Other Treatments, Tips for Maintaining a Healthy Digestive Tract, a Glossary, and Directory of Digestive Diseases Organizations

Edited by Karen Bellenir. 323 pages. 2000. 978-0-7808-0327-5.

"An excellent addition to all public or patient-research libraries."
—American Reference Books Annual, 2001

"Recommended reference source."
—Booklist, May '00

SEE ALSO *Gastrointestinal Diseases and Disorders Sourcebook, 2nd Edition*

Disabilities Sourcebook

Basic Consumer Health Information about Physical and Psychiatric Disabilities, Including Descriptions of Major Causes of Disability, Assistive and Adaptive Aids, Workplace Issues, and Accessibility Concerns

Along with Information about the Americans with Disabilities Act, a Glossary, and Resources for Additional Help and Information

Edited by Dawn D. Matthews. 602 pages. 2000. 978-0-7808-0389-3.

"A must for libraries with a consumer health section."
—American Reference Books Annual, 2002

"A much needed addition to the Omnigraphics Health Reference Series. A current reference work to provide people with disabilities, their families, caregivers or those who work with them, a broad range of information in one volume, has not been available until now... It is recommended for all public and academic library reference collections."
—E-Streams, May '01

"An excellent source book in easy-to-read format covering many current topics; highly recommended for all libraries."
—CHOICE, Jan '01

Disease Management Sourcebook

Basic Consumer Health Information about Coping with Chronic and Serious Illnesses, Navigating the Health Care System, Communicating with Health Care Providers, Assessing Health Care Quality, and Making Informed Health Care Decisions, Including Facts about Second Opinions, Hospitalization, Surgery, and Medications

Along with a Section about Children with Chronic Conditions, Information about Legal, Financial, and Insurance Issues, a Glossary of Related Terms, and Directories of Additional Resources

Edited by Joyce Brennfleck Shannon. 621 pages. 2008. 978-0-7808-1002-0.

"Consumers need to know how to manage their health care the same way they manage anything else in their lives. The text is very readable and is written for the layperson and consumer. The cost is not prohibitive. This book should be in all collections of health care libraries and public libraries."
— American Reference Books Annual, 2009

"The information is very current, and the selection of font and layout make the book easy to read. A hardback that will stand up to much usage, this is an excellent resource for consumers... Recommended. General readers."
—CHOICE, Nov '08

"Intended for lay readers, this resource clarifies the many confusing and overwhelming details associated with chronic disease care. Meticulous and clearly explained, the book even includes diagrams intended to ease comprehension of over-the-counter medication labels. An essential guide to navigating the health-care rapids."
—Library Journal, Aug '08

Domestic Violence Sourcebook, 3rd Edition

Basic Consumer Health Information about Warning Signs, Risk Factors, and Health Consequences of Intimate Partner Violence, Sexual Violence and Rape, Stalking, Human Trafficking, Child Maltreatment, Teen Dating Violence, and Elder Abuse

Along with Facts about Victims and Perpetrators, Strategies for Violence Prevention, and Emergency Interventions, Safety Plans, and Financial and Legal Tips for Victims, a Glossary of Related Terms, and Directories of Resources for Additional Information and Support

Edited by Joyce Brennfleck Shannon. 634 pages. 2009. 978-0-7808-1038-9.

"A recommended pick for any library interested in consumer health and social issues... A 'must' for any serious health collection."
—California Bookwatch, Jul '09

SEE ALSO Child Abuse Sourcebook, 2nd Edition

Drug Abuse Sourcebook, 3rd Edition

Basic Consumer Health Information about the Abuse of Cocaine, Club Drugs, Hallucinogens, Heroin, Inhalants, Marijuana, and Other Illicit Substances, Prescription Medications, and Over-the-Counter Medicines

Along with Facts about Addiction and Related Health Effects, Drug Abuse Treatment and Recovery, Drug Testing, Prevention Programs, Glossaries of Drug-Related Terms, and Directories of Resources for More Information

Edited by Joyce Brennfleck Shannon. 600 pages. 2010. 978-0-7808-1079-2.

SEE ALSO Alcoholism Sourcebook, 3rd Edition

Ear, Nose, and Throat Disorders Sourcebook, 2nd Edition

Basic Consumer Health Information about Disorders of the Ears, Hearing Loss, Vestibular Disorders, Nasal and Sinus Problems, Throat and Vocal Cord Disorders, and Otolaryngologic Cancers, Including Facts about Ear Infections and Injuries, Genetic and Congenital Deafness, Sensorineural Hearing Disorders, Tinnitus, Vertigo, Ménière Disease, Rhinitis, Sinusitis, Snoring, Sore Throats, Hoarseness, and More

Along with Reports on Current Research Initiatives, a Glossary of Related Medical Terms, and a Directory of Sources for Further Help and Information

Edited by Sandra J. Judd. 631 pages. 2007. 978-0-7808-0872-0.

"A resource book for the general public that provides comprehensive coverage of basic up-to-date medical information about the causes, symptoms, diagnosis, and treatment of diseases and disorders that affect the ears, nose, sinuses, throat, and voice... The majority of information is presented in question and answer format, much like questions a patient might ask of a health care provider. An extensive index facilitates the reader's ability to easily access information on any specific topic."
—*Journal of Dental Hygiene, Oct '07*

"A handy compilation of information on common and some not so common ailments of the ears, nose, and throat."
—*Doody's Review Service, 2007*

Eating Disorders Sourcebook, 2nd Edition

Basic Consumer Health Information about Anorexia Nervosa, Bulimia, Binge Eating, Compulsive Exercise, Female Athlete Triad, and Other Eating Disorders, Including Facts about Body Image and Other Cultural and Age-Related Risk Factors, Prevention Efforts, Adverse Health Effects, Treatment Options, and the Recovery Process

Along with Guidelines for Healthy Weight Control, a Glossary, and Directories of Additional Resources

Edited by Joyce Brennfleck Shannon. 557 pages. 2007. 978-0-7808-0948-2.

"Recommended for the reference collection of large public libraries."
—*American Reference Books Annual, 2008*

"A basic health reference any health or general library needs."
—*Internet Bookwatch, Jun '07*

SEE ALSO Diet and Nutrition Sourcebook, 3rd Edition, Mental Health Disorders Sourcebook, 4th Edition

Emergency Medical Services Sourcebook

Basic Consumer Health Information about Preventing, Preparing for, and Managing Emergency Situations, When and Who to Call for Help, What to Expect in the Emergency Room, the Emergency Medical Team,

Patient Issues, and Current Topics in Emergency Medicine

Along with Statistical Data, a Glossary, and Sources of Additional Help and Information

Edited by Jenni Lynn Colson. 472 pages. 2002. 978-0-7808-0420-3.

"Handy and convenient for home, public, school, and college libraries. Recommended."
—*CHOICE, Apr '03*

"This reference can provide the consumer with answers to most questions about emergency care in the United States, or it will direct them to a resource where the answer can be found."
—*American Reference Books Annual, 2003*

SEE ALSO Injury and Trauma Sourcebook

Endocrine and Metabolic Disorders Sourcebook, 2nd Edition

Basic Consumer Health Information about Hormonal and Metabolic Disorders that Affect the Body's Growth, Development, and Functioning, Including Disorders of the Pancreas, Ovaries and Testes, and Pituitary, Thyroid, Parathyroid, and Adrenal Glands, with Facts about Growth Disorders, Addison Disease, Cushing Syndrome, Conn Syndrome, Diabetic Disorders, Multiple Endocrine Neoplasia, Inborn Errors of Metabolism, and More

Along with Information about Endocrine Functioning, Diagnostic and Screening Tests, a Glossary of Related Terms, and Directories of Additional Resources

Edited by Joyce Brennfleck Shannon. 597 pages. 2007. 978-0-7808-0952-9.

SEE ALSO Diabetes Sourcebook, 4th Edition

Environmental Health Sourcebook, 3rd Edition

Basic Consumer Health Information about the Environment and Its Effects on Human Health, Including Facts about Air, Water, and Soil Contamination, Hazardous Chemicals, Foodborne Hazards and Illnesses, Household Hazards Such as Radon, Mold, and Carbon Monoxide, Consumer Hazards from Toxic Products and Imported Goods, and Disorders

Linked to Environmental Causes, Including Chemical Sensitivity, Cancer, Allergies, and Asthma

Along with Information about the Impact of Environmental Hazards on Specific Populations, a Glossary of Related Terms, and Resources for Additional Help and Information.

Edited by Laura Larsen. 600 pages. 2010. 978-0-7808-1078-5

Ethnic Diseases Sourcebook

Basic Consumer Health Information for Ethnic and Racial Minority Groups in the United States, Including General Health Indicators and Behaviors, Ethnic Diseases, Genetic Testing, the Impact of Chronic Diseases, Women's Health, Mental Health Issues, and Preventive Health Care Services

Along with a Glossary and a Listing of Additional Resources

Edited by Joyce Brennfleck Shannon. 648 pages. 2001. 978-0-7808-0336-7.

"Not many books have been written on this topic to date, and the Ethnic Diseases Sourcebook is a strong addition to the list. It will be an important introductory resource for health consumers, students, health care personnel, and social scientists. It is recommended for public, academic, and large hospital libraries."
— American Reference Books Annual, 2002

"Will prove valuable to any library seeking to maintain a current, comprehensive reference collection of health resources... An excellent source of health information about genetic disorders which affect particular ethnic and racial minorities in the U.S."
—The Bookwatch, Aug '01

Eye Care Sourcebook, 3rd Edition

Basic Consumer Health Information about Eye Care and Eye Disorders, Including Facts about the Diagnosis, Prevention, and Treatment of Refractive Disorders, Cataracts, Glaucoma, Macular Degeneration, and Problems Affecting the Cornea, Retina, and Lacrimal Glands

Along with Advice about Preventing Eye Injuries and Tips for Living with Low Vision or Blindness, a Glossary of Related Terms, and Directories of Resources for More Help and Information

Edited by Amy L. Sutton. 646 pages. 2008. 978-0-7808-1000-6.

"A solid reference tool for eye care and a valuable addition to a collection."
—American Reference Books Annual, 2009

Family Planning Sourcebook

Basic Consumer Health Information about Planning for Pregnancy and Contraception, Including Traditional Methods, Barrier Methods, Hormonal Methods, Permanent Methods, Future Methods, Emergency Contraception, and Birth Control Choices for Women at Each Stage of Life

Along with Statistics, a Glossary, and Sources of Additional Information

Edited by Amy Marcaccio Keyzer. 503 pages. 2001. 978-0-7808-0379-4.

"Recommended for public, health, and undergraduate libraries as part of the circulating collection."
—E-Streams, Mar '02

"Will prove valuable to any library seeking to maintain a current, comprehensive reference collection of health resources... Excellent reference."
—The Bookwatch, Aug '01

SEE ALSO Pregnancy and Birth Sourcebook, 3rd Edition

Fitness and Exercise Sourcebook, 3rd Edition

Basic Consumer Health Information about the Physical and Mental Benefits of Fitness, Including Cardiorespiratory Endurance, Muscular Strength, Muscular Endurance, and Flexibility, with Facts about Sports Nutrition and Exercise-Related Injuries and Tips about Physical Activity and Exercises for People of All Ages and for People with Health Concerns

Along with Advice on Selecting and Using Exercise Equipment, Maintaining Exercise Motivation, a Glossary of Related Terms, and a Directory of Resources for More Help and Information

Edited by Amy L. Sutton. 635 pages. 2007. 978-0-7808-0946-8.

"Updates the consumer information on the physical and mental benefits of physical activity throughout the lifespan offered in earlier editions... Recommended. All readers; all levels."

—*CHOICE, Oct '07*

"An exceptionally well-rounded coverage perfect for any concerned about developing and understanding a fitness program."

—*California Bookwatch, Jun '07*

SEE ALSO *Sports Injuries Sourcebook, 3rd Edition*

Food Safety Sourcebook

Basic Consumer Health Information about the Safe Handling of Meat, Poultry, Seafood, Eggs, Fruit Juices, and Other Food Items, and Facts about Pesticides, Drinking Water, Food Safety Overseas, and the Onset, Duration, and Symptoms of Foodborne Illnesses, Including Types of Pathogenic Bacteria, Parasitic Protozoa, Worms, Viruses, and Natural Toxins

Along with the Role of the Consumer, the Food Handler, and the Government in Food Safety, a Glossary, and Resources for Additional Help and Information

Edited by Dawn D. Matthews. 327 pages. 1999. 978-0-7808-0326-8.

"Recommended reference source."

—*Booklist, May '00*

"This book takes the complex issues of food safety and foodborne pathogens and presents them in an easily understood manner. [It does] an excellent job of covering a large and often confusing topic."

— *American Reference Books Annual, 2000*

Forensic Medicine Sourcebook

Basic Consumer Information for the Layperson about Forensic Medicine, Including Crime Scene Investigation, Evidence Collection and Analysis, Expert Testimony, Computer-Aided Criminal Identification, Digital Imaging in the Courtroom, DNA Profiling, Accident Reconstruction, Autopsies, Ballistics, Drugs and Explosives Detection, Latent Fingerprints,

Product Tampering, and Questioned Document Examination

Along with Statistical Data, a Glossary of Forensics Terminology, and Listings of Sources for Further Help and Information

Edited by Annemarie S. Muth. 574 pages. 1999. 978-0-7808-0232-2.

"Given the expected widespread interest in its content and its easy to read style, this book is recommended for most public and all college and university libraries."

—*E-Streams, Feb '01*

"A wealth of information, useful statistics, references are up-to-date and extremely complete. This wonderful collection of data will help students who are interested in a career in any type of forensic field. It is a great resource for attorneys who need information about types of expert witnesses needed in a particular case. It also offers useful information for fiction and nonfiction writers whose work involves a crime. A fascinating compilation. All levels."

—*CHOICE, Jan '00*

"There are several items that make this book attractive to consumers who are seeking certain forensic data... This is a useful current source for those seeking general forensic medical answers."

—*American Reference Books Annual, 2000*

Gastrointestinal Diseases and Disorders Sourcebook, 2nd Edition

Basic Consumer Health Information about the Upper and Lower Gastrointestinal (GI) Tract, Including the Esophagus, Stomach, Intestines, Rectum, Liver, and Pancreas, with Facts about Gastroesophageal Reflux Disease, Gastritis, Hernias, Ulcers, Celiac Disease, Diverticulitis, Irritable Bowel Syndrome, Hemorrhoids, Gastrointestinal Cancers, and Other Diseases and Disorders Related to the Digestive Process

Along with Information about Commonly Used Diagnostic and Surgical Procedures, Statistics, Reports on Current Research Initiatives and Clinical Trials, a Glossary, and Resources for Additional Help and Information

Edited by Sandra J. Judd. 654 pages. 2006. 978-0-7808-0798-3.

"The text is designed for the general reader seeking information on prevention, disease warning signs, diagnostic and therapeutic questions... It is an excellent resource for the general reader to conveniently locate credible, coordinated and indexed information... The sourcebook will prove very helpful for patients, caregivers and should be available in every physician waiting room."
—*Doody's Review Service, 2006*

SEE ALSO *Diet and Nutrition Sourcebook, 3rd Edition, Digestive Diseases and Disorders Sourcebook*

Genetic Disorders Sourcebook, 4th Edition

Basic Consumer Health Information about Hereditary Diseases and Disorders, Including Facts about the Human Genome, Genetic Inheritance Patterns, Disorders Associated with Specific Genes, Such as Sickle Cell Disease, Hemophilia, and Cystic Fibrosis, Chromosome Disorders, Such as Down Syndrome, Fragile X Syndrome, and Turner Syndrome, and Complex Diseases and Disorders Resulting from the Interaction of Environmental and Genetic Factors, Such as Allergies, Cancer, and Obesity

Along with Facts about Genetic Testing, Suggestions for Parents of Children with Special Needs, Reports on Current Research Initiatives, a Glossary of Genetic Terminology, and Resources for Additional Help and Information

Edited by Sandra J. Judd. 600 pages. 2010. 978-0-7808-1076-1.

Head Trauma Sourcebook

Basic Information for the Layperson about Open-Head and Closed-Head Injuries, Treatment Advances, Recovery, and Rehabilitation

Along with Reports on Current Research Initiatives

Edited by Karen Bellenir. 414 pages. 1997. 978-0-7808-0208-7.

Headache Sourcebook

Basic Consumer Health Information about Migraine, Tension, Cluster, Rebound and Other Types of Headaches, with Facts about

the Cause and Prevention of Headaches, the Effects of Stress and the Environment, Headaches during Pregnancy and Menopause, and Childhood Headaches

Along with a Glossary and Other Resources for Additional Help and Information

Edited by Dawn D. Matthews. 342 pages. 2002. 978-0-7808-0337-4.

"Highly recommended for academic and medical reference collections."
—*Library Bookwatch, Sep '02*

SEE ALSO *Pain Sourcebook, 3rd Edition*

Healthy Aging Sourcebook

Basic Consumer Health Information about Maintaining Health through the Aging Process, Including Advice on Nutrition, Exercise, and Sleep, Help in Making Decisions about Midlife Issues and Retirement, and Guidance Concerning Practical and Informed Choices in Health Consumerism

Along with Data Concerning the Theories of Aging, Different Experiences in Aging by Minority Groups, and Facts about Aging Now and Aging in the Future; and Featuring a Glossary, a Guide to Consumer Help, Additional Suggested Reading, and Practical Resource Directory

Edited by Jenifer Swanson. 537 pages. 1999. 978-0-7808-0390-9.

"Recommended reference source."
—*Booklist, Feb '00*

SEE ALSO *Adult Health Sourcebook, Physical and Mental Issues in Aging Sourcebook*

Healthy Children Sourcebook

Basic Consumer Health Information about the Physical and Mental Development of Children between the Ages of 3 and 12, Including Routine Health Care, Preventative Health Services, Safety and First Aid, Healthy Sleep, Dental Care, Nutrition, and Fitness, and Featuring Parenting Tips on Such Topics as Bedwetting, Choosing Day Care, Monitoring TV and Other Media, and Establishing a Foundation for Substance Abuse Prevention

Along with a Glossary of Commonly Used Pediatric Terms and Resources for Additional Help and Information.

Edited by Chad T. Kimball. 624 pages. 2003. 978-0-7808-0247-6.

"Should be required reading for parents and teachers."
—*E-Streams, Jun '04*

"It is hard to imagine that any other single resource exists that would provide such a comprehensive guide of timely information on health promotion and disease prevention for children aged 3 to 12."
—*American Reference Books Annual, 2004*

"This easy-to-read volume is a tremendous resource."
—*AORN Journal, May '05*

SEE ALSO Childhood Diseases and Disorders Sourcebook, 2nd Edition

---

Healthy Heart Sourcebook for Women

Basic Consumer Health Information about Cardiac Issues Specific to Women, Including Facts about Major Risk Factors and Prevention, Treatment and Control Strategies, and Important Dietary Issues

Along with a Special Section Regarding the Pros and Cons of Hormone Replacement Therapy and Its Impact on Heart Health, and Additional Help, Including Recipes, a Glossary, and a Directory of Resources

Edited by Dawn D. Matthews. 321 pages. 2000. 978-0-7808-0329-9.

"A good reference source and recommended for all public, academic, medical, and hospital libraries."
—*Medical Reference Services Quarterly, Summer '01*

"Contains very important information about coronary artery disease that all women should know. The information is current and presented in an easy-to-read format. The book will make a good addition to any library."
—*American Medical Writers Association Journal, Summer '00*

SEE ALSO Cardiovascular Diseases and Disorders Sourcebook, 4th Edition, Women's Health Concerns Sourcebook, 3rd Edition

---

Hepatitis Sourcebook

Basic Consumer Health Information about Hepatitis A, Hepatitis B, Hepatitis C, and Other Forms of Hepatitis, Including Autoimmune Hepatitis, Alcoholic Hepatitis, Nonalcoholic Steatohepatitis, and Toxic Hepatitis, with Facts about Risk Factors, Screening Methods, Diagnostic Tests, and Treatment Options

Along with Information on Liver Health, Tips for People Living with Chronic Hepatitis, Reports on Current Research Initiatives, a Glossary of Terms Related to Hepatitis, and a Directory of Sources for Further Help and Information

Edited by Sandra J. Judd. 570 pages. 2006. 978-0-7808-0749-5.

"The breadth of information found in this one book would not be readily found in another source. Highly recommended."
—*American Reference Books Annual, 2006*

SEE ALSO Contagious Diseases Sourcebook, 2nd Edition

Household Safety Sourcebook

Basic Consumer Health Information about Household Safety, Including Information about Poisons, Chemicals, Fire, and Water Hazards in the Home

Along with Advice about the Safe Use of Home Maintenance Equipment, Choosing Toys and Nursery Furniture, Holiday and Recreation Safety, a Glossary, and Resources for Further Help and Information

Edited by Dawn D. Matthews. 587 pages. 2002. 978-0-7808-0338-1.

"As a sourcebook on household safety this book meets its mark. It is encyclopedic in scope and covers a wide range of safety issues that are commonly seen in the home."
—*E-Streams, Jul '02*

Hypertension Sourcebook

Basic Consumer Health Information about the Causes, Diagnosis, and Treatment of High Blood Pressure, with Facts about Consequences, Complications, and Co-Occurring Disorders, Such as Coronary Heart Disease, Diabetes, Stroke, Kidney Disease, and Hypertensive Retinopathy, and Issues in Blood Pressure

Control, Including Dietary Choices, Stress Management, and Medications

Along with Reports on Current Research Initiatives and Clinical Trials, a Glossary, and Resources for Additional Help and Information

Edited by Dawn D. Matthews and Karen Bellenir. 588 pages. 2004. 978-0-7808-0674-0.

"Academic, public, and medical libraries will want to add the Hypertension Sourcebook to their collections."
—E-Streams, Aug '05

"The strength of this source is the wide range of information given about hypertension."
—American Reference Books Annual, 2005

SEE ALSO Stroke Sourcebook, 2nd Edition

Immune System Disorders Sourcebook, 2nd Edition

Basic Consumer Health Information about Disorders of the Immune System, Including Immune System Function and Response, Diagnosis of Immune Disorders, Information about Inherited Immune Disease, Acquired Immune Disease, and Autoimmune Diseases, Including Primary Immune Deficiency, Acquired Immunodeficiency Syndrome (AIDS), Lupus, Multiple Sclerosis, Type 1 Diabetes, Rheumatoid Arthritis, and Graves' Disease

Along with Treatments, Tips for Coping with Immune Disorders, a Glossary, and a Directory of Additional Resources

Edited by Joyce Brennfleck Shannon. 643 pages. 2005. 978-0-7808-0748-8.

"Highly recommended for academic and public libraries."
—American Reference Books Annual, 2006

"The updated second edition is a 'must' for any consumer health library seeking a solid resource covering the treatments, symptoms, and options for immune disorder sufferers... An excellent guide."
—MBR Bookwatch, Jan '06

SEE ALSO AIDS Sourcebook, 4th Edition, Arthritis Sourcebook, 3rd Edition

Infant and Toddler Health Sourcebook

Basic Consumer Health Information about the Physical and Mental Development of Newborns, Infants, and Toddlers, Including Neonatal Concerns, Nutrition Recommendations, Immunization Schedules, Common Pediatric Disorders, Assessments and Milestones, Safety Tips, and Advice for Parents and Other Caregivers

Along with a Glossary of Terms and Resource Listings for Additional Help

Edited by Jenifer Swanson. 570 pages. 2000. 978-0-7808-0246-9.

"As a reference for the general public, this would be useful in any library."
—E-Streams, May '01

"Recommended reference source."
—Booklist, Feb '01

Infectious Diseases Sourcebook

Basic Consumer Health Information about Non-Contagious Bacterial, Viral, Prion, Fungal, and Parasitic Diseases Spread by Food and Water, Insects and Animals, or Environmental Contact, Including Botulism, E. Coli, Encephalitis, Legionnaires' Disease, Lyme Disease, Malaria, Plague, Rabies, Salmonella, Tetanus, and Others, and Facts about Newly Emerging Diseases, Such as Hantavirus, Mad Cow Disease, Monkeypox, and West Nile Virus

Along with Information about Preventing Disease Transmission, the Threat of Bioterrorism, and Current Research Initiatives, with a Glossary and Directory of Resources for More Information

Edited by Karen Bellenir. 610 pages. 2004. 978-0-7808-0675-7.

"This reference continues the excellent tradition of the Health Reference Series in consolidating a wealth of information on a selected topic into a format that is easy to use and accessible to the general public."
—American Reference Books Annual, 2005

"Recommended for public and academic libraries."
—E-Streams, Jan '05

SEE ALSO Environmental Health Sourcebook, 3rd Edition

Injury and Trauma Sourcebook

Basic Consumer Health Information about the Impact of Injury, the Diagnosis and Treatment of Common and Traumatic Injuries, Emergency Care, and Specific Injuries Related to Home, Community, Workplace, Transportation, and Recreation

Along with Guidelines for Injury Prevention, a Glossary, and a Directory of Additional Resources

Edited by Joyce Brennfleck Shannon. 675 pages. 2002. 978-0-7808-0421-0.

"Practitioners should be aware of guides such as this in order to facilitate their use by patients and their families."
—*Doody's Health Sciences Book Review Journal, Sep-Oct '02*

"Recommended reference source."
—*Booklist, Sep '02*

"Highly recommended for academic and medical reference collections."
—*Library Bookwatch, Sep '02*

SEE ALSO *Emergency Medical Services Sourcebook, Sports Injuries Sourcebook, 3rd Edition*

▓

Learning Disabilities Sourcebook, 3rd Edition

Basic Consumer Health Information about Dyslexia, Auditory and Visual Processing Disorders, Communication Disorders, Dyscalculia, Dysgraphia, and Other Conditions That Impede Learning, Including Attention Deficit/ Hyperactivity Disorder, Autism Spectrum Disorders, Hearing and Visual Impairments, Chromosome-Based Disorders, and Brain Injury

Along with Facts about Brain Function, Assessment, Therapy and Remediation, Accommodations, Assistive Technology, Legal Protections, and Tips about Family Life, School Transitions, and Employment Strategies, a Glossary of Related Terms, and Directories of Additional Resources

Edited by Joyce Brennfleck Shannon. 613 pages. 2009. 978-0-7808-1039-6.

"Intended to be a starting point for people who need to know about learning disabilities. Each chapter on a specific disability includes readable,

well-organized descriptions... The book is well indexed and a glossary is included. Chapters on organizations and helpful websites will aid the reader who needs more information."
—*American Reference Books Annual, 2009*

"This book provides the necessary information to better understand learning disabilities and work with children who have them... It would be difficult to find another book that so comprehensively explains learning disabilities without becoming incomprehensible to the average parent who needs this information."
—*Doody's Review Service, 2009*

SEE ALSO *Attention Deficit Disorder Sourcebook, Autism and Pervasive Developmental Disorders Sourcebook*

▓

Leukemia Sourcebook

Basic Consumer Health Information about Adult and Childhood Leukemias, Including Acute Lymphocytic Leukemia (ALL), Chronic Lymphocytic Leukemia (CLL), Acute Myelogenous Leukemia (AML), Chronic Myelogenous Leukemia (CML), and Hairy Cell Leukemia, and Treatments Such as Chemotherapy, Radiation Therapy, Peripheral Blood Stem Cell and Marrow Transplantation, and Immunotherapy

Along with Tips for Life During and After Treatment, a Glossary, and Directories of Additional Resources

Edited by Joyce Brennfleck Shannon. 564 pages. 2003. 978-0-7808-0627-6.

"Unlike other medical books for the layperson... the language does not talk down to the reader... This volume is highly recommended for all libraries."
—*American Reference Books Annual, 2004*

"A fine title which ranges from diagnosis to alternative treatments, staging, and tips for life during and after diagnosis."
—*The Bookwatch, Dec '03*

SEE ALSO *Blood & Circulatory Disorders Sourcebook, 3rd Edition, Cancer Sourcebook, 5th Edition*

▓

Liver Disorders Sourcebook

Basic Consumer Health Information about the Liver and How It Works; Liver Diseases, Including Cancer, Cirrhosis, Hepatitis, and

Toxic and Drug Related Diseases; Tips for Maintaining a Healthy Liver; Laboratory Tests, Radiology Tests, and Facts about Liver Transplantation

Along with a Section on Support Groups, a Glossary, and Resource Listings

Edited by Joyce Brennfleck Shannon. 580 pages. 2000. 978-0-7808-0383-1.

"This title is recommended for health sciences and public libraries with consumer health collections."
—E-Streams, Oct '00

"Recommended reference source."
—Booklist, Jun '00

SEE ALSO *Gastrointestinal Diseases and Disorders Sourcebook, 2nd Edition, Hepatitis Sourcebook*

Lung Disorders Sourcebook

Basic Consumer Health Information about Emphysema, Pneumonia, Tuberculosis, Asthma, Cystic Fibrosis, and Other Lung Disorders, Including Facts about Diagnostic Procedures, Treatment Strategies, Disease Prevention Efforts, and Such Risk Factors as Smoking, Air Pollution, and Exposure to Asbestos, Radon, and Other Agents

Along with a Glossary and Resources for Additional Help and Information

Edited by Dawn D. Matthews. 657 pages. 2002. 978-0-7808-0339-8.

"Highly recommended for academic and medical reference collections."
—Library Bookwatch, Sep '02

SEE ALSO *Asthma Sourcebook, 2nd Edition, Respiratory Disorders Sourcebook, 2nd Edition*

Medical Tests Sourcebook, 3rd Edition

Basic Consumer Health Information about X-Rays, Blood Tests, Stool and Urine Tests, Biopsies, Mammography, Endoscopic Procedures, Ultrasound Exams, Computed Tomography, Magnetic Resonance Imaging (MRI), Nuclear Medicine, Genetic Testing, Home-Use Tests, and More

Along with Facts about Preventive Care and Screening Test Guidelines, Screening and

---

Assessment Tests Associated with Such Specific Concerns as Cancer, Heart Disease, Allergies, Diabetes, Thyroid Disfunction, and Infertility, a Glossary of Related Terms, and a Directory of Resources for Additional Help and Information

Edited by Karen Bellenir. 627 pages. 2008. 978-0-7808-1040-2

"This volume has a wide scope that makes it useful... Can be a valuable reference guide."
—American Reference Books Annual, 2009

"Would be a valuable contribution to any consumer health or public library."
—Doody's Book Review Service, 2009

Men's Health Concerns Sourcebook, 3rd Edition

Basic Consumer Health Information about Wellness in Men and Gender-Related Differences in Health, With Facts about Heart Disease, Cancer, Traumatic Injury, and Other Leading Causes of Death in Men, Reproductive Concerns, Sexual Dysfunction, Disorders of the Prostate, Penis, and Testes, Sex-Linked Genetic Disorders, and Other Medical and Mental Concerns of Men

Along with Statistical Data, a Glossary of Related Terms, and a Directory of Resources for Additional Information

Edited by Sandra J. Judd. 632 pages. 2009. 978-0-7808-1033-4.

"A good addition to any reference shelf in academic, consumer health, or hospital libraries."
—ARBAOnline, Oct '09

SEE ALSO *Prostate and Urological Disorders Sourcebook*

Mental Health Disorders Sourcebook, 4th Edition

Basic Consumer Health Information about the Causes and Symptoms of Mental Health Problems, Including Depression, Bipolar Disorder, Anxiety Disorders, Posttraumatic Stress Disorder, Obsessive-Compulsive Disorder, Eating Disorders, Addictions, and Personality and Psychotic Disorders

Along with Information about Medications and Treatments, Mental Health Concerns in

Children, Adolescents, and Adults, Tips on Living with Mental Health Disorders, a Glossary of Related Terms, and a Directory of Resources for Additional Help and Information

Edited by Amy L. Sutton. 680 pages. 2009. 978-0-7808-1041-9.

"Mental health concerns are presented in everyday language and intended for patients and their families as well as the general public... This resource is comprehensive and up to date... The easy-to-understand writing style helps to facilitate assimilation of needed facts and specifics on often challenging topics."
—*ARBAOnline, Oct '09*

"No health collection should be without this resource, which will reach into many a general lending library as well."
—*Internet Bookwatch, Oct '09*

SEE ALSO Depression Sourcebook, 2nd Edition, Stress-Related Disorders Sourcebook, 2nd Edition

---

Mental Retardation Sourcebook

Basic Consumer Health Information about Mental Retardation and Its Causes, Including Down Syndrome, Fetal Alcohol Syndrome, Fragile X Syndrome, Genetic Conditions, Injury, and Environmental Sources

Along with Preventive Strategies, Parenting Issues, Educational Implications, Health Care Needs, Employment and Economic Matters, Legal Issues, a Glossary, and a Resource Listing for Additional Help and Information

Edited by Joyce Brennfleck Shannon. 627 pages. 2000. 978-0-7808-0377-0.

"Public libraries will find the book useful for reference and as a beginning research point for students, parents, and caregivers."
—*American Reference Books Annual, 2001*

"The strength of this work is that it compiles many basic fact sheets and addresses for further information in one volume. It is intended and suitable for the general public."
—*E-Streams, Nov '00*

"An invaluable overview."
—*Reviewer's Bookwatch, Jul '00*

Movement Disorders Sourcebook, 2nd Edition

Basic Consumer Health Information about the Symptoms and Causes of Movement Disorders, Including Parkinson Disease, Amyotrophic Lateral Sclerosis, Cerebral Palsy, Muscular Dystrophy, Multiple Sclerosis, Myasthenia, Myoclonus, Spina Bifida, Dystonia, Essential Tremor, Choreatic Disorders, Huntington Disease, Tourette Syndrome, and Other Disorders That Cause Slowed, Absent, or Excessive Movements

Along with Information about Surgical and Nonsurgical Interventions, Physical Therapies, Strategies for Independent Living, a Glossary of Related Terms, and a Directory of Resources for Additional Help and Information

Edited by Amy L. Sutton. 618 pages. 2009. 978-0-7808-1034-1.

"The second updated edition of Movement Disorders Sourcebook is a winner, providing the latest research and health findings on all kinds of movement disorders in children and adults... a top pick for any health or general lending library's health reference collection."
—*California Bookwatch, Aug '09*

SEE ALSO Muscular Dystrophy Sourcebook

Multiple Sclerosis Sourcebook

Basic Consumer Health Information about Multiple Sclerosis (MS) and Its Effects on Mobility, Vision, Bladder Function, Speech, Swallowing, and Cognition, Including Facts about Risk Factors, Causes, Diagnostic Procedures, Pain Management, Drug Treatments, and Physical and Occupational Therapies

Along with Guidelines for Nutrition and Exercise, Tips on Choosing Assistive Equipment, Information about Disability, Work, Financial, and Legal Issues, a Glossary of Related Terms, and a Directory of Additional Resources

Edited by Joyce Brennfleck Shannon. 553 pages. 2007. 978-0-7808-0998-7.

Muscular Dystrophy Sourcebook

Basic Consumer Health Information about Congenital, Childhood-Onset, and Adult-Onset

Forms of Muscular Dystrophy, Such as Duchenne, Becker, Emery-Dreifuss, Distal, Limb-Girdle, Facioscapulohumeral (FSHD), Myotonic, and Ophthalmoplegic Muscular Dystrophies, Including Facts about Diagnostic Tests, Medical and Physical Therapies, Management of Co-Occurring Conditions, and Parenting Guidelines

Along with Practical Tips for Home Care, a Glossary, and Directories of Additional Resources

Edited by Joyce Brennfleck Shannon. 552 pages. 2004. 978-0-7808-0676-4.

"This book is highly recommended for public and academic libraries as well as health care offices that support the information needs of patients and their families."
—E-Streams, Apr '05

"Excellent reference."
—The Bookwatch, Jan '05

SEE ALSO Movement Disorders Sourcebook, 2nd Edition

Obesity Sourcebook

Basic Consumer Health Information about Diseases and Other Problems Associated with Obesity, and Including Facts about Risk Factors, Prevention Issues, and Management Approaches

Along with Statistical and Demographic Data, Information about Special Populations, Research Updates, a Glossary, and Source Listings for Further Help and Information

Edited by Wilma Caldwell and Chad T. Kimball. 360 pages. 2001. 978-0-7808-0333-6.

"The book synthesizes the reliable medical literature on obesity into one easy-to-read and useful resource for the general public."
—American Reference Books Annual, 2002

"Well suited for the health reference collection of a public library or an academic health science library that serves the general population."
—E-Streams, Sep '01

Osteoporosis Sourcebook

Basic Consumer Health Information about Primary and Secondary Osteoporosis and Juvenile Osteoporosis and Related Conditions, Including Fibrous Dysplasia, Gaucher Disease, Hyperthyroidism, Hypophosphatasia,

Myeloma, Osteopetrosis, Osteogenesis Imperfecta, and Paget's Disease

Along with Information about Risk Factors, Treatments, Traditional and Non-Traditional Pain Management, a Glossary of Related Terms, and a Directory of Resources

Edited by Allan R. Cook. 568 pages. 2001. 978-0-7808-0239-1.

"This resource is recommended as a great reference source for public, health, and academic libraries, and is another triumph for the editors of Omnigraphics."
—American Reference Books Annual, 2002

"Will prove valuable to any library seeking to maintain a current, comprehensive reference collection of health resources... From prevention to treatment and associated conditions, this provides an excellent survey."
—The Bookwatch, Aug '01

SEE ALSO Healthy Aging Sourcebook, Women's Health Concerns Sourcebook, 3rd Edition

Pain Sourcebook, 3rd Edition

Basic Consumer Health Information about Acute and Chronic Pain, Including Nerve Pain, Bone Pain, Muscle Pain, Cancer Pain, and Disorders Characterized by Pain, Such as Arthritis, Temporomandibular Muscle and Joint (TMJ) Disorder, Carpal Tunnel Syndrome, Headaches, Heartburn, Sciatica, and Shingles, and Facts about Diagnostic Tests and Treatment Options for Pain, Including Over-the-Counter and Prescription Drugs, Physical Rehabilitation, Injection and Infusion Therapies, Implantable Technologies, and Complementary Medicine

Along with Tips for Living with Pain, a Glossary of Related Terms, and a Directory of Additional Resources

Edited by Joyce Brennfleck Shannon. 644 pages. 2008. 978-0-7808-1006-8.

"Excellent for ready-reference users and can be used for beginning students in health fields... appropriate for the consumer health collection in both public and academic libraries."
—American Reference Books Annual, 2009

SEE ALSO Arthritis Sourcebook, 3rd Edition; Back and Neck Sourcebook, 2nd Edition;

Headache Sourcebook; Sports Injuries Sourcebook, 3rd Edition

Pediatric Cancer Sourcebook

Basic Consumer Health Information about Leukemias, Brain Tumors, Sarcomas, Lymphomas, and Other Cancers in Infants, Children, and Adolescents, Including Descriptions of Cancers, Treatments, and Coping Strategies

Along with Suggestions for Parents, Caregivers, and Concerned Relatives, a Glossary of Cancer Terms, and Resource Listings

Edited by Edward J. Prucha. 575 pages. 1999. 978-0-7808-0245-2.

"An excellent source of information. Recommended for public, hospital, and health science libraries with consumer health collections."
—*E-Streams, Jun '00*

"A valuable addition to all libraries specializing in health services and many public libraries."
—*American Reference Books Annual, 2000*

SEE ALSO *Childhood Diseases and Disorders Sourcebook, 2nd Edition, Healthy Children Sourcebook*

Physical and Mental Issues in Aging Sourcebook

Basic Consumer Health Information on Physical and Mental Disorders Associated with the Aging Process, Including Concerns about Cardiovascular Disease, Pulmonary Disease, Oral Health, Digestive Disorders, Musculoskeletal and Skin Disorders, Metabolic Changes, Sexual and Reproductive Issues, and Changes in Vision, Hearing, and Other Senses

Along with Data about Longevity and Causes of Death, Information on Acute and Chronic Pain, Descriptions of Mental Concerns, a Glossary of Terms, and Resource Listings for Additional Help

Edited by Jenifer Swanson. 660 pages. 1999. 978-0-7808-0233-9.

"This is a treasure of health information for the layperson."
—*CHOICE Health Sciences Supplement, May '00*

"Recommended for public libraries."
—*American Reference Books Annual, 2000*

SEE ALSO *Healthy Aging Sourcebook*

Podiatry Sourcebook, 2nd Edition

Basic Consumer Health Information about Disorders, Diseases, and Deformities that Affect the Foot and Ankle, Including Sprains, Corns, Calluses, Bunions, Plantar Warts, Plantar Fasciitis, Neuromas, Clubfoot, Flat Feet, Achilles Tendonitis, and Much More

Along with Information about Selecting a Foot Care Specialist, Foot Fitness, Shoes and Socks, Diagnostic Tests and Corrective Procedures, Financial Assistance for Corrective Devices, a Glossary of Related Terms, and a Directory of Resources for Additional Help and Information

Edited by Ivy L. Alexander. 516 pages. 2007. 978-0-7808-0944-4.

"An excellent resource... Although there have been various types of 'foot books' published in the past, none are as comprehensive as this one. 5 Stars (out of 5)!"
—*Doody's Review Service, 2007*

"Perfect for both health libraries and general-interest lending collections."
—*Internet Bookwatch, Jul '07*

Pregnancy and Birth Sourcebook, 3rd Edition

Basic Consumer Health Information about Pregnancy and Fetal Development, Including Facts about Fertility and Conception, Physical and Emotional Changes during Pregnancy, Prenatal Care and Diagnostic Tests, High-Risk Pregnancies and Complications, Labor, Delivery, and the Postpartum Period

Along with Tips on Maintaining Health and Wellness during Pregnancy and Caring for Newborn Infants, a Glossary of Related Terms, and Directories of Resources for Additional Help and Information

Edited by Amy L. Sutton. 645 pages. 2009. 978-0-7808-1074-7.

SEE ALSO *Breastfeeding Sourcebook, Congenital Disorders Sourcebook, 2nd Edition, Family Planning Sourcebook, Women's Health Concerns Sourcebook, 3rd Edition*

Prostate and Urological Disorders Sourcebook

Basic Consumer Health Information about Urogenital and Sexual Disorders in Men, Including Prostate and Other Andrological Cancers, Prostatitis, Benign Prostatic Hyperplasia, Testicular and Penile Trauma, Cryptorchidism, Peyronie Disease, Erectile Dysfunction, and Male Factor Infertility, and Facts about Commonly Used Tests and Procedures, Such as Prostatectomy, Vasectomy, Vasectomy Reversal, Penile Implants, and Semen Analysis

Along with a Glossary of Andrological Terms and a Directory of Resources for Additional Information

Edited by Karen Bellenir. 604 pages. 2006. 978-0-7808-0797-6.

"Certain to be a popular pick among library reference holdings... No prior knowledge is assumed for any of the conditions or terms herein, making it a most accessible general-interest reference."
—California Bookwatch, Apr '06

SEE ALSO *Men's Health Concerns Sourcebook, 3rd Edition, Urinary Tract and Kidney Diseases and Disorders Sourcebook, 2nd Edition*

Prostate Cancer Sourcebook

Basic Consumer Health Information about Prostate Cancer, Including Information about the Associated Risk Factors, Detection, Diagnosis, and Treatment of Prostate Cancer

Along with Information on Non-Malignant Prostate Conditions, and Featuring a Section Listing Support and Treatment Centers and a Glossary of Related Terms

Edited by Dawn D. Matthews. 340 pages. 2001. 978-0-7808-0324-4.

"Recommended reference source."
—Booklist, Jan '02

"A valuable resource for health care consumers seeking information on the subject... All text is written in a clear, easy-to-understand language that avoids technical jargon. Any library that collects consumer health resources would strengthen their collection with the addition of the Prostate Cancer Sourcebook."
—American Reference Books Annual, 2002

SEE ALSO *Cancer Sourcebook, 5th Edition, Men's Health Concerns Sourcebook, 3rd Edition*

Rehabilitation Sourcebook

Basic Consumer Health Information about Rehabilitation for People Recovering from Heart Surgery, Spinal Cord Injury, Stroke, Orthopedic Impairments, Amputation, Pulmonary Impairments, Traumatic Injury, and More, Including Physical Therapy, Occupational Therapy, Speech/Language Therapy, Massage Therapy, Dance Therapy, Art Therapy, and Recreational Therapy

Along with Information on Assistive and Adaptive Devices, a Glossary, and Resources for Additional Help and Information

Edited by Dawn D. Matthews. 519 pages. 2000. 978-0-7808-0236-0.

"This is an excellent resource for public library reference and health collections."
—American Reference Books Annual, 2001

"Recommended reference source."
—Booklist, May '00

Respiratory Disorders Sourcebook, 2nd Edition

Basic Consumer Health Information about Infectious, Inflammatory, and Chronic Conditions Affecting the Lungs and Respiratory System, Including Pneumonia, Bronchitis, Influenza, Tuberculosis, Sarcoidosis, Asthma, Cystic Fibrosis, Chronic Obstructive Pulmonary Disease, Lung Abscesses, Pulmonary Embolism, Occupational Lung Diseases, and Other Bacterial, Viral, and Fungal Infections

Along with Facts about the Structure and Function of the Lungs and Airways, Methods of Diagnosing Respiratory Disorders, and Treatment and Rehabilitation Options, a Glossary of Related Terms, and a Directory of Resources for Additional Help and Information

Edited by Sandra L. Judd. 638 pages. 2008. 978-0-7808-1007-5.

"An excellent book for patients, their families, or for those who are just curious about respiratory disease. Public libraries and physician offices would find this a valuable resource as well. 4 Stars! (out of 5)"
—Doody's Review Service, 2009

"A great addition for public and school libraries because it provides concise health information... readers can start with this reference source and get satisfactory answers before proceeding to other medical reference tools for

more in depth information... A good guide for health education on lung disorders."
—*American Reference Books Annual, 2009*

SEE ALSO *Asthma Sourcebook, 2nd Edition, Lung Disorders Sourcebook*

■

Sexually Transmitted Diseases Sourcebook, 4th Edition

Basic Consumer Health Information about Chlamydial Infections, Gonorrhea, Hepatitis, Herpes, HIV/AIDS, Human Papillomavirus, Pubic Lice, Scabies, Syphilis, Trichomoniasis, Vaginal Infections, and Other Sexually Transmitted Diseases, Including Facts about Risk Factors, Symptoms, Diagnosis, Treatment, and the Prevention of Sexually Transmitted Infections

Along with Updates on Current Research Initiatives, a Glossary of Related Terms, and Resources for Additional Help and Information

Edited by Laura Larsen. 623 pages. 2009. 978-0-7808-1073-0.

"Extremely beneficial... The question-and-answer format along with the index and table of contents make this well-organized resource extremely easy to reference, read, and comprehend... an invaluable medical reference source for lay readers, and a highly appropriate addition for public library collections, health clinics, and any library with a consumer health collection"
—*ARBAOnline, Oct '09*

SEE ALSO *AIDS Sourcebook, 4th Edition, Contagious Diseases Sourcebook, 2nd Edition, Men's Health Concerns Sourcebook, 3rd Edition, Women's Health Concerns Sourcebook, 3rd Edition*

■

Sleep Disorders Sourcebook, 3rd Edition

Basic Consumer Health Information about Sleep Disorders, Including Insomnia, Sleep Apnea and Snoring, Jet Lag and Other Circadian Rhythm Disorders, Narcolepsy, and Parasomnias, Such as Sleep Walking and Sleep Talking, and Featuring Facts about Other Health Problems that Affect Sleep, Why Sleep Is Necessary, How Much Sleep Is Needed, the Physical and Mental Effects of Sleep Deprivation, and Pediatric Sleep Issues

Along with Tips for Diagnosing and Treating Sleep Disorders, a Glossary of Related Terms, and a List of Resources for Additional Help and Information

Edited by Sandra J. Judd. 600 pages. 2010. 978-0-7808-1084-6.

■

Smoking Concerns Sourcebook

Basic Consumer Health Information about Nicotine Addiction and Smoking Cessation, Featuring Facts about the Health Effects of Tobacco Use, Including Lung and Other Cancers, Heart Disease, Stroke, and Respiratory Disorders, Such as Emphysema and Chronic Bronchitis

Along with Information about Smoking Prevention Programs, Suggestions for Achieving and Maintaining a Smoke-Free Lifestyle, Statistics about Tobacco Use, Reports on Current Research Initiatives, a Glossary of Related Terms, and Directories of Resources for Additional Help and Information

Edited by Karen Bellenir. 595 pages. 2004. 978-0-7808-0323-7.

"Provides everything needed for the student or general reader seeking practical details on the effects of tobacco use."
—*The Bookwatch, Mar '05*

"Public libraries and consumer health care libraries will find this work useful."
—*American Reference Books Annual, 2005*

SEE ALSO *Respiratory Disorders Sourcebook, 2nd Edition*

■

Sports Injuries Sourcebook, 3rd Edition

Basic Consumer Health Information about Sprains and Strains, Fractures, Growth Plate Injuries, Overtraining Injuries, and Injuries to the Head, Face, Shoulders, Elbows, Hands, Spinal Column, Knees, Ankles, and Feet, and with Facts about Heat-Related Illness, Steroids and Sport Supplements, Protective Equipment, Diagnostic Procedures, Treatment Options, and Rehabilitation

Along with a Glossary of Related Terms and a Directory of Resources for Additional Help and Information

Edited by Sandra J. Judd. 623 pages. 2007. 978-0-7808-0949-9.

SEE ALSO Fitness and Exercise Sourcebook, 3rd Edition, Podiatry Sourcebook, 2nd Edition

■

Stress-Related Disorders Sourcebook, 2nd Edition

Basic Consumer Health Information about Stress and Stress-Related Disorders, Including Types of Stress, Sources of Acute and Chronic Stress, the Impact of Stress on the Body's Systems, and Mental and Emotional Health Problems Associated with Stress, Such as Depression, Anxiety Disorders, Substance Abuse, Posttraumatic Stress Disorder, and Suicide

Along with Advice about Getting Help for Stress-Related Disorders, Information about Stress Management Techniques, a Glossary of Stress-Related Terms, and a Directory of Resources for Additional Help and Information

Edited by Amy L. Sutton. 608 pages. 2007. 978-0-7808-0996-3.

"Accessible to the lay reader. Highly recommended for medical and psychiatric collections."
—*Library Journal, Mar '08*

"Well-written for a general readership, the 2nd Edition of Stress-Related Disorders Sourcebook is a useful addition to the health reference literature."
—*American Reference Books Annual, 2008*

SEE ALSO Mental Health Disorders Sourcebook, 4th Edition

■

Stroke Sourcebook, 2nd Edition

Basic Consumer Health Information about Stroke, Including Ischemic, Hemorrhagic, and Mini Strokes, as Well as Risk Factors, Prevention Guidelines, Diagnostic Tests, Medications and Surgical Treatments, and Complications of Stroke

Along with Rehabilitation Techniques and Innovations, Tips on Staying Healthy and Maintaining Independence after Stroke, a Glossary of Related Terms, and a Directory of Resources for Stroke Survivors and Their Families

Edited by Amy L. Sutton. 626 pages. 2008. 978-0-7808-1035-8.

"An encyclopedic handbook on stroke that is written in a language the layperson can understand... This is one of the most helpful, readable books on stroke. This volume is highly recommended and should be in every medical, hospital and public library; in addition, every family practitioner should have a copy in his or her office."
—*American Reference Books Annual, 2009*

SEE ALSO Brain Disorders Sourcebook, 3rd Edition, Hypertension Sourcebook

■

Surgery Sourcebook, 2nd Edition

Basic Consumer Health Information about Common Inpatient and Outpatient Surgeries, Including Critical Care and Trauma, Gastrointestinal, Gynecologic and Obstetric, Cardiac and Vascular, Neurologic, Ophthalmologic, Orthopedic, Reconstructive and Cosmetic, and Other Major and Minor Surgeries

Along with Information about Anesthesia and Pain Relief Options, Risks and Complications, Postoperative Recovery Concerns, and Innovative Surgical Techniques and Tools, a Glossary of Related Terms, and a Directory of Additional Resources

Edited by Amy L. Sutton. 645 pages. 2008. 978-0-7808-1004-4.

"Large public libraries and medical libraries would benefit from this material in their reference collections."
—*American Reference Books Annual, 2009*

SEE ALSO Cosmetic and Reconstructive Surgery Sourcebook, 2nd Edition

■

Thyroid Disorders Sourcebook

Basic Consumer Health Information about Disorders of the Thyroid and Parathyroid Glands, Including Hypothyroidism, Hyperthyroidism, Graves Disease, Hashimoto Thyroiditis, Thyroid Cancer, and Parathyroid Disorders, Featuring Facts about Symptoms, Risk Factors, Tests, and Treatments

Along with Information about the Effects of Thyroid Imbalance on Other Body Systems, Environmental Factors That Affect the Thyroid Gland, a Glossary, and a Directory of Additional Resources

Edited by Joyce Brennfleck Shannon. 573 pages. 2005. 978-0-7808-0745-7.

"Recommended for consumer health collections."
—*American Reference Books Annual, 2006*

"Highly recommended pick for Basic Consumer health reference holdings at all levels."
—*The Bookwatch, Aug '05*

SEE ALSO *Endocrine and Metabolic Disorders Sourcebook, 2nd Edition*

■

Transplantation Sourcebook
Basic Consumer Health Information about Organ and Tissue Transplantation, Including Physical and Financial Preparations, Procedures and Issues Relating to Specific Solid Organ and Tissue Transplants, Rehabilitation, Pediatric Transplant Information, the Future of Transplantation, and Organ and Tissue Donation

Along with a Glossary and Listings of Additional Resources

Edited by Joyce Brennfleck Shannon. 610 pages. 2002. 978-0-7808-0322-0.

"Recommended for libraries with an interest in offering consumer health information."
—*E-Streams, Jul '02*

"This is a unique and valuable resource for patients facing transplantation and their families."
—*Doody's Review Service, Jun '02*

■

Traveler's Health Sourcebook
Basic Consumer Health Information for Travelers, Including Physical and Medical Preparations, Transportation Health and Safety, Essential Information about Food and Water, Sun Exposure, Insect and Snake Bites, Camping and Wilderness Medicine, and Travel with Physical or Medical Disabilities

Along with International Travel Tips, Vaccination Recommendations, Geographical Health Issues, Disease Risks, a Glossary, and a Listing of Additional Resources

Edited by Joyce Brennfleck Shannon. 619 pages. 2000. 978-0-7808-0384-8.

"Recommended reference source."
—*Booklist, Feb '01*

"This book is recommended for any public library, any travel collection, and especially any collection for the physically disabled."
—*American Reference Books Annual, 2001*

SEE ALSO *Worldwide Health Sourcebook*

■

Urinary Tract and Kidney Diseases and Disorders Sourcebook, 2nd Edition
Basic Consumer Health Information about the Urinary System, Including the Bladder, Urethra, Ureters, and Kidneys, with Facts about Urinary Tract Infections, Incontinence, Congenital Disorders, Kidney Stones, Cancers of the Urinary Tract and Kidneys, Kidney Failure, Dialysis, and Kidney Transplantation

Along with Statistical and Demographic Information, Reports on Current Research in Kidney and Urologic Health, a Summary of Commonly Used Diagnostic Tests, a Glossary of Related Terms, and a Directory of Resources for Additional Help and Information

Edited by Ivy L. Alexander. 621 pages. 2005. 978-0-7808-0750-1.

"A good choice for a consumer health information library or for a medical library needing information to refer to their patients."
—*American Reference Books Annual, 2006*

SEE ALSO *Prostate and Urological Disorders Sourcebook*

■

Vegetarian Sourcebook
Basic Consumer Health Information about Vegetarian Diets, Lifestyle, and Philosophy, Including Definitions of Vegetarianism and Veganism, Tips about Adopting Vegetarianism, Creating a Vegetarian Pantry, and Meeting Nutritional Needs of Vegetarians, with Facts Regarding Vegetarianism's Effect on Pregnant and Lactating Women, Children, Athletes, and Senior Citizens

Along with a Glossary of Commonly Used Vegetarian Terms and Resources for Additional Help and Information

Edited by Chad T. Kimball. 337 pages. 2002. 978-0-7808-0439-5.

"Organizes into one concise volume the answers to the most common questions concerning vegetarian diets and lifestyles. This title is recommended for public and secondary school libraries."

—E-Streams, Apr '03

"Invaluable reference for public and school library collections alike."

—Library Bookwatch, Apr '03

"The articles in this volume are easy to read and come from authoritative sources. The book does not necessarily support the vegetarian diet but instead provides the pros and cons of this important decision... Recommended for public libraries and consumer health libraries."

—American Reference Books Annual, 2003

SEE ALSO Diet and Nutrition Sourcebook, 3rd Edition

Women's Health Concerns Sourcebook, 3rd Edition

Basic Consumer Health Information about Issues and Trends in Women's Health and Health Conditions of Special Concern to Women, Including Endometriosis, Uterine Fibroids, Menstrual Irregularities, Menopause, Sexual Dysfunction, Infertility, Cancer in Women, and Other Such Chronic Disorders as Lupus, Fibromyalgia, and Thyroid Disease

Along with Statistical Data, Tips for Maintaining Wellness, a Glossary, and a Directory of Resources for Further Help and Information

Edited by Sandra J. Judd. 679 pages. 2009. 978-0-7808-1036-5.

"This useful resource provides information about a wide range of topics that will help women understand their bodies, prevent or treat disease, and maintain health... A detailed index helps readers locate information. This is a useful addition to public and consumer health library collections"

—ARBAOnline, Jun '09

SEE ALSO Breast Cancer Sourcebook, 3rd Edition, Cancer Sourcebook for Women, 4th Edition, Healthy Heart Sourcebook for Women

Workplace Health and Safety Sourcebook

Basic Consumer Health Information about Workplace Health and Safety, Including the Effect of Workplace Hazards on the Lungs,

Skin, Heart, Ears, Eyes, Brain, Reproductive Organs, Musculoskeletal System, and Other Organs and Body Parts

Along with Information about Occupational Cancer, Personal Protective Equipment, Toxic and Hazardous Chemicals, Child Labor, Stress, and Workplace Violence

Edited by Chad T. Kimball. 610 pages. 2000. 978-0-7808-0231-5.

"As a reference for the general public, this would be useful in any library."

—E-Streams, Jun '01

"Provides helpful information for primary care physicians and other caregivers interested in occupational medicine... General readers; professionals."

—CHOICE, May '01

Worldwide Health Sourcebook

Basic Information about Global Health Issues, Including Malnutrition, Reproductive Health, Disease Dispersion and Prevention, Emerging Diseases, Risky Health Behaviors, and the Leading Causes of Death

Along with Global Health Concerns for Children, Women, and the Elderly, Mental Health Issues, Research and Technology Advancements, and Economic, Environmental, and Political Health Implications, a Glossary, and a Resource Listing for Additional Help and Information

Edited by Joyce Brennfleck Shannon. 597 pages. 2001. 978-0-7808-0330-5.

"Named an Outstanding Academic Title."

—CHOICE, Jan '02

"Yet another handy but also unique compilation in the extensive Health Reference Series, this is a useful work because many of the international publications reprinted or excerpted are not readily available. Highly recommended."

—CHOICE, Nov '01

SEE ALSO Traveler's Health Sourcebook

Teen Health Series
Complete Catalog
List price $69 per volume. School and library price $62 per volume.

Abuse and Violence Information for Teens
Health Tips about the Causes and Consequences of Abusive and Violent Behavior
Including Facts about the Types of Abuse and Violence, the Warning Signs of Abusive and Violent Behavior, Health Concerns of Victims, and Getting Help and Staying Safe

Edited by Sandra Augustyn Lawton. 411 pages. 2008. 978-0-7808-1008-2.

"A useful resource for schools and organizations providing services to teens and may also be a starting point in research projects."
—*Reference and Research Book News, Aug '08*

"Violence is a serious problem for teens... This resource gives teens the information they need to face potential threats and get help—either for themselves or for their friends."
—*American Reference Books Annual, 2009*

Accident and Safety Information for Teens
Health Tips about Medical Emergencies, Traumatic Injuries, and Disaster Preparedness
Including Facts about Motor Vehicle Accidents, Burns, Poisoning, Firearms, Natural Disasters, National Security Threats, and More

Edited by Karen Bellenir. 420 pages. 2008. 978-0-7808-1046-4.

"Aimed at teenage audiences, this guide provides practical information for handling a comprehensive list of emergencies, from sport injuries and auto accidents to alcohol poisoning and natural disasters."
—*Library Journal, Apr 1, '09*

"Useful in the young adult collections of public libraries as well as high school libraries."
—*American Reference Books Annual, 2009*

SEE ALSO *Sports Injuries Information for Teens, 2nd Edition*

Alcohol Information for Teens, 2nd Edition
Health Tips about Alcohol and Alcoholism
Including Facts about Alcohol's Effects on the Body, Brain, and Behavior, the Consequences of Underage Drinking, Alcohol Abuse Prevention and Treatment, and Coping with Alcoholic Parents

Edited by Lisa Bakewell. 410 pages. 2009. 978-0-7808-1043-3.

"This handbook, written for a teenage audience, provides information on the causes, effects, and preventive measures related to alcohol abuse among teens... The chapters are quick to make a connection to their teenage reading audience. The prose is straightforward and the book lends itself to spot reading. It should be useful both for practical information and for research, and it is suitable for public and school libraries."
—*ARBAOnline, Jun '09*

SEE ALSO *Drug Information for Teens, 2nd Edition*

Allergy Information for Teens
Health Tips about Allergic Reactions Such as Anaphylaxis, Respiratory Problems, and Rashes
Including Facts about Identifying and Managing Allergies to Food, Pollen, Mold, Animals, Chemicals, Drugs, and Other Substances

Edited by Karen Bellenir. 410 pages. 2006. 978-0-7808-0799-0.

"This is a comprehensive, readable text on the subject of allergic diseases in teenagers. 5 Stars (out of 5)!"
—*Doody's Review Service, Jun '06*

"This authoritative and useful self-help title is a solid addition to YA collections, whether for personal interest or reports."
—*School Library Journal, Jul '06*

Asthma Information for Teens, 2nd Ed.
Health Tips about Managing Asthma and Related Concerns

Including Facts about Asthma Causes, Triggers and Symptoms, Diagnosis, and Treatment

Edited by Kim Wohlenhaus. 400 pages. 2010. 978-0-7808-1086-0.

Body Information for Teens
Health Tips about Maintaining Well-Being for a Lifetime

Including Facts about the Development and Functioning of the Body's Systems, Organs, and Structures and the Health Impact of Lifestyle Choices

Edited by Sandra Augustyn Lawton. 458 pages. 2007. 978-0-7808-0443-2.

Cancer Information for Teens, 2nd Edition
Health Tips about Cancer Awareness, Symptoms, Prevention, Diagnosis, and Treatment

Including Facts about Common Cancers Affecting Teens, Causes, Detection, Coping Strategies, Clinical Trials, Nutrition and Exercise, Cancer in Friends or Family, and More

Edited by Karen Bellenir and Lisa Bakewell. 445 pages. 2010. 978-0-7808-1085-3.

Complementary and Alternative Medicine Information for Teens
Health Tips about Non-Traditional and Non-Western Medical Practices

Including Information about Acupuncture, Chiropractic Medicine, Dietary and Herbal Supplements, Hypnosis, Massage Therapy, Prayer and Spirituality, Reflexology, Yoga, and More

Edited by Sandra Augustyn Lawton. 407 pages. 2007. 978-0-7808-0966-6.

"This volume covers CAM specifically for teenagers but of general use also. It should be a welcome addition to both public and academic libraries."
—*American Reference Books Annual, 2008*

"This volume provides a solid foundation for further investigation of the subject, making it useful for both public and high school libraries."
—*VOYA: Voice of Youth Advocates, Jun '07*

Diabetes Information for Teens
Health Tips about Managing Diabetes and Preventing Related Complications

Including Information about Insulin, Glucose Control, Healthy Eating, Physical Activity, and Learning to Live with Diabetes

Edited by Sandra Augustyn Lawton. 410 pages. 2006. 978-0-7808-0811-9.

"A comprehensive instructional guide for teens... some of the material may also be directed towards parents or teachers. 5 stars (out of 5)!"
—*Doody's Review Service, 2006*

"Students dealing with their own diabetes or that of a friend or family member or those writing reports on the topic will find this a valuable resource."
—*School Library Journal, Aug '06*

"This text is directed to the teen population and would be an excellent library resource for a health class or for the teacher as a reference for class preparation. It can, however, serve a much wider audience. The clinical educator on diabetes may find it valuable to educate the newly diagnosed client regardless of age. It also would be an excellent reference and education tool for a preventive medicine seminar on diabetes."
—*Physical Therapy, Mar '07*

Diet Information for Teens, 2nd Edition
Health Tips about Diet and Nutrition

Including Facts about Dietary Guidelines, Food Groups, Nutrients, Healthy Meals, Snacks, Weight Control, Medical Concerns Related to Diet, and More

Edited by Karen Bellenir. 432 pages. 2006. 978-0-7808-0820-1.

"A very quick and pleasant read in spite of the fact that it is very detailed in the information it gives... A book for anyone concerned about diet and nutrition."
—*American Reference Books Annual, 2007*

SEE ALSO *Eating Disorders Information for Teens, 2nd Edition*

648

Drug Information for Teens, 2nd Edition
Health Tips about the Physical and Mental Effects of Substance Abuse

Including Information about Marijuana, Inhalants, Club Drugs, Stimulants, Hallucinogens, Opiates, Prescription and Over-the-Counter Drugs, Herbal Products, Tobacco, Alcohol, and More

Edited by Sandra Augustyn Lawton. 468 pages. 2006. 978-0-7808-0862-1.

"As with earlier installments in Omnigraphics' Teen Health Series, Drug Information for Teens is designed specifically to meet the needs and interests of middle and high school students... Strongly recommended for both academic and public libraries."
—American Reference Books Annual, 2007

"Solid thoughtful advice is given about how to handle peer pressure, drug-related health concerns, and treatment strategies."
—School Library Journal, Dec '06

SEE ALSO Alcohol Information for Teens, 2nd Edition, Tobacco Information for Teens, 2nd Edition

Eating Disorders Information for Teens, 2nd Edition
Health Tips about Anorexia, Bulimia, Binge Eating, And Other Eating Disorders

Including Information about Risk Factors, Diagnosis and Treatment, Prevention, Related Health Concerns, and Other Issues

Edited by Sandra Augustyn Lawton. 377 pages. 2009. 978-0-7808-1044-0.

"This handy reference offers basic information and addresses specific disorders, consequences, prevention, diagnosis and treatment, healthy eating, and more. It is written in a conversational style that is easy to understand... Will provide plenty of facts for reports as well as browsing potential for students with an interest in the topic.
—School Library Journal, Jun '09

"Written in a straightforward style that will appeal to its teenage audience. The author does not play down the danger of living with an eating disorder and urges those struggling with this problem to seek professional help.

This work, as well as others in this series, will be a welcome addition to high school and undergraduate libraries."
—American Reference Books Annual, 2009

SEE ALSO Diet Information for Teens, 2nd Edition

Fitness Information for Teens, 2nd Edition
Health Tips about Exercise, Physical Well-Being, and Health Maintenance

Including Facts about Conditioning, Stretching, Strength Training, Body Shape and Body Image, Sports Nutrition, and Specific Activities for Athletes and Non-Athletes

Edited by Lisa Bakewell. 432 pages. 2009. 978-0-7808-1045-7.

"This no-nonsense guide packs a great deal into its pages... This is a helpful reference for basic diet and exercise information for health reports or personal use."
—School Library Journal, April 2009

"An excellent source for general information on why teens should be active, making time to exercise, the equipment people might need, various types of activities to try, how to maintain health and wellness, and how to avoid barriers to becoming healthier... This would still be an excellent addition to a public library ready-reference collection or a high school health library collection."
—American Reference Books Annual, 2009

"This easy to read, well-written, up-to-date overview of fitness for teenagers provides excellent wellness and exercise tips, information, and directions... It is a useful tool for them to obtain a base knowledge in fitness topics and different sports."
—Doody's Review Service, 2009

SEE ALSO Diet Information for Teens, 2nd Edition, Sports Injuries Information for Teens, 2nd Edition

Learning Disabilities Information for Teens
Health Tips about Academic Skills Disorders and Other Disabilities That Affect Learning

649

Including Information about Common Signs of Learning Disabilities, School Issues, Learning to Live with a Learning Disability, and Other Related Issues

Edited by Sandra Augustyn Lawton. 400 pages. 2006. 978-0-7808-0796-9.

"This book provides a wealth of information for any reader interested in the signs, causes, and consequences of learning disabilities, as well as related legal rights and educational interventions... Public and academic libraries should want this title for both students and general readers."
—American Reference Books Annual, 2006

Mental Health Information for Teens, 3rd Edition
Health Tips about Mental Wellness and Mental Illness
Including Facts about Mental and Emotional Health, Depression and Other Mood Disorders, Anxiety Disorders, Behavior Disorders, Self-Injury, Psychosis, Schizophrenia, and More

Edited by Karen Bellenir. 400 pages. 2010. 978-0-7808-1087-7.

SEE ALSO Stress Information for Teens, Suicide Information for Teens, 2nd Edition

Pregnancy Information for Teens
Health Tips about Teen Pregnancy and Teen Parenting
Including Facts about Prenatal Care, Pregnancy Complications, Labor and Delivery, Postpartum Care, Pregnancy-Related Lifestyle Concerns, and More

Edited by Sandra Augustyn Lawton. 434 pages. 2007. 978-0-7808-0984-0.

Sexual Health Information for Teens, 2nd Edition
Health Tips about Sexual Development, Reproduction, Contraception, and Sexually Transmitted Infections
Including Facts about Puberty, Sexuality, Birth Control, Chlamydia, Gonorrhea, Herpes, Human Papillomavirus, Syphilis, and More

Edited by Sandra Augustyn Lawton. 430 pages. 2008. 978-0-7808-1010-5.

"This offering represents the most up-to-date information available on an array of topics including abstinence-only sexual education and pregnancy-prevention methods... The range of coverage—from puberty and anatomy to sexually transmitted diseases—is thorough and extensive. Each chapter includes a bibliographic citation, and the three back sections containing additional resources, further reading, and the index are all first-rate... This volume will be well used by students in need of the facts, whether for educational or personal reasons."
—School Library Journal, Nov '08

"Presents information related to the emotional, physical, and biological development of both males and females that occurs during puberty. It also strives to address some of the issues and questions that may arise... The text is easy to read and understand for young readers, with satisfactory definitions within the text to explain new terms."
—American Reference Books Annual, 2009

Skin Health Information for Teens, 2nd Edition
Health Tips about Dermatological Concerns and Skin Cancer Risks
Including Facts about Acne, Warts, Hives, and Other Conditions and Lifestyle Choices, Such as Tanning, Tattooing, and Piercing, That Affect the Skin, Nails, Scalp, and Hair

Edited by Edited by Kim Wohlenhaus. 418 pages. 2009. 978-0-7808-1042-6.

"The material in this work will be easily understood by teenagers and young adults. The publisher has liberally used bulleted lists and sidebars to keep the reader's attention... A useful addition to school and public library collections."
—ARBAOnline, Oct '09

Sleep Information for Teens
Health Tips about Adolescent Sleep Requirements, Sleep Disorders, and the Effects of Sleep Deprivation
Including Facts about Why People Need Sleep, Sleep Patterns, Circadian Rhythms, Dreaming, Insomnia, Sleep Apnea, Narcolepsy, and More

Edited by Karen Bellenir. 355 pages. 2008. 978-0-7808-1009-9.

"Clear, concise, and very readable and would be a good source of sleep information for anyone—not just teenagers. This work is highly recommended for medical libraries, public school libraries, and public libraries."
—*American Reference Books Annual, 2009*

SEE ALSO Body Information for Teens

▓

Sports Injuries Information for Teens, 2nd Edition
Health Tips about Acute, Traumatic, and Chronic Injuries in Adolescent Athletes
Including Facts about Sprains, Fractures, and Overuse Injuries, Treatment, Rehabilitation, Sport-Specific Safety Guidelines, Fitness Suggestions, and More

Edited by Karen Bellenir. 429 pages. 2008. 978-0-7808-1011-2.

"An engaging selection of informative articles about the prevention and treatment of sports injuries... The value of this book is that the articles have been vetted and are often augmented with inserts of useful facts, definitions of technical terms, and quick tips. Sensitive topics like injuries to genitalia are discussed openly and responsibly. This revised edition contains updated articles and defines sport more broadly than the first edition."
—*School Library Journal, Nov '08*

"This work will be useful in the young adult collections of public libraries as well as high school libraries... A useful resource for student research."
—*American Reference Books Annual, 2009*

SEE ALSO Accident and Safety Information for Teens

▓

Stress Information for Teens
Health Tips about the Mental and Physical Consequences of Stress
Including Information about the Different Kinds of Stress, Symptoms of Stress, Frequent Causes of Stress, Stress Management Techniques, and More

Edited by Sandra Augustyn Lawton. 392 pages. 2008. 978-0-7808-1012-9.

"Understanding what stress is, what causes it, how the body and the mind are impacted by it, and what teens can do are the general categories addressed here... The chapters are brief but informative, and the list of community-help organizations is exhaustive. Report writers will find information quickly and easily, as will those who have personal concerns. The print is clear and the format is readable, making this an accessible resource for struggling readers and researchers."
—*School Library Journal, Dec '08*

"The articles selected will specifically appeal to young adults and are designed to answer their most common questions."
— *American Reference Books Annual, 2009*

SEE ALSO Mental Health Information for Teens, 3rd Edition

▓

Suicide Information for Teens, 2nd Edition
Health Tips about Suicide Causes and Prevention
Including Facts about Depression, Risk Factors, Getting Help, Survivor Support, and More

Edited by Kim Wohlenhaus. 400 pages. 2010. 978-0-7808-1088-4.

SEE ALSO Mental Health Information for Teens, 3rd Edition

▓

Tobacco Information for Teens, 2nd Edition
Health Tips about the Hazards of Using Cigarettes, Smokeless Tobacco, and Other Nicotine Products
Including Facts about Nicotine Addiction, Nicotine Delivery Systems, Secondhand Smoke, Health Consequences of Tobacco Use, Related Cancers, Smoking Cessation, and Tobacco Use Statistics

Edited by Karen Bellenir. 400 pages. 2010. 978-0-7808-1153-9.

SEE ALSO Drug Information for Teens, 2nd Edition

Health Reference Series